Core Topics in Airway Management

Second Edition

Core Topics in Airway Management

Second Edition

Edited by

Ian Calder
Consultant Anaesthetist, The National Hospital for Neurology and Neurosurgery, and The Royal Free Hospital, London, UK

Adrian Pearce
Consultant Anaesthetist, Guy's and St. Thomas' Hospital, London, UK

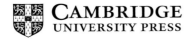
CAMBRIDGE
UNIVERSITY PRESS

CAMBRIDGE UNIVERSITY PRESS
Cambridge, New York, Melbourne, Madrid, Cape Town, Singapore,
São Paulo, Delhi, Dubai, Tokyo, Mexico City

Cambridge University Press
The Edinburgh Building, Cambridge CB2 8RU, UK

Published in the United States of America by
Cambridge University Press, New York

www.cambridge.org
Information on this title: www.cambridge.org/9780521111881

© Cambridge University Press 2011

First published 2011

Printed in the United Kingdom at the University Press, Cambridge

A catalogue record for this publication is available from the British Library

Library of Congress Cataloguing-in-Publication Data

Core topics in airway management / [edited by] Ian Calder, Adrian
Pearce. – 2nd ed.
    p. ; cm.
    Includes bibliographical references and index.
    ISBN 978-0-521-11188-1 (Hardback)
1. Airway (Medicine)   2. Respiratory therapy.   3. Inhalation
anesthesia.   4. Trachea–Intubation.   I. Calder, Ian, 1948–   II. Pearce,
Adrian C.   III. Title.
    [DNLM: 1. Airway Obstruction–prevention & control.   2. Anesthesia.
3. Intubation, Intratracheal–methods. WO 250]
    RC732.C67 2010
    616.2–dc22
                                                                    2010027605

ISBN 978-0-521-11188-1 Hardback

Contents

Section 4 – Ethics and the law

Section 5 – Examination questions

Contributors

Derek Barrett
Chief Specialist Anaesthesiologist and
Honorary Lecturer,
Ngwelezane Hospital,
Empangeni, South Africa, and
Department of Anaesthesia and Critical Care,
Nelson R. Mandela School of Medicine,
University of Kwa Zulu Natal,
Durban, South Africa

Mark C. Bellamy
Professor of Critical Care Anaesthesia,
Intensive Care Unit,
St. James' University Hospital,
Leeds, UK

Andrew R. Bodenham
Consultant in Anaesthesia and
Intensive Care Medicine,
Leeds General Infirmary, Leeds, UK

Pieter A.J. Borg
Consultant Anaesthetist, Afd. Anesthesiologie,
Maastricht Universitair Medisch Centrum,
Maastricht, The Netherlands

Ian Calder
Consultant Anaesthetist,
The National Hospital for Neurology and
Neurosurgery, Queen Square, and
The Royal Free Hospital, London, UK

Tim Cook
Consultant in Anaesthesia and
Intensive Care, Royal United Hospital,
Bath, UK

Joy E. Curran
Consultant Anaesthetist,
The Queen Victoria NHS Foundation Trust,
East Grinstead, West Sussex, UK

Philippa Evans
Consultant Anaesthetist,
Great Ormond Street Hospital, London, UK

Andrew D. Farmery
Consultant Anaesthetist,
The John Radcliffe Hospital, Oxford, UK

Chris Frerk
Consultant Anaesthetist,
Northampton General Hospital,
Northampton, UK

Priya Gauthama
Airway Fellow,
Northampton General Hospital,
Northampton, UK

Ankie E.W. Hamaekers
Consultant Anaesthetist,
Maastrict Universitair Medisch Centrum,
Maastricht, The Netherlands

John Henderson
Consultant Anaesthetist,
The Western Infirmary, Glasgow, UK

Eric Hodgson
Principal Specialist and Honorary Lecturer,
Department of Anaesthesia,
Critical Care and Pain Control,
Addington Hospital and
Nelson R. Mandela Medical School,
University of Kwa Zulu Natal,
Durban, South Africa

Jeremy A. Langton
Honorary Reader in Anaesthesia,
Peninsula College of Medicine and
Dentistry and Consultant Anaesthetist,
Derriford Hospital, Plymouth, UK

Andrew D.M. McLeod
Consultant Anaesthetist,
Royal Marsden NHS Foundation Trust,
London, UK

Abhiram Mallick
Consultant Anaesthetist,
Anaesthesia and Intensive Care Medicine,
Leeds General Infirmary, Leeds, UK

Viki Mitchell
Consultant Anaesthetist,
University College London Hospitals,
London, UK

James Nicholson
Specialist Registrar,
The Queen Victoria NHS Foundation Trust,
East Grinstead, West Sussex, UK

Anil Patel
Consultant Anaesthetist,
Department of Anaesthesia,
The Royal National ENT Hospital,
London, UK

Adrian Pearce
Consultant Anaesthetist,
Guy's and St. Thomas' Hospital, London, UK

Will Peat
Specialist Registrar,
St James' University Hospital,
Leeds, UK

John Picard
Consultant Anaesthetist,
Imperial College Healthcare NHS Trust and
Honorary Senior Lecturer,
Imperial College, London, UK

Mansukh Popat
Consultant Anaesthetist and
Regional Advisor in Anaesthesia,
The John Radcliffe Hospital, Oxford, UK

Brian Prater
Consultant Anaesthetist,
King's College Hospital,
London, UK

Mridula Rai
Consultant Anaesthetist,
The John Radcliffe Hospital,
Oxford, UK

Om Sanehi
Consultant in Anaesthetist,
Trafford Healthcare NHS Trust,
Manchester, UK

Jane Stanford
Consultant Anaesthetist,
St. George's Hospital,
London, UK

Richard Vanner
Consultant Anaesthetist,
Department of Anaesthesia,
Gloucestershire Hospitals
NHS Foundation Trust,
Gloucester, UK

Peter J.H. Venn
Consultant Anaesthetist,
The Sleep Disorder Centre,
East Grinstead,
West Sussex, UK

Steven M. Yentis
Consultant Anaesthetist,
Chelsea and Westminster Hospital and
Honorary Senior Lecturer,
Imperial College,
London, UK

Preface to the second edition – Calder and Pearce

In the preface to the first edition we wrote that there was *"an uneasy combination of art and science in airway management"*, and six years later opinions continue to diverge on how best to manage various problems. However, there has been considerable progress in both equipment and policy and we hope that readers will find this update helpful. There are some new chapters and most of the original material has been extensively revised.

One important issue is the growth of interest in the concept of "human factors" in the causation of problems. Medicine is following aviation's lead in recognising that human errors and omissions during stressful (or tedious) procedures can be as important as faulty technology, and whilst this edition was in preparation there has been a national (UK) audit of airway management (NAP 4), which looks likely to show that incidents are not as rare as we would wish.

Airway management remains literally a life or death issue. In the developed world there has been a welcome reduction in morbidity in some conditions, such as childhood epiglottitis, but the increasing age and associated co-morbidity of the population adds layers of difficulty. Obesity is a modern day scourge in many affluent societies, affecting even the youngest patients, and has important consequences for airway management. In contrast, the new chapter by Barrett and Hodgson on solutions to problems when resources are scarce makes sobering reading.

Both of us are approaching the end of our careers in anaesthesia and we would like to record our appreciation of the outstanding contributions of two individuals – Andranik "Andy" Ovassapian and Archie Brain. Andy Ovassapian (1936–2010) died during the European Society of Anaesthesiology Meeting in Helsinki. Andy was Iranian by birth but will always be associated with Chicago, where he worked in various positions for thirty six years. He was a pioneer of flexible fibreoptic intubation and his textbook on the subject remains the definitive publication. Andy founded the Society for Airway Management in 1995, and established the first and best-known Airway Study and Training Center in 1998. He was devoted to education, selfless with his time and a great friend.

Archie Brain was born in 1942 in Japan. Most would agree that Archie's invention of the laryngeal mask airway has been the greatest contribution to airway management since the tracheal tube (see Chapter 9). He was awarded the Magill Gold Medal in 1995.

Ian Calder
Adrian Pearce
2010

Andranik Ovassapian 1936–2010

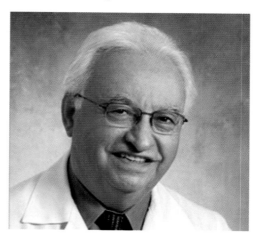

Anatomy

John Picard

Fine lingerie itself is rather tedious: it is the context that makes it exciting. The same is true for anatomy: topology alone is for *idiots savants*. The following lines instead offer a selective account of the functional anatomy of the adult head, neck and airway as it applies to anaesthetic clinical practice.

The mouth

The mouth is dominated by the tongue, a muscular instrument of pleasure – gastronomic and linguistic. For anaesthetists, little else counts but its size. It may be swollen acutely (as in angioneurotic oedema), but is also susceptible to disproportionate enlargement in trisomy 21, myxoedema, acromegaly and glycogen storage diseases, among others.

Angioneurotic oedema can cause such swelling as to fill the entire pharynx, preventing both nasal and mouth breathing and making a percutaneous subglottic airway necessary for survival. Less dramatically, a large tongue (relative to the submandibular space) can hinder direct laryngoscopy. That is, manoeuvered with reasonable force, the laryngoscope blade should squeeze the posterior tongue so as to allow a direct view of the glottis. If the tongue is too large, or the jaw hypotrophied, it may not be possible to see the glottis over the compressed tongue.

Within the mouth, the tongue is like a thrust stage in a theatre. It is surrounded by two tiers of teeth (stalls and royal circle), and a series of trapdoors, wings and flies (Figure 1.1).

Each tooth consists of calcified dentine, cementum and enamel surrounding a cavity filled (if the tooth is alive) with vessels and nerves. Each tooth is held in its socket in the jaw by a periodontal ligament. If a tooth is inadvertently knocked out, the sooner it is returned to its socket the better. If the root is clean, the tooth can simply be put back in; if dirty, the root should first be rinsed with saline or whole milk. A dentist will then be able to splint the tooth in place. If a displaced tooth cannot be immediately replaced, whole milk is the best storage medium; a dental cavity exposed too long to saline, or worse water, dies. Calcification of the periodontal ligament is then inevitable, and the tooth will become brittle and discoloured, and may fracture, loosen or fall out again.

The floor of the mouth can be opened like a trap by a surgeon. During maxillofacial surgery, for example, oral and nasal tubes may both obstruct surgical access. (Fractures may further relatively contraindicate nasal intubation.) If long-term ventilatory support is unlikely, then a tracheostomy can be avoided by a submandibular intubation: a plane is developed from the submandibular triangle (between anterior and posterior bellies of digastric) to the floor of the mouth, avoiding the salivary apparatus and the lingual nerve, and a tracheal tube passed from the oral cavity despite the closed mouth.

The stage's side wings are formed by mucosal folds running over palatoglossal and palatopharyngeal muscles (from anterior backwards). Between the two folds on each side lie the tonsils (which may be invisible in adults, but in children may be so large as to kiss in the midline, hampering laryngoscopy). The glossopharyngeal nerve runs under the mucosa of the base of the palatoglossal arch (towards the posterior tongue) and can be blocked there. (Just as in the theatre, so in the mouth: confusion surrounds the wings. Properly called the palatoglossal and palatopharyngeal arches, they are also commonly called *fauces and pillars*. They are all the same thing.)

Core Topics in Airway Management, Second Edition, ed. Ian Calder and Adrian Pearce. Published by Cambridge University Press.
© Cambridge University Press 2011.

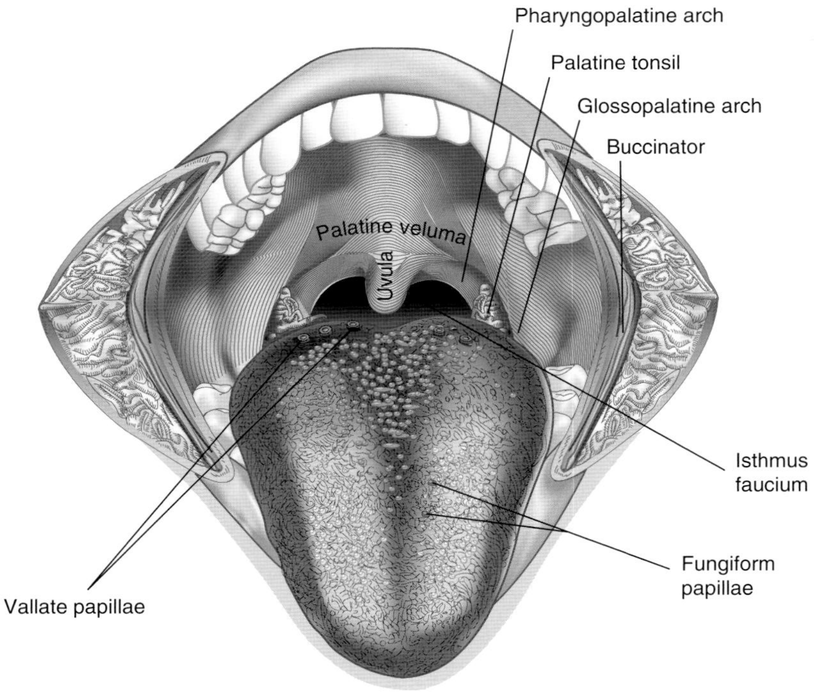

Figure 1.1. The mouth.

Pharyngopalatine arch
Palatine tonsil
Glossopalatine arch
Buccinator
Palatine velum
Uvula
Isthmus faucium
Fungiform papillae
Vallate papillae

Access to the stage's flies is controlled by the soft palate, a flap of soft tissue which can move up to separate the nasopharynx from the mouth and oropharynx (during swallowing), or move down to separate/shield the pharynx from mouth (during chewing).

The soft tissues which surround the pharyngeal airway are themselves contained by boney structures (the maxilla, the mandible, the vertebrae and the base of the skull). When awake, tone in the pharyngeal musculature maintains airway patency. But once a patient's asleep, sedated or anaesthetised, muscular tone falls, and airway patency may depend on the balance between the bones and the volume of the soft tissues within them. Patients with more soft tissue, a shorter mandible or squatter cervical vertebrae may be at particular risk of obstructive sleep apnoea.

The nose

The nose has evolved to humidify and warm air before directing it to the nasopharynx and thence towards the lungs; all roles likely to be subverted by anaesthetists. Nevertheless the anatomy of both inside and outside of the nose has anaesthetic relevance.

The nose encases the two nasal cavities which each lead from nostril to nasopharynx. Each cavity is lined by a mucous membrane of peculiar vascularity; luxurient perfusion limits local cooling and dessication despite evaporation. It also means minimal trauma can cause profuse bleeding.

The mucosa's innervation is so complex as to make topical anaesthesia the most practical option for even the most ardent regional anaesthetist (no less than nine nerves innervate each cavity). That said, simply pouring a local anaesthetic solution down the nostrils of a supine anaesthetised patient is profoundly unanatomical: the solution can be directed to its target by gravity. Before functional endoscopic sinus surgery, for example, if the solution is to reach the cephalad reaches of the nasal cavity, the head must be tilted back (with Trendelenburg tilt and a pillow below the shoulders). To direct solution along the projected path of a fibrescope, less Trendelenburg is necessary. Moreover, some sensory fibres pass through the contralateral sphenopalatine ganglion. It is therefore sensible to apply local anaesthetic to both nostrils, even if only one is to be subjected to a foreign body.

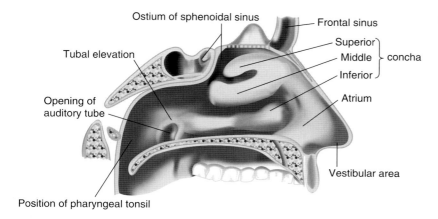

Figure 1.2. The lateral nose.

Ostium of sphenoidal sinus

Tubal elevation

Opening of
auditory tube

Position of pharyngeal tonsil

Frontal sinus

Superior
Middle } concha
Inferior

Atrium

Vestibular area

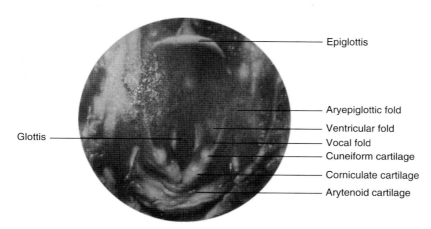

Figure 1.3. Anatomic specimen of adult human larynx.

Glottis

Epiglottis

Aryepiglottic fold

Ventricular fold

Vocal fold

Cuneiform cartilage

Corniculate cartilage

Arytenoid cartilage

Each nasal cavity is divided by three turbinates (more properly conchae) which extend laterally from the midline (Figure 1.2). The space between the floor of the nose and the inferior concha is larger than that between inferior and middle conchae. Moreover the more caudad a fibrescope's path, the less acutely it must turn past the soft palate towards the glottis. For both reasons, keeping a 'scope to the floor' of the nose should facilitate its passage. Furthermore, the ostia (holes) through which the sinuses drain into the nose are all cephalad to the inferior concha. A foreign body running caudad to it may therefore be less likely to obstruct drainage or cause sinusitis.

The damage that can be done by tubes passed blindly through the nose is remarkable; entire conchae have been amputated, and the brain directly oxygenated by tubes passed into it through fractures in the skull base. Clearly endotracheal tubes should be of as small a diameter as possible while bleeding diatheses and basal skull fractures are contraindications to nasal intubation. The nose's profile also determines how tightly a facemask can fit. Too large a nasal bone, gas escapes around the mask's sides, and too small, gas escapes at the midline.

Glottis and epiglottis

The human larynx is often declared the organ of speech (Figure 1.3). More extraordinary still, it allows singing. Its intrinsic musculature is accordingly complex, but not always relevant to the anaesthetist simply aiming for the cavity the muscles surround. That said, a naming of the parts seen on laryngoscopy allows accurate description of abnormality. Just as for a glutton before fancy chocolates, only a few details of the box are relevant; the key is to get in, past the epiglottis and past the cords themselves.

3

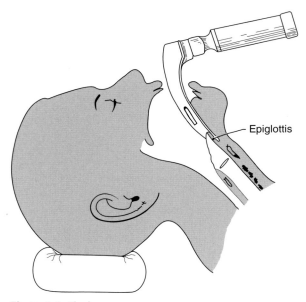

Epiglottis

Figure 1.4. The laryngoscope.

The epiglottis has evolved to shield the glottis not from anaesthetists, but from nutrients headed towards the stomach. It works like the flexible lid of a pedal bin. Generally it is half open, to allow respiration. But on swallowing the epiglottis and larynx come together. Like the lid closing on the bin, the larger and more flexible the epiglottis, the better it can fit the glottis, but the more it can frustrate direct laryngoscopy. Given adequate anaesthesia, the tip of a laryngoscope placed in the vallecula and drawn anteriorly will generally also pull the epiglottis sufficiently far anteriorly to reveal the glottis. But if an anaesthetised patient is in the supine position, and the epiglottis is long and flaccid, it may fall to hide the cords unless it too is scooped above the laryngoscope's blade (Figure 1.4). Alternatively, the tip of a McCoy laryngoscope blade can be deployed to apply anterior pressure at the root of the epiglottis (perhaps this has more to do with airway management, and less to do with anatomy). Conversely, if the tissue around the epiglottis is incompliant (after radiotherapy, for instance), deploying the McCoy blade's tip may simply push the blade posteriorly, hindering direct laryngoscopy rather than making it easier.

A hypertrophied lingual tonsil at the root of the tongue may also push the epiglottis posteriorly to obstruct the glottis, just as a bin's lid may be pushed down. While asymptomatic and imperceptible during a standard examination, such an enlarged tonsil may severely hamper airway control.

The mucosa of the larynx above the cords is supplied by the internal laryngeal nerve; below the cords, the mucosa is innervated by the recurrent laryngeal nerve, which also supplies all the intrinsic muscles of the larynx (bar cricothyroid, innervated by the external laryngeal nerve). As it is purely sensory, the internal laryngeal nerve can be blocked without fear of attendant paresis. But transection of the recurrent laryngeal nerve partially adducts the cord, and – worse – less extreme surgical damage of the nerve can cause the cord to adduct more extremely, across the midline. So anatomy dictates that the mucosa below the cords is anaesthetised topically, if at all.

Subglottic airway: cricothyroid puncture and tracheostomy

'If you cannot go through it, go round it': if teeth, tongue, epiglottis or glottis obstruct the path to the cords, then it may be easier to reach the trachea directly through skin, either by cricothyroid puncture or tracheostomy.

As the trachea must run posteriorly from the glottis to reach the carina in the mediastinum, it is most superficial at its start. Indeed, the defect between the thyroid cartilage and the first tracheal ring (the cricoid) is easily palpable in a normal neck, and is covered only by skin, loose areolar tissue and the fibrous cricothyroid membrane (Figure 1.5). So, in theory, a needle or cannula can be passed into the trachea here without risk of haemorrhage from anterior structures. But posteriorly the oesophagus runs directly behind the trachea, and the needle can perforate the posterior wall of the trachea. Moreover, the gap between cricoid and thyroid cartilages will not admit a tube wide enough to allow conventional ventilation: some form of jetting device must be used.

More caudally a larger tube can be passed into the trachea without undue force (either surgically or with a percutaneous technique). But again the oesophagus runs directly behind the trachea, and can be damaged through the posterior wall in a percutaneous approach. Moreover, the trachea is far from subcutaneous as it approaches the sternum: the thyroid isthmus lies over the second, third and fourth tracheal rings; from there the inferior thyroid veins drain the gland running close to the midline towards the chest – and in a short neck, the left brachiocephalic vein may poke above the sternum as it crosses the trachea. The position of this vein and other vessels, and

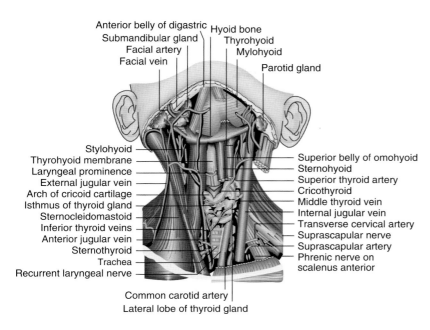

Anterior belly of digastric
Submandibular gland
Facial artery
Facial vein
Hyoid bone
Thyrohyoid
Mylohyoid
Parotid gland

Stylohyoid
Thyrohyoid membrane
Laryngeal prominence
External jugular vein
Arch of cricoid cartilage
Isthmus of thyroid gland
Sternocleidomastoid
Inferior thyroid veins
Anterior jugular vein
Sternothyroid
Trachea
Recurrent laryngeal nerve

Superior belly of omohyoid
Sternohyoid
Superior thyroid artery
Cricothyroid
Middle thyroid vein
Internal jugular vein
Transverse cervical artery
Suprascapular nerve
Suprascapular artery
Phrenic nerve on
scalenus anterior

Common carotid artery
Lateral lobe of thyroid gland

Figure 1.5. Thyroid gland and the front of the neck.

indeed the trachea, can usefully be identified by ultrasound before cricothyroidotomy or tracheostomy (see Chapter 28).

Trachea and bronchial tree

Like a jetliner's wing, the trachea's apparent simplicity belies its complexity. It is held open by the tracheal cartilages. The most cephalad of these (the cricoid) forms a complete ring. (Indeed, cricoid means *like a ring*.) The remainder are each shaped like a C, with the curve facing anteriorly. Not only does this help disorientated bronchoscopists, it also allows the tracheal bore to vary. The two ends of each C are joined by the trachealis muscle which forms the posterior wall of the trachea. If the muscle tightens the trachea's radius is reduced (as the points of the C are drawn together), airway resistance rises and the volume of the dead space falls; conversely, airway resistance falls and the dead space swells as the muscle relaxes. So, just as in a wing, the trachea's shape can be optimized for different flow rates (Figure 1.6).

As the bronchial tree ramifies beyond the trachea, its initial divisions are crucially asymmetric. The carina itself is on the left of the midline; the left main bronchus is narrower and runs off closer to the horizontal than the right; all conspire to send aspirated material towards the right main bronchus. Moreover,

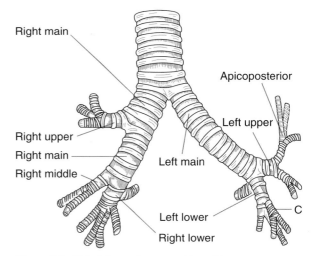

Right main

Apicoposterior

Left upper

Right upper
Right main
Right middle

Left main

Left lower

Right lower

C

Figure 1.6. Main, lobar and segmental bronchi.

in an adult the left main bronchus is some 4.5 cm long while the right main bronchus runs just 2.5 cm before giving off the bronchus to the right upper lobe. Clearly a larger target is easier to hit. It is therefore easier to isolate the lungs without occluding a lobar bronchus, if the left rather than the right main bronchus is the target.

The trachea is shortened by cervical flexion, and lengthened by cervical extension. If an endotracheal tube is anchored at the mouth, and rests above the carina when the neck is in the neutral position, it may stimulate the carina or even pass into a bronchus if the neck is flexed.

Mouth opening and the temporomandibular joint

Hominids evolved before cutlery: so, until the Stone Age, biting hard and opening the mouth wide were both advantageous.

A strong bite and a wide gape may seem to be conflicting ambitions. A firm bite, for instance, depends on a single-fused mandible, and on muscles inserting some way from the joint to gain greater leverage, as in humans (Figure 1.7). (In snakes, in contrast, each of the two halves of the mandible and the maxilla move independently from the skull and from each other, and their muscles insert close to the relevant joints, to give an enormous gape, but weak bite.)

An adequate gape is nevertheless achieved in most humans by subluxation. When the jaw is closed, the head of the mandible rests in the mandibular fossa in the temporal bone. But as the jaw opens, the head of the mandible is pulled out of the fossa by the lateral pterygoids. Rather than turning on its head, the mandible swivels on an axis which runs through the mandibular foramina (i.e., close to the insertion sites of temporalis and masseter). This shift in the axis of rotation allows both strong bite and wide gape: at the limit of closure, as the molars meet, the jaw is turning on the temporomandibular joint, and masseter and temporalis are working with leverage. But at the jaw's widest opening, it turns about their insertion sites; they are not so passively stretched and the bones of the joint do not so impinge on one another. The lower limit of normal inter-incisor distance has been found to be 37 mm in young adults. Mouth opening declines with age and in general females have slightly smaller inter-incisor distances.

Mouth opening ability also depends on craniocervical flexion/extension. Head extension facilitates opening. Normal humans extend about 26 degrees from the neutral position at the craniocervical junction to achieve maximal mouth opening. If extension from the neutral position is prevented a subject can be expected to lose about one-third of their normal inter-dental distance. Patients with poor craniocervical extension therefore suffer a 'double whammy' in terms of airway management.

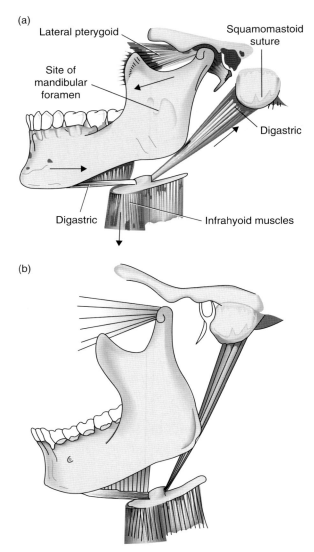

Figure 1.7. (a) Mandible and muscle actions. (b) Mandibular movement for opening the mouth wide.

Cervical spine

Mobility and strength also characterize the cervical spine. The mobility stems from the arrangement of so many bones over a comparatively short distance (as at the wrist); the strength from the geometry of the joints' articular surfaces and from the ligaments which bind them.

The joints between occiput, atlas (C1) and axis (C2) are unlike others in the vertebral column. Working caudad, the occipital condyles rest on the lateral masses of atlas like the rails of a rocking horse

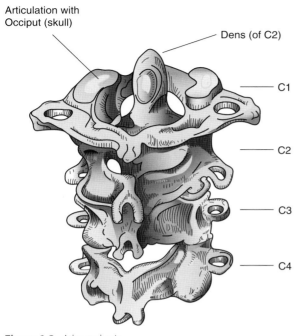

Articulation with
Occiput (skull)

Dens (of C2)

C1

C2

C3

C4

Figure 1.8. Atlas and axis.

stuck in tram tracks: the head can flex forward at the joint (until the odontoid hits the skull) and extend backwards; some abduction is allowed, but rotation is not possible. Atlas, however, turns around the axial odontoid peg. Posterior movement of atlas over axis is obviously limited by the axial anterior arch impinging on the peg (Figure 1.8).

Otherwise ligaments are responsible for the stability of the joints:

- The alar ligaments run from the sides of the peg to the foramen magnum – depending on which way the head is turned, one or other tightens and so limits rotation.
- The transverse band of the cruciform ligament runs behind the peg, from one side of atlas to the other – it stops atlas moving anteriorly over axis.
- The tectorial membrane runs as a fibrous sheet from the back of the body of the peg to insert around the anterior half of the foramen magnum – running anterior to the axis around which the head nods, it tightens as the head is extended.

The functional unit formed by the base of the skull, the atlas and the axis, is often known as the occipito-atlanto-axial complex. Normal movement at this complex permits easy airway management, both for mask anaesthesia ('chin lift') and direct laryngoscopy. Quantification of the movements of the cervical spine is not simple. There is considerable variation in the population, and the range of all movements declines with age. Wilson suggested the use of a pencil placed on, and at right angles to, the forehead. The angle swept by the pencil during flexion/extension should be more than 80 degrees. Another method is to compare the movement of a line between the canthus of the eye and tragus of the ear and also a horizontal or vertical line. The normal range of extension from the neutral position is about 60 degrees. An attractive but sadly, generally impractical, test is to ask the subject to drink from a narrow champagne flute. The rim of a flute will impinge on even a delicate nose, and the head must be tilted if the wine is to be had. Patients with poor craniocervical movement can find this inconvenient.

Below the axis, in the 'subaxial' spine, the vertebrae assume a more conventional form. They articulate at the zygoapophyseal joints between each bone's facets. Extension and flexion are both limited by the bones impinging on one another, either at the facet joints, or in the anterior midline.

Like the other subjects in this chapter, the normal cervical spine is largely relevant only to the extent that it obstructs anaesthetists' access to the airway. Direct laryngoscopy is classically facilitated by bringing oral, pharyngeal and laryngeal axes into line. In practice that means extension at the occipito-atlanto-axial complex and minimal movement in the subaxial cervical spine.

Key points

- The landmarks associated with the cricothyroid membrane offer the easiest emergency site for percutaneous airway access.
- The oesophagus lies behind the trachea and is easily perforated by needles introduced into the trachea.
- Normal mouth opening is a complex phenomenon.
- The occipito-atlanto-axial complex has a profound influence on airway management.

Further reading

Calder I, Picard J, Chapman M, O'Sullivan C, Crockard HA. 2003. Mouth opening – a new angle. *Anesthesiology*, **99**, 799–801.

Crosby ET. 2002. Airway management after upper cervical spine injury: What have we learned? *Canadian Journal of Anaesthesia*, **49**, 733–744.

Greenland KB, Cumpston PH, Huang J. 2009. Magnetic resonance scanning of the upper airway following difficult intubation reveals an unexpected lingual tonsil. *Anaesthesia Intensive Care*, **37**, 301–304.

Hernández AF. 1986. The submental route for endotracheal intubation. A new technique. *Journal of Maxillofacial Surgery*, **14**, 64–65.

Pemberton P, Calder I, O'Sullivan C, Crockard HA. 2002. The champagne angle. *Anaesthesia*, **57**, 402–403.

Sawin PD, Todd MM, Traynelis VC, et al. 1996. Cervical spine motion with direct laryngoscopy and orotracheal intubation: An *in vivo* cinefluoroscopic study of subjects without cervical abnormality. *Anesthesiology*, **85**, 26–36.

Sinnatamby CS. 1999. *Last's Anatomy: Regional and Applied*. Edinburgh: Churchill Livingstone.

Wong DT, Weng H, Lam E, Song HB, Liu J. 2008. Lengthening of the trachea during neck extension: Which part of the trachea is stretched? *Anesthesia and Analgesia*, **107**, 989–993.

Chapter 2

Physiology of apnoea and hypoxia

Andrew D. Farmery

Ethical constraints make the study of these all important topics very difficult. Simple questions, such as *How long will an apnoeic patient survive?* cannot be answered with precision.

Classification of hypoxia

'Cellular respiration' occurs at the level of the mitochondria, when electrons are passed from an electron donor (reduced nicotinamide adenine dinucleotide (NADH)) via the mitochondrial respiratory cytochromes to 'reduce' molecular oxygen (O_2). The energy from this redox reaction is used to phosphorylate adenosine diphosphate (ADP), thereby generating the universal energy source, adenosine triphosphate (ATP), which powers all biological processes. If molecular O_2 cannot be reduced in this way, this bit of biochemistry fails and cellular hypoxia occurs. Based on Barcroft's original classification, four separate causes of cellular hypoxia can be considered.

Three of these four factors affect O_2 delivery to the tissues ($\dot{D}O_2$), which is described mathematically by the equation in Box 2.1. Derangements of each of the terms on the right-hand side of this equation will reduce O_2 delivery to tissues.

The fourth cause of cellular hypoxia in our classification is *histotoxic hypoxia*. An example of this is cyanide or carbon monoxide poisoning. In histotoxic hypoxia, there is not (or there need not be) any deficit in O_2 delivery. Cellular and mitochondrial partial pressure of O_2 (PO_2) may be more than adequate, but the deficit lies in the reduction of molecular O_2 due to a failure of electron transfer. In order to fully understand the classification of hypoxia, it is useful to consider the example of carbon monoxide poisoning.

What is the mechanism of death in severe carbon monoxide poisoning?

After an unsuccessful suicide attempt involving motor exhaust-gas inhalation, a patient is taken to hospital. He is alert and breathing O_2-enriched air via a Hudson mask. His haemoglobin concentration is 15 g dl^{-1}, and his carboxyhaemoglobin fraction is 33%. The patient later dies. What is the mechanism of his death?

Let us consider each of the factors of Barcroft's classification in Box 2.1.

Hypoxaemic hypoxia is not likely to be the cause. Assuming no lung damage has occurred, this patient's arterial PO_2 (P_aO_2) is likely to be normal if breathing air, or elevated if breathing O_2. P_aO_2 is determined by the gas-exchanging properties of the lung, and is unaffected by haemoglobin concentration or by the nature of the haemoglobin species present.

A common (and erroneous) answer to this question is that, since carbon monoxide has a very high affinity for haemoglobin, and that since carboxyhaemoglobin has no O_2 carrying capacity, O_2 delivery to tissues is compromised, resulting in cellular hypoxia and death. This is clearly erroneous since, if the total haemoglobin concentration is 15 g dl^{-1} and the carboxyhaemoglobin fraction is 33%, then there is 10 g dl^{-1} of normal haemoglobin which, since the P_aO_2 is normal, is fully saturated. While this does constitute a form of functional anaemia, an *anaemic hypoxia* mechanism cannot realistically be implicated as a cause of death, since having a haemoglobin concentration of 10 g dl^{-1} is hardly fatal.

Stagnant hypoxia is unlikely to be a cause, since the cardiac output is likely to be elevated as a compensatory mechanism.

The underlying mechanism of cellular death in this case is *histotoxic hypoxia*. Just as carbon monoxide has a high affinity for the haem group in haemoglobin, it also has a high affinity for the

Core Topics in Airway Management, Second Edition, ed. Ian Calder and Adrian Pearce. Published by Cambridge University Press.
© Cambridge University Press 2011.

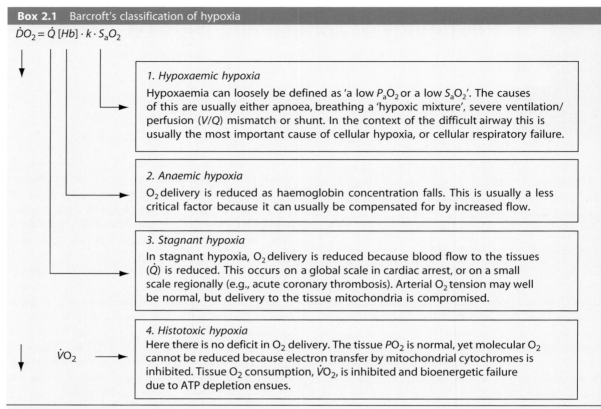

Box 2.1 Barcroft's classification of hypoxia

$$\dot{D}O_2 = \dot{Q}\,[Hb] \cdot k \cdot S_aO_2$$

1. Hypoxaemic hypoxia

Hypoxaemia can loosely be defined as 'a low P_aO_2 or a low S_aO_2'. The causes of this are usually either apnoea, breathing a 'hypoxic mixture', severe ventilation/perfusion (V/Q) mismatch or shunt. In the context of the difficult airway this is usually the most important cause of cellular hypoxia, or cellular respiratory failure.

2. Anaemic hypoxia

O_2 delivery is reduced as haemoglobin concentration falls. This is usually a less critical factor because it can usually be compensated for by increased flow.

3. Stagnant hypoxia

In stagnant hypoxia, O_2 delivery is reduced because blood flow to the tissues ($\dot{Q}$) is reduced. This occurs on a global scale in cardiac arrest, or on a small scale regionally (e.g., acute coronary thrombosis). Arterial O_2 tension may well be normal, but delivery to the tissue mitochondria is compromised.

4. Histotoxic hypoxia

Here there is no deficit in O_2 delivery. The tissue PO_2 is normal, yet molecular O_2 cannot be reduced because electron transfer by mitochondrial cytochromes is inhibited. Tissue O_2 consumption, $\dot{V}O_2$, is inhibited and bioenergetic failure due to ATP depletion ensues.

$\dot{Q}$ is the cardiac output, $[Hb]$ is the haemoglobin concentration and S_aO_2 is the arterial oxyhaemoglobin saturation. The constant, k, can be ignored in this analysis. Deficiencies in $\dot{Q}$, $[Hb]$ and S_aO_2 produce *stagnant, anaemic and hypoxaemic* hypoxia, respectively.

iron-containing haem flavoprotein in mitochondrial respiratory cytochromes. Once bound, electron transfer is interrupted and tissue O_2, albeit in abundant supply, cannot be reduced and bioenergetic failure supervenes. In carbon monoxide poisoning, the presence of carboxyhaemoglobin merely serves as a marker of carbon monoxide exposure. It is not usually part of the mechanism of death.

Differential effects of deficits in O_2 delivery

The equation in Box 2.1 shows that $\dot{D}O_2$ is simply proportional to the product of the three Barcroft variables. It would, therefore, appear at first sight that any given deficit in $\dot{D}O_2$ should cause identical degrees of cellular hypoxia regardless of whether the deficit in $\dot{D}O_2$ is due to anaemia, low flow or

hypoxaemia. We shall see below that, whereas $\dot{D}O_2$ deficits due to anaemic and stagnant hypoxia have virtually identical consequences, $\dot{D}O_2$ deficits due to hypoxaemic hypoxia are very distinct and uniquely important.

Anaemic and stagnant $\dot{D}O_2$ deficits

Experimental and theoretical models show that the variables $[Hb]$ and $\dot{Q}$ are not uniquely independent variables; it is merely the product, $\dot{Q}[Hb]$ which determines O_2 delivery and cellular oxygenation. For example, if haemoglobin concentration is halved and blood flow doubled, O_2 delivery and cellular oxygenation remain unchanged. It also follows that the degree of cellular hypoxia caused by a reduction in haemoglobin concentration (while blood flow remains constant) is identical to the degree of cellular hypoxia caused by a proportionally equal reduction in

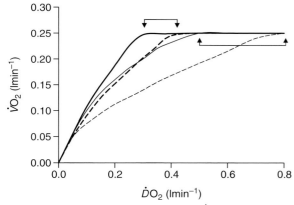

Figure 2.1. Plot of cellular O_2 consumption ($\dot{V}O_2$) versus bulk O_2 delivery ($\dot{D}O_2$). Solid lines represent stagnant/anaemic hypoxia. Broken lines represent hypoxaemic hypoxia. Bold lines show normal relationship for tissue without significant barrier to O_2 diffusion from capillary to cell. Feint lines represent tissue with significant diffusional resistance, as in oedema or shock. As $\dot{D}O_2$ falls, $\dot{V}O_2$ initially remains constant and satisfies the normal metabolic requirement (0.25 litre min^{-1}). When $\dot{D}O_2$ falls to a critical value, $\dot{D}_{crit}$ (shown by arrows), cellular O_2 consumption falls and cellular hypoxia begins. The difference in $\dot{D}_{crit}$ between hypoxaemic and stagnant/anaemic hypoxia is shown to increase when a diffusional barrier exists. (Redrawn from Farmery and Whiteley (2001).)

blood flow (while haemoglobin concentration remains fixed). This is because these variables simply determine the flux of O_2 to the tissues, and they have no other significance beyond this point.

Hypoxaemic $\dot{D}O_2$ deficits

If $\dot{D}O_2$ is reduced because of hypoxaemia, the effects on tissue hypoxia are (under certain circumstances) greater than if an equal $\dot{D}O_2$ reduction were due to anaemic or stagnant causes. This seems counterintuitive if considered in terms of Barcroft's classification. This is because Barcroft's classification focuses on O_2 delivery (bulk O_2 flux) to the tissue capillaries, and not on events beyond this; namely transfer of O_2 from capillary to cell and mitochondrion.

While it is true that the term arterial saturation of O_2 (S_aO_2) determines O_2 delivery in the same way as do $\dot{Q}$ and $[Hb]$, it is the P_aO_2 in the capillary which drives the diffusion of O_2 from capillary to cell. So the effects of hypoxaemia are twofold: not only does it reduce O_2 flux along the arterial tree (via a reduced S_aO_2), but it also impairs O_2 delivery beyond the tissue capillary (via a reduced PO_2).

The PO_2 at the cellular level is around 3–10 mmHg, and at the mitochondrion it is around 1 mmHg. The

PO_2 in tissue capillaries may be around 40 mmHg and this PO_2 gradient drives O_2 from capillary to mitochondrion according to Fick's law of diffusion. Figure 2.1 shows the effect of reducing $\dot{D}O_2$ on the cell's ability to take-up and consume O_2 ($\dot{V}O_2$), and how this differs depending on whether the fall in $\dot{D}O_2$ is achieved via anaemic/stagnant or hypoxaemic mechanisms. It can be seen that as $\dot{D}O_2$ falls, $\dot{V}O_2$ remains constant until a critical $\dot{D}O_2$, $\dot{D}O_{2crit}$, is reached, below which cellular O_2 uptake and utilization are diminished. $\dot{D}O_{2crit}$ represents the O_2 delivery at which cellular hypoxia begins. In normal tissue (bold lines), cellular hypoxia is seen to begin when $\dot{D}O_2$ falls to 0.4 litre min^{-1} for hypoxaemic hypoxia, whereas the cell can tolerate a lower $\dot{D}O_2$ if the mechanism is anaemic or stagnant. In other words, cells are more vulnerable to hypoxaemic hypoxia.

According to Fick's law, diffusive O_2 flux depends not only on the partial pressure gradient, but also on the distance between capillary and cell, and this may be increased in oedematous states (where the interstitium occupies a greater volume, separating capillary from cell), and in capillary de-recruitment due to shock (where, if a cell's nearest capillary is de-recruited, it's new nearest patent capillary will now be a greater distance away). This may explain why the difference between stagnant/anaemic and hypoxaemic hypoxia on cellular O_2 uptake is exaggerated in states of reduced diffusive conductance. This effect is also shown in Figure 2.1 (feint curves).

The rate of arterial desaturation in apnoea

We have seen that hypoxaemic hypoxia is of particular importance in the development of cellular hypoxia and it goes without saying that, in the context of the difficult airway, the principal cause of hypoxaemia is airway obstruction. It is important to understand the mechanisms by which hypoxaemia develops, and the factors which determine the rate of this process.

As soon as apnoea (with an obstructed airway) occurs, alveolar and hence pulmonary capillary PO_2 begins to fall. In apnoea, the process of gas exchange between alveolus and pulmonary capillary becomes non-linear. The rising partial pressure of carbon dioxide (PCO_2) and falling pH associated with CO_2 accumulation continually shifts the O_2–haemoglobin dissociation curve adding yet more non-linearity to the process of arterial desaturation. The time lag

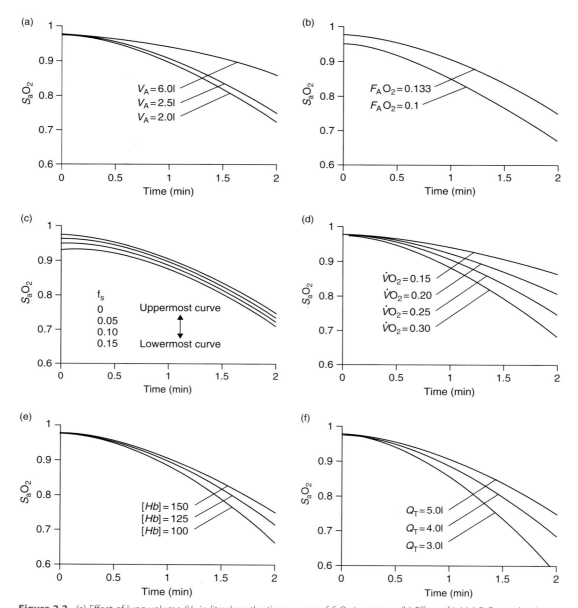

Figure 2.2. (a) Effect of lung volume (V_A in litres) on the time course of S_aO_2 in apnoea. (b) Effect of initial F_AO_2 on the time course of S_aO_2 in apnoea. (c) Effect of shunt fraction (f_s) ranging from 0% to 15% on the time course of S_aO_2 in apnoea. (d) Effect of O_2 consumption rate ($\dot{V}O_2$) ranging from 0.15 to 0.3 litre min^{-1} on the time course of S_aO_2 in apnoea. (e) Effect of haemoglobin concentration ([Hb] in g litre^{-1}) on the time course of S_aO_2 in apnoea. (f) Effect of total blood volume (Q_T) on the time course of S_aO_2 in apnoea. (Reproduced with permission from Farmery and Roe (1996).)

between changes in PO_2 feeding through into changes in mixed venous PO_2 enhances the complexity of the mathematical model further. Figure 2.2 shows the effects of six different physiological derangements on the rate of arterial desaturation in obstructed apnoea. Figure 2.2(a) shows that desaturation is exaggerated in small lung volumes (as might occur in supine anaesthetised patients). Figure 2.2(b) shows that the value of the initial alveolar O_2 concentration at the onset of apnoea is also important. Due to the various mathematical non-linearities in the system, the lower the initial alveolar O_2 tension, the greater the rate of desaturation. This has important implications for patients who have periods of partial airway

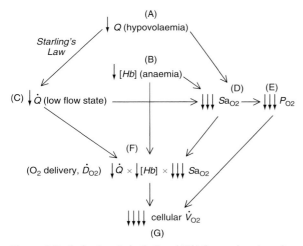

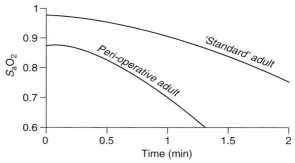

Figure 2.4. Rate of arterial oxyhaemoglobin desaturation with combination of small derangements in pathophysiological variables as might be seen in a peri-operative adult. Haemoglobin = 10 g dl^{-1}, cardiac output = 4 litre min^{-1}, initial P_AO_2 = 10 kPa, initial P_ACO_2 = 8 kPa, alveolar volume = 2.0 litre, shunt fraction (f_s) = 0.1. (Reproduced with permission from Farmery and Roe (1996).)

Figure 2.3. Reductions in both Q and $[Hb]$ (hypovolaemia and anaemia) independently increase the rate of desaturation in apnoea via pathways A-D and B-D respectively. Since hypovolaemia results in reduced cardiac output, it independently contributes further to reduced arterial saturation via pathway A-C-D. Oxygen delivery is consequently very sensitive to derangements in these variables by both direct (C-F and B-F) and indirect (A-D-F, B-D-F, A-C-D-F) pathways. The reduced oxygen delivery may reduce cellular O_2 uptake (via pathway F-G), as predicted by the unbroken lines in figure 2.1. In addition, hypoxaemia (with a low capillary driving P_{O2}) may independently compound the reduction of cellular O_2 uptake (via pathway E-G) as predicted by the broken lines in figure 2.1.

obstruction (and hence diminished alveolar PO_2 (P_AO_2)) before obstructing completely. Figure 2.2(c) shows that, while shunt diminishes the value of S_aO_2 at any given time during apnoea, the rate of desaturation is unaltered. Figure 2.2(d) shows that increased metabolic rates (as may occur in sepsis, or when struggling to breathe in severe airway obstruction) increase the rate of arterial desaturation, and this effect is exaggerated as desaturation proceeds. Figure 2.2(e) and (f) show how both hypovolaemia and reduced haemoglobin concentrations increase the rate of arterial desaturation in apnoea. This is partly because haemoglobin acts as an oxygen reservoir, and the total body mass of haemoglobin is reduced in anaemic and hypovolaemic states. Hypovolaemia has another effect in that it also results in reduced stroke volume and cardiac output. The reduced cardiac output results in lower mixed venous saturation, and if shunt is present, this increasingly desaturated venous admixture causes further arterial desaturation. So, not only does arterial hypoxaemia have a unique importance in terms of cellular hypoxia (as discussed above and also Figure 2.1), but in apnoea, anaemia, hypovolaemia and low flow states

compound the reduction in S_aO_2 and also markedly exaggerate the reduction in O_2 delivery, which is the product of all three of these terms. The interplay of these factors is depicted in Figure 2.3.

Also of note is the fact that small derangements in each of the physiological factors in Figure 2.2 combine to produce a larger overall effect on the rate of arterial desaturation. An example of this might be a 'typical' sick patient about to undergo induction of anaesthesia. This is shown in Figure 2.4.

Hypoxaemia during anaesthesia

Causes of hypoxaemia occurring during anaesthesia can be divided into the following three categories:

1. *Problems with O_2 supply*: This usually involves equipment failure resulting in the delivery of a hypoxic mixture. Meticulous pre-anaesthetic checks, and use of O_2 monitoring at the common gas outlet or in the inspired limb of the breathing system will eliminate this cause.
2. *Problems with O_2 delivery from lips to lung*: The causes of hypoventilation are numerous, but the commonest are central respiratory depression, intrinsic airway obstruction and breathing system obstruction. It is important to note that, if patients are breathing high inspired O_2 fractions, hypoxaemia will be a very late (possibly too late) feature of hypoventilation. Figure 2.5 demonstrates how, as alveolar ventilation falls to even very low levels, P_AO_2 is preserved if the inspired O_2 fraction is >30%. This clearly emphasizes the fact that pulse oximeters have no

13

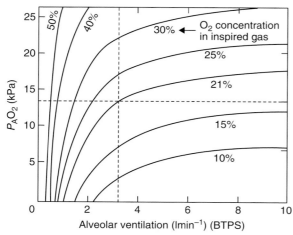

Figure 2.5. Relationship between F_iO_2, alveolar ventilation and P_AO_2.

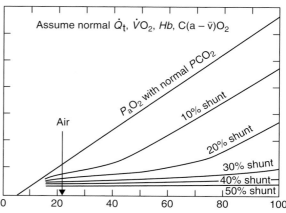

Figure 2.6. Effect of changes in inspired O_2 concentration on P_aO_2 for various right-to-left transpulmonary true shunts. Cardiac output, haemoglobin, O_2 consumption and arteriovenous O_2 content differences were assumed to be normal. (Reproduced with permission from Nunn JF. (1987) *Applied Respiratory Physiology*, 3rd ed. London, Boston: Butterworths.)

Causes of hypoventilation	Causes of V/Q mismatch
Obstructed airway	Anaesthesia
Pneumothorax	Bronchial intubation
Obstructed tube/breathing system, defective ventilator	Oesophageal intubation
Central respiratory depression	Aspiration lung disease
Peripheral weakness	Embolism

place in monitoring the adequacy of ventilation in the critical care setting.

3. *Problems with O_2 transfer from lung to blood*: Under anaesthesia considerable V/Q mismatch occurs. The mechanisms for this are not fully understood but are thought to include inhibition of hypoxic pulmonary vasoconstriction (HPV) by anaesthetic agents. Changes in posture, cephalad movement of the diaphragm and increased thoracic blood volume are also implicated. V/Q mismatching produces hypoxaemia which to a large extent can be restored by increasing the inspired O_2 fraction. This distinguishes it from shunt. 'Shunt' is a term used to describe regions of lung with perfusion but no ventilation as may occur in acute respiratory distress syndrome (ARDS) or pneumonia. Increasing the inspired O_2

fraction has little effect on oxygenation here if the shunt fraction (f_s) is >30% (Figure 2.6). Oxygenation can often be improved in shunt and V/Q abnormalities by increasing the cardiac output. There are two mechanisms for this effect. The first is that by increasing cardiac output there may be a differential increase in perfusion to ventilated lung regions greater than to unventilated lung regions, thereby reducing the shunt fraction. The second mechanism is that by increasing cardiac output, the tissues extract less oxygen per unit volume of blood and so mixed venous saturation increases, and so these same degree of venous admixture (i.e. shunt fraction) produces less arterial desaturation. Application of positive end-expiratory pressure (PEEP) or continuous positive airway pressure (CPAP) may recruit more alveoli and reduce V/Q mismatch.

Pre-oxygenation

Pre-oxygenation aims to increase body O_2 stores to their maximum, so that periods of apnoea are tolerated for longer before critical desaturation occurs. There are two elements within the practice of pre-oxygenation:

- *Supplying 100% inspired O_2*: Good pre-oxygenation technique involves a close-fitting facemask so that the patient breathes the delivered fresh gas rather than entraining air around the mask. Correct facemask application can be confirmed by seeing a full reservoir bag which moves with respiration. The bag is an essential component of the circuit because it provides the reservoir necessary when the patient's peak inspiratory flow ($\sim$30 litres min^{-1}) exceeds the fresh gas flow. The fresh gas flow should be high enough to prevent any rebreathing within the circuit, a problem with the Bain circuit particularly. The circle absorber system is much less affected by rebreathing but the circuit itself has a high volume which may be filled with air initially. It is reasonable, therefore, to pre-oxygenate always with maximal inflow of O_2 into the circuit, preferably at least 10 litres min^{-1}. If the inspired O_2 is <100%, the time to critical desaturation will be reduced.

- *Time required for effective de-nitrogenation with 100% O_2:* The aim is to maximise O_2 stores within the lung and the blood. The blood stores of O_2 do *not* change dramatically with pre-oxygenation. If the haemoglobin is 98% saturated on room air and rises to 100% with pre-oxygenation, then the increase is minimal. The amount of O_2 dissolved in the plasma is increased by the rise in partial pressure, but this is trivial.

O_2 content of blood

- O_2 carried by Hb = [Hb] conc $\times$ saturation $\times$ 1.39 ml 100 ml^{-1} blood
- O_2 dissolved in plasma = O_2 partial pressure (kPa) $\times$ 0.022 ml 100 ml^{-1} plasma

The major change during pre-oxygenation is in the amount of O_2 in the lungs. At the end of a quiet expiration the lung volume at functional residual capacity (FRC) is normally about 2500 ml. This will be affected by patient position or disease processes and may be much reduced by obesity, pregnancy or a distended bowel. On breathing 100% O_2, the wash-in of O_2 is exponential. The time constant (t) of this wash-in process is the ratio of FRC or alveolar volume to alveolar ventilation ($V_A/\dot{V}_A$). Given an alveolar ventilation of 4 litres min^{-1} and FRC volume of 2.5 litres we can estimate the time constant to be 2.5/4 = 0.625 minutes. After three time constants (1.9 minutes) the exponential process will be 95% complete.

Exponential wash-in of O_2 during pre-oxygenation (typical values)

- Time constant (t) of exponential process $= V_A/\dot{V}_A$
  $=2.5/4$
  $=0.63$ minutes
- After 1 time constant (0.63 minutes) pre-oxygenation is 37% complete
- After two time constants (1.25 minutes) pre-oxygenation is 68% complete
- After three time constants (1.9 minutes) pre-oxygenation is 95% complete

It is, therefore, reasonable to continue pre-oxygenation for at least three time constants to ensure maximal pre-oxygenation. It should be noted that patients with a small FRC will pre-oxygenate more quickly than normal but the O_2 store contained in the FRC will be reduced. Increasing alveolar minute ventilation (four to eight deep or vital capacity breaths) increases the rapidity of increase in P_AO_2 and is extremely useful when time for pre-oxygenation is limited. Administering opioids such as fentanyl before pre-oxygenation may lengthen the time required to achieve a high P_AO_2.

In any particular patient, the magnitude of the alveolar minute ventilation and FRC are unknown. It is, therefore, useful to monitor the process of de-nitrogenation by measuring end-tidal FO_2. An end-tidal FO_2 of 90–91% indicates maximal pre-oxygenation and a store of O_2 in the FRC of >2000 ml. In order to use the end-tidal O_2 to guide pre-oxygenation, gas sampling must be reliable (tight-fitting facemask) and gas should not have bi-directional flow over the capnograph sampling line (use a circle absorber circuit not a Bain system). The overall increase in O_2 stores in the blood and lungs with pre-oxygenation is from 1200 ml (air) to 3500 ml.

Desaturation following the use of succinylcholine

The American Society of Anesthesiologists (ASA) difficult airway algorithm recommends that, if initial attempts at tracheal intubation after the induction of general anaesthesia are unsuccessful, the anaesthetist should 'consider the advisability of awakening the patient'. 'Awakening' more realistically means allowing return to an unparalysed state that permits spontaneous ventilation. This is considered to be safe practice.

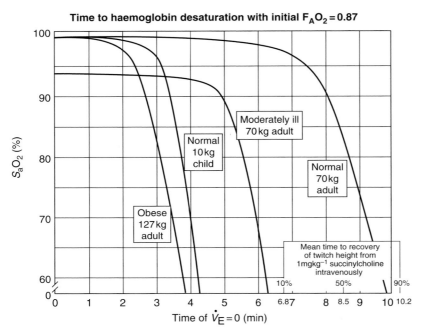

Figure 2.7. S_aO_2 versus time of apnoea for various types of patients. (Reproduced with permission from Benumof et al (1997).)

However to what level might arterial saturation fall before spontaneous ventilation resumes? Using a combination of clinical data and a theoretical model, Benumof demonstrated that during complete obstructive apnoea, and in the 'can't intubate, can't ventilate' situation, critical haemoglobin desaturation occurs before the time to functional recovery for various patients receiving 1 mg kg^{-1} of intravenous succinylcholine.

Figure 2.7 shows that, in all but the 'normal' adult, critical desaturation occurs long before recovery of even 10% of neuromuscular function.

From this analysis it is clear that, in a complete 'can't ventilate, can't intubate' situation, it is not appropriate to wait for the return of spontaneous ventilation, but rather a rescue option should be pursued immediately. Benumof points out that this analysis ignores the central respiratory depressant effects of the concomitantly administered general anaesthetics, and so this should be regarded as an underestimation of the time to functional recovery.

The final common pathway of cellular hypoxia: membrane potential and cell death

Venous PO_2 is a reasonable indicator of *capillary* and hence *tissue* PO_2. In many respects, measuring venous PO_2 (either mixed venous, or organ specific venous such as jugular venous) is more useful in evaluating tissue oxygenation than measuring P_aO_2. Experimental and clinical evidence suggests that consciousness is lost when jugular venous PO_2 (and hence 'tissue PO_2' in the watershed of this drainage) falls below 20 mmHg. It is this PO_2 which drives diffusion of O_2 to its final destination in the mitochondria, where the PO_2 may be a fraction of a mmHg. With this degree of mitochondrial hypoxia, electron transfer cannot proceed (there is insufficient available molecular O_2 to accept electrons). This redox reaction falters and there is insufficient energy production to power the generation of ATP. We discuss the events which follow the onset of cellular bioenergetic failure.

Tissues vary in their sensitivity to hypoxia, but cortical neurones are particularly sensitive. They (along with the myocardium) are perhaps the most clinically important and are therefore the most studied. It is said that 'hypoxia stops the machine and wrecks the machinery'. As far as neurones and the myocardium are concerned this aphorism means that hypoxia initially arrests cellular function. For a period of time the integrity of the cell and its viability remain intact. If hypoxia is reversed, function will resume. However sustained hypoxia wrecks the machinery. Via numerous and complex mechanisms, and in neurones particularly, an accelerating series of

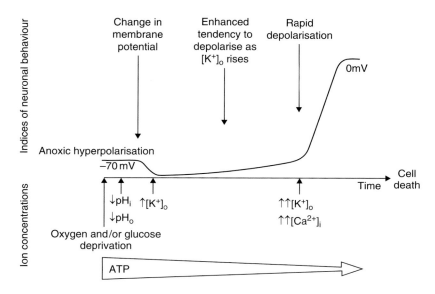

Figure 2.8. Membrane potential changes induced by cellular hypoxia. Intra- and extracellular pH changes are the first to be observed. Changes in membrane potential occur between 15 and 90 seconds. This is usually hyperpolarisation due to increased K^+ channel conductance. K^+ then leaks from within the cell. This causes an increase in extracellular $[K^+]$, especially if perfusion is limited (as in ischaemia), since the extracellular space is not washed-out of ions and metabolites. The increasing extracellular $[K^+]$ causes gradual membrane depolarisation which in turn activates voltage-sensitive Ca^{2+} channels, contributing further to the depolarisation. The increasing acidosis and increasing depolarisation triggers Ca^{2+} release from intracellular stores, which in turn triggers synaptic release of glutamate. The release of this massive amount of glutamate stimulates ligand-gated cation channels whose opening coincides with a very rapid phase of membrane depolarisation. At this point, the Na^+–K^+–ATPase pump has ceased to operate and membrane potential is lost irretrievably.

destructive events ensues, which results in cell death. The length of this process is highly variable depending on the tissue, the metabolic rate, blood flow and many other factors. However it may be as short as 4 minutes for some neurones.

Anoxia and membrane potential

In general, living cells can be characterised by possession of a resting membrane potential whereas dead cells have no resting membrane potential. The effect of anoxia on resting membrane potential depends on the nature of the anoxic insult. In ischaemia (as in stroke), the tissue is deprived of O_2 and blood flow, whereas in airway obstruction, hypoxaemia occurs while blood flow (and glucose supply) continues, and this may have more deleterious effects.

One of the first metabolic features of mitochondrial bioenergetic failure is the depletion in ATP and accumulation of NADH. Small amounts of ATP can be generated from the glycolytic pathway, but this requires oxidized nicotinamide adenine dinucleotide (NAD^+) which is in short supply. However the necessary NAD^+ can be generated by converting pyruvate to lactate, thus facilitating limited ATP production

anaerobically. The intracellular acidosis which results from anaerobic metabolism is one of the first changes to be detected following cellular anoxia. If the nature of the hypoxia is *hypoxaemic hypoxia*, then blood flow will be preserved and there will be an abundant supply of glucose which will exacerbate the acidosis. Hyperglycaemic patients are particularly at risk.

Shortly after the onset of intracellular acidosis, the membrane potential of neurones begins to change. This is shown in Figure 2.8. The effect is variable, but the majority hyperpolarize. It is thought that this is due to an increase in K^+ channel conductance. The mechanisms are not clear but possibilities include activation of ATP-sensitive K^+ channels (increased conductance in low ATP states), activation of direct O_2-sensitive K^+ channels or activation of pH-sensitive K^+ channels. Hyperpolarisation of neurones renders them less susceptible to synaptic activation, and this may manifest as loss of consciousness (i.e., 'the machine stops').

From this point, membrane potential changes from hyperpolarisation to slow depolarisation. The mechanism of this is thought to be that the increased K^+ conductance (which initially hyperpolarised the

17

membrane) allows K^+ efflux out of the cell down its concentration gradient. This escaped K^+ is normally removed from the extracellular space by the Na^+–K^+-ATPase, but as this pump begins to fail, extracellular $[K^+]$ increases and, as can be predicted by the Nernst equation, resting membrane potential begins to depolarise. As the membrane potential depolarises further, Ca^{2+} channels are activated and Ca^{2+} influx contributes to an acceleration of the depolarisation.

At this point, these electrophysiological effects are reversible if oxygenation is restored. If not, a cascade of irreversible events ensues.

Within a short time, membrane depolarisation becomes very rapid. This coincides with a number of cellular events: the failure of the Na^+–K^+-ATPase pump, massive release of Ca^{2+} from intracellular stores triggering massive release of excitatory neurotransmitters (principally glutamate) from synaptic vesicles, which in turn stimulates glutamate receptor-linked ion channels triggering further cation influx into the cell. Beyond this point, cell survival is unlikely. The machine is wrecked.

The time course for these events is variable. It is quickest for neurones exposed to ischaemia (arrested flow) under hyperglycaemic and hyperthermic conditions, where the process may be a matter of only 1–4 minutes. Under hypoxaemic conditions with preserved flow and normoglycaemia, the process may take between 4 and 15 minutes depending on the degree and abruptness of the insult.

Key points

- Tissue hypoxia can be fatal despite normoxaemia (cyanide and CO poisoning).
- Hypoxaemic hypoxia (airway obstruction) is more damaging to cells than anaemic or stagnant hypoxia.
- Oximeters measure saturation not ventilation. A normal saturation does not mean that ventilation is not dangerously depressed.
- Oxygen saturation will fall more quickly in an apnoeic sick patient. Waiting for spontaneous ventilation to return may not be a sensible option.
- An end-tidal oxygen of >90% indicates maximum pre-oxygenation.
- Pre-oxygenation achieves its end by increasing the amount of oxygen in the lung.

Further reading

Benumof JL. (1999). Preoxygenation. *Anesthesiology*, **91**, 603–605.

Benumof JL, Dagg R, Benumof R. (1997). Critical hemoglobin desaturation will occur before return to an unparalyzed state following 1 mg/kg intravenous succinylcholine. *Anesthesiology*, **87**, 979–982.

Farmery AD, Roe PG. (1996). A model to describe the rate of oxyhaemoglobin desaturation during apnoea. *British Journal of Anaesthesia*, **76**, 284–291.

Farmery AD, Whiteley JP. (2001). A mathematical model of electron transfer within the mitochondrial respiratory cytochromes. *Journal of Theoretical Biology*, **213**, 197–207.

Chapter 3

Physics and physiology

Andrew D. Farmery

Physics of airflow

Gas flowing through tubes can be characterised by possessing either *laminar* or *turbulent* flow, or more usually, a mixture of both. Before we explore these we need to familiarise ourselves with a fundamental thermodynamic concept detailed below.

Laminar flow

In laminar flow, although gas molecules in different parts of the 'stream' have different velocities, the vectors of these velocities are parallel, as shown in Figure 3.1.

For a viscous Newtonian fluid such as air, molecules can be thought of as being arranged in slippery sheets or layers and these have been schematically labelled 1, 2, 3 in Figure 3.1. The sheet of molecules closest to the wall of the tube (sheet 1) is stationary and bound to the wall of the tube. Each sheet of molecules can exert a force on its neighbour ('shear' force) so that a slow moving sheet will tend to retard a quicker moving neighbour, and quicker moving sheets will tend to drag slower neighbours along. For example, the shear forces exerted on sheet 2 by the stationary sheet 1 would tend to retard it, but the shear force exerted by its other neighbour, the faster moving sheet 3, would tend to increase its velocity.

The sheets of molecules in the middle of the stream (e.g., sheet 3) are the least influenced by the static layers at the edges, and so these have the highest velocity.

The amount of 'grip' which one sheet has on another (the shear force) is a property of the *viscosity* of the fluid. For low viscosity (i.e., slippery) fluids the stationary boundary layer has little 'grip' on its neighbour and so the velocity of subsequent layers rises very quickly as one moves towards the centre of the stream. For high viscosity (sticky) fluids the stationary boundary layer grips its neighbour and retards it. This layer, in turn, retards the next innermost layer, and so on. The result is that successive layers increase in velocity towards the centre only slowly.

'Pressure-drop' and 'flow' are linearly related in laminar flow

For laminar flow, pressure and flow are analogous to electrical voltage and current. The relationship is described by Poiseuille's law, which is analogous to Ohm's law, and is shown in Figure 3.2.

For a gas moving in a tube such as shown in Figure 3.1, the friction (or shear forces) created as layers slide over each other will generate heat and so

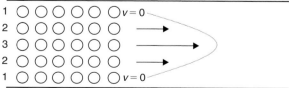

Numbers represent 'layers' of molecules. Arrows represent velocity vectors.

Figure 3.1. Laminar flow.

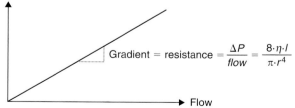

Pressure gradient

$$\text{Gradient} = \text{resistance} = \frac{\Delta P}{flow} = \frac{8 \cdot \eta \cdot l}{\pi \cdot r^4}$$

Flow

Figure 3.2. Pressure gradient versus flow diagram. $\eta =$ viscosity, $l =$ length, $r =$ radius.

Core Topics in Airway Management, Second Edition, ed. Ian Calder and Adrian Pearce. Published by Cambridge University Press.
© Cambridge University Press 2011.

energy will be lost from the gas as it passes down the tube (energy lost = mean friction force × distance down the tube). Given that the mean friction force is constant at any point along the tube there must be a constant (or linear) loss of energy with distance travelled down the tube. What effect will this have on the gas pressure down the tube?

From the equation in Box 3.1, the 'kinetic term' must be constant, because the mean velocity of the layers of molecules is the same at any point along the tube. So by deduction, this must mean that the linear drop in energy (as heat is liberated by friction as the gas flows down the tube) must be manifest as a linear drop in *pressure* along the tube. This explains the obedience to Ohm's/Poiseuille's law as shown in Figure 3.2.

The key feature of laminar flow is that the velocity vectors of all the sheets are parallel, and although each layer has a different velocity to its neighbour, each sheet retains its own velocity and so there is no change in the relative velocities, and the *mean* velocity at any point remains constant. Laminar flow is favoured for viscous fluids at low velocities in long narrow tubes with smooth sides. These properties are quantified by the Reynold's number, N_R, which is given by:

$$N_R = \frac{\rho \cdot \bar{V} \cdot D}{\eta}$$

Where ρ is density, $\bar{V}$ is mean linear velocity, D is pipe diameter, η is viscosity.

For Reynold's numbers below 2000, laminar flow is favoured and above 2000 turbulent flow dominates.

Turbulent flow

In turbulent flow, molecules do not move as sheets slipping over each other with parallel velocity vectors

in such an orderly way, but rather swirl and eddy in a seemingly random way. So in turbulent flow, molecules not only have a linear velocity down the length of the pipe, but also a turbulent or rotational velocity as they swirl around in eddies and vortices (Figure 3.3).

'Pressure-drop' and 'flow' have a quadratic relationship in turbulent flow

Turbulent kinetic energy (due to the velocity of molecules swirling round eddies) amounts to a few percent of the linear kinetic energy, and is a fixed proportion of it. As these molecules swirl around, their turbulent kinetic energy is dissipated as they collide with each other and the pipe wall, and so energy is lost at a greater rate than compared to laminar flow. The rate at which energy is lost is proportional to the turbulent kinetic energy which the molecules possess and this in turn is proportional to the mean linear kinetic energy. This energy loss is 'paid for' by a drop in static pressure. The above can be summarised as follows:

$$\Delta P = \text{energy dissipated} \ \alpha \ \text{turbulent kinetic energy} \ \alpha$$
$$\text{linear kinetic energy} \ \alpha \ \rho.\text{flow}^2$$

The relative importance of *viscosity* and *density* in *upper* and *lower* airway obstruction.

Acute bronchospasm is characterised by narrowing, due to bronchial smooth muscle contraction and mucosal inflammation, of the distal airways. This process occurs to some extent throughout the bronchial tree, but its effect on small distal airways has the biggest contribution to the increased airways resistance. This can be appreciated by considering the Poiseuille equation:

Resistance (R) α $1/r^4$

From this we see that the *change* in resistance, *R*, per unit change in airway radius, *r* (d*R*/d*r*) is proportional to $1/r^5$. In other words, the smaller the airway, the greater will be the increase in resistance resulting from a further reduction in radius.

Is it possible to increase airflow in acute bronchospasm by giving a low density gas such as Heliox?

The total cross-sectional area of the 11th generation of the bronchial tree is believed to be about seven times larger than at the lobar bronchi, so that flow is characteristically laminar. In this region molecules

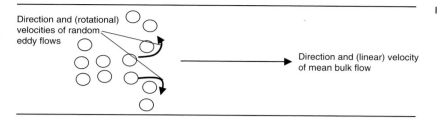

Figure 3.3. Turbulent flow.

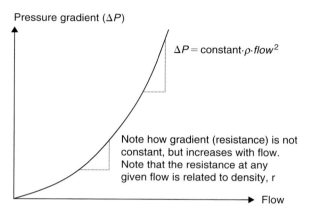

Figure 3.4. Pressure–flow relationship for turbulent flow.

move as orderly sheets sliding over each other and the friction between these sheets, which is responsible for the energy loss and pressure drop, is a function of the *viscosity* of the gas and not its *density*. So reducing the density of the gas will have no effect on the pressure gradient required to achieve the same flow. Heliox at 70%/30% (helium/oxygen) is about one-fifth of the density of 70%/30% (nitrogen/oxygen), but its *viscosity* is about the same. For this reason, its use makes little difference to *total* airways resistance because the site of predominant resistance is the small airways where laminar flow predominates. However turbulence may occur in acute asthma, where the entire bronchial tree may be affected. Whether Heliox is helpful is debated, but a recent review concluded that there is some evidence of benefit, particularly in severe cases.

Is Heliox useful in upper airway obstruction?

Wherever turbulent flow prevails, the flow for a given pressure gradient is a function of the *density* of the gas. This is because the kinetic energy lost as molecules whiz around eddies is a property of their speed and mass (i.e., density), rather than their 'stickiness'. So if the site of maximum airways resistance is a site at which turbulent flow occurs, then using Heliox will greatly increase flow

for a given pressure gradient, or allow the same flow for a smaller pressure gradient. Clinical examples of this include:

- Upper airway obstruction from haematoma, tissue swelling or tumour
- Laryngeal obstruction from oedema/infection, nerve palsy, tumour
- Large airway obstruction from tumour or extrinsic vascular compression

The benefits of Heliox however are double-edged. The higher the concentration of helium in the mixture, the lower, by definition, will be the F_IO_2. For most patients with critical airflow obstruction, the decision to give any gas other than 100% oxygen (O_2) needs to be made very carefully. It would be difficult to justify giving nitrous oxide, which has a higher density than O_2.

Physics of distensible airways
Anatomy

The anatomy of the upper airway is depicted in Figure 3.5. The nasopharynx is a rigid bony structure and is therefore not liable to collapse. Likewise the trachea, with its supporting cartilaginous structure is rigid and resistant to collapse. However the intervening segment, the pharynx, is not supported by bone or cartilage and is therefore potentially collapsible. In adults, the commonest site for airway collapse in sleep and anaesthesia is the velopharynx (where the soft palate meets the posterior pharyngeal wall). This has been shown in radiological studies during both inhalational and intravenous anaesthesia. This contradicts the previously commonly held view that the principal site of airway obstruction was retrolingual, and caused by posterior displacement of the tongue. In one study of isoflurane anaesthesia, retrolingual obstruction accounted for only 2 of 16 subjects, the remaining obstructed at the level of the velopharynx and larynx.

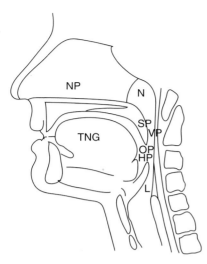

Figure 3.5. Anatomy of the upper airway. NP: nasopharynx; TNG: tongue; SP: soft palate; VP: velopharynx; OP: oropharynx; HP: hypopharynx; L: larynx.

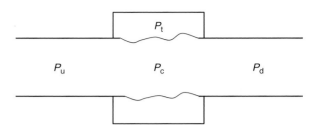

Figure 3.6. Functional anatomy of the upper airway between the segments. P_t: tissue pressure; P_u: upstream pressure; P_d: downstream pressure; P_c: pressure at site of collapsible segment.

The Starling resistor

The *functional* anatomy of the upper airway can be reduced to a consideration of a collapsible segment (the pharynx) between two rigid segments (the nasopharynx and the trachea) as shown in Figure 3.6. This system behaves as a 'Starling resistor' and airflow can become limited or completely abolished during spontaneous ('negative intrathoracic pressure') breathing as described below. A Starling resistor is one whose characteristics can be ohmic (i.e., flow is simply dependent on the difference between upstream pressure, P_u, and downstream pressure, P_d) under certain conditions, and non-ohmic under other circumstances (when flow becomes independent of downstream pressure, yet dependent on transmural pressure at the site of the distensible segment).

The value of pressure at the site of a collapsible segment (P_c) lies somewhere between P_u and P_d, tending towards P_u at the upstream end and P_d at the downstream end. This resistor can exist in one of the three states as depicted in Figure 3.7.

The Starling resistor is analogous to water flowing over a weir where the heights of the upstream and downstream sections are analogous to P_u and P_d, and the height of the weir is analogous to tissue pressure (P_t). This is shown is Figure 3.7.

Figure 3.7 shows that

1. When P_t always exceeds P_u, P_c and P_d, the distensible segment will move inwards and occlude the airway completely. Here flow = 0.
2. When P_u, P_c and P_d always exceed P_t, the distensible segment will always be open and the tube behaves as a simple ohmic resistor where flow $\propto$ ($P_u - P_d$).
3. When $P_u > P_t > P_d$, the airway remains patent at its upstream end (where P_c is close to P_u and greater than P_t) and tends to partially collapse at its downstream end where P_c tends toward P_d. Here flow is proportional to ($P_u - P_t$) rather than ($P_u - P_d$). Note how flow over the weir cannot be increased by merely lowering the height of the downstream weir-pool.

Similarly in the upper airway under these conditions, flow cannot be increased by lowering P_d (i.e., by increasing inspiratory effort) because by doing so the distensible segment moves further in, thus buffering the effect of this drop in P_d at the site of the constriction, so that P_c remains in equilibrium with P_t and hence remains constant. As flow is proportional to $P_u - P_t$ it too remains constant despite increasing inspiratory effort. In this state flow can only be increased by increasing upstream pressure with, for example, continuous positive airway pressure (CPAP).

Critical instability at points of narrowing

Points of narrowing within the upper airway such as enlarged tonsils or partial posterior displacement of the tongue can potentially lead to critical instability in upper airway patency. Consider a narrowing such as shown in Figure 3.7c. Here the airway wall has moved inwards until the pressure at the site of constriction has equilibrated with the tissue pressure, thus buffering the fall in P_c which would have otherwise resulted from the lowering of P_d. However this has created a constriction at this site with a resultant forced increase in the velocity of the gas at this point. According to Bernoulli's principle (Box 3.1) this will result in a fall in pressure P_c which will be buffered to some extent

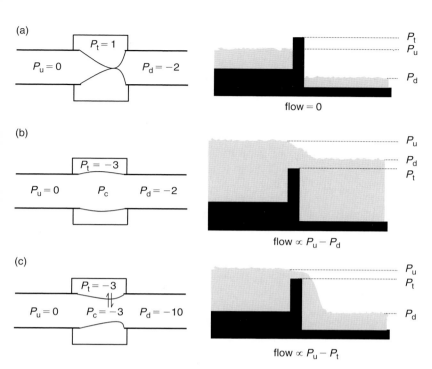

Figure 3.7. Three states in a Starling resistor.

by further inward movement of the airway wall. This unstable cycle repeats itself until collapse occurs.

Needle cricothyrotomy

In the event of complete airway collapse despite attempted application of CPAP or positive pressure mask ventilation, oxygenation can be facilitated via a needle cricothyrotomy. Reasonable 'tidal volumes' of O_2 can be passed via a relatively fine bore needle because we are able to apply great driving pressure either via a bag or direct intermittent connection to the wall-mounted rotameter. However there is a theoretical risk that since the upper airway is obstructed, gas may not be able to leave the lungs resulting in dangerous hyperinflation.

Figure 3.8 shows how, due to the properties of a Starling resistor, this risk is small and mostly unrealised.

Passage of O_2 into the trachea, downstream of the obstruction, increases P_d such that it now exceeds P_t. Excess gas can now easily escape without risk of hyperinflation. With the airway now partially open, application of CPAP via a facemask may now aid convection and diffusion of O_2 down the trachea, and excess retrograde O_2 leak (from the cricothyrotomy site to the upper airway) can be controlled.

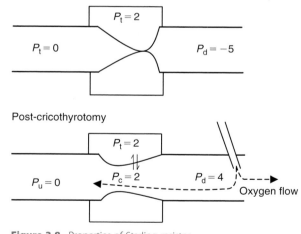

Figure 3.8. Properties of Starling resistor.

Flow-volume loops

We will restrict our discussions to analysis of flow-volume (FV) loops seen in *extrathoracic* airway obstruction, as opposed to the more familiar FV loops seen in intrathoracic airway obstruction, such as asthma and emphysema. Extrathoracic obstructions are classified in Box 3.2.

23

FV loop patterns for extrathoracic airway obstruction are distinctive, and furthermore, fixed and variable obstructions can also be distinguished. Figure 3.9 shows these patterns for fixed and variable extrathoracic obstructions compared with a normal FV loop.

Normal FV loops are characterised by the rapid emptying of the lung from total lung capacity (TLC); peak-flow being achieved early in the breath. Thereafter there is a linear decay in flow as the lung empties (the so-called 'effort independent' part of the loop). The inspiratory limb is almost 'semi-circular'.

Fixed extrathoracic obstructions produce a FV loop whose inspiratory and expiratory limbs are almost symmetrical. The loop is more 'box-like' than 'loop-like' on account of the maximum inspiratory and expiratory flows being held constant for most of the breath duration.

What physical properties of the lung account for these differences in the FV loop? To understand this we need to consider some lung mechanics for normal airway emptying. Figure 3.10 shows pressures at various points in the airway during expiration. During breath-holding (Figure 3.10a) with an open glottis there is no flow and pressure = 0 (atmospheric) at all points. Note how the intrapleural pressure is sub-atmospheric (-7 cmH$_2$O) as this pressure must equal and oppose the recoil pressure of the lung ($+7$ cmH$_2$O) which would tend to collapse the lung. The alveolar pressure therefore always exceeds pleural pressure by an amount equal to the recoil pressure ($P_A = P_{Pl} + P_R$).

During maximal forced expiration (Figure 3.10b) if the pleural pressure is raised say to 12 cmH$_2$O, then the alveolar pressure will equal 19 cmH$_2$O and flow will occur along the airway. Flow through the airway resistance causes pressure to drop along its passage until at a certain point (the 'equal pressure point', or EPP) the intraluminal pressure equals the pleural pressure which in this example is 12 cmH$_2$O. At this point, for the first time, transmural pressure becomes positive and causes airway narrowing. This narrowing causes airflow to accelerate and approach the critical wave speed (i.e., the speed of sound). So beyond this point, gas travels at a higher velocity than the speed at which pressure waves can travel. This being the case, the downstream pressure caused by (or causing) this airflow cannot be transmitted upstream and so *downstream* pressure can have no influence on it. Therefore the only influence on airflow is the 'pressure gradient' ΔP, *upstream* of the EPP which equals $19 - 12 = 7$ cmH$_2$O. In other words, the driving pressure for airflow, ΔP, is simply equal to the recoil pressure which is a *constant*. It therefore follows that airflow will reach a maximal value which is uninfluenced by expiratory effort. The only reason flow decays throughout the breath is that, as the lung empties and gets smaller, the calibre of the airways also gets smaller and so flow falls in proportion to lung *volume* and not *effort*. This lack of effort dependency is demonstrated by the fact that the maximal and submaximal dotted curves shown on Figure 3.9 share the same envelope for most of the latter part of the breath.

In extrathoracic airway obstruction (Figure 3.10c), no equal pressure point within the intrathoracic airways exists because the site of maximal airflow limitation is the *extrathoracic* resistance. Upstream of this, intraluminal pressure always exceeds the intrapleural pressure and so the driving pressure to flow, ΔP, is simply the alveolar pressure, P_A and hence it is 'effort-dependent'. This is evidenced by the fact that the maximal and submaximal expiratory curves on Figure 3.9 have distinctly different envelopes.

Because the intraluminal pressure always exceeds the intrapleural pressure, the tendency for the airway calibre to reduce as the lung gets smaller is reduced (*c.f.* the normal situation). For this reason, although flow is dependent on effort, it is independent of lung volume, and this accounts for the long flat plateau in the expiratory curve.

Variable versus fixed obstruction

Figure 3.9b shows a FV loop in variable obstruction as may occur during sleep, and following anaesthesia

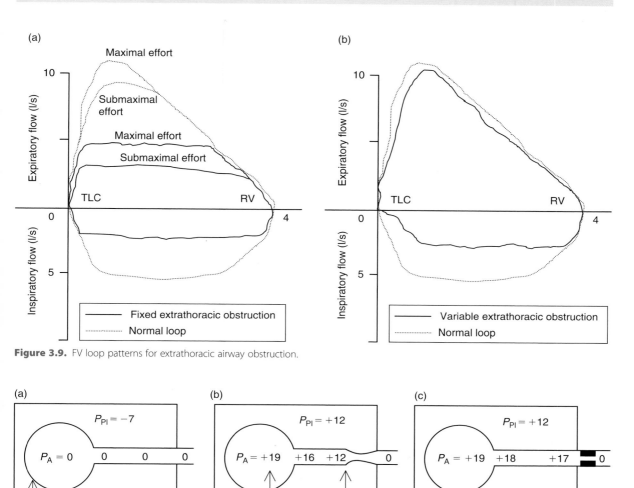

Figure 3.9. FV loop patterns for extrathoracic airway obstruction.

Figure 3.10. Pressures at various points in the airway during expiration (a) breath-holding, (b) maximal forced-expiration: normal lung mechanics, (c) maximal forced-expiration: extrathoracic obstruction.

without necessarily any airway pathology. The dominant characteristic of this loop is that expiration is essentially normal, whereas inspiration is markedly impaired for reasons discussed in the Physics of distensible airways section (see Figure 3.7).

Physics of the Sanders injector

In 1967 Sanders described a device which permitted ventilation of patients during bronchoscopy. This comprised a 16-gauge needle mounted axially at the proximal end of the bronchoscope and through which high pressure oxygen could be intermittently passed. This mode of ventilation is a form of what later became known as 'jet ventilation' and has a number of uses beyond ventilation during rigid bronchoscopy. Details of the use of jet ventilation in the context of the difficult airway are provided elsewhere in this book. The purpose of this section is to describe the physics and function of the device.

There are a number of misconceptions regarding the operating principles of the Sanders injector. The

25

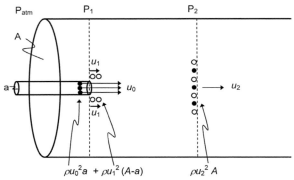

$$\rho u_0{}^2 a + \rho u_1{}^2 (A-a) \qquad\qquad \rho u_2{}^2 A$$

Figure 3.11. Oxygen molecules (filled dots) are injected via a narrow pipe of cross-sectional area a at velocity u_0 into a wider bore pipe of cross-sectional area A. The friction and shear forces between the high velocity oxygen molecules and the nearly static air molecules drag the latter to a velocity of u_1 at the level of the tip of the injector. From this point onwards, air molecules are dragged to a higher velocity and oxygen molecules are reciprocally dragged to a slower velocity until their velocities are common and equal to u_2, at which point the oxygen and entrained air are mixed and uniform. The momentum rates of the injected gas, the air about to be entrained, and the mixed gas are shown. P_{atm}, P_1 and P_2 are atmospheric pressure, and pressures at the point of entrainment and post entrainment respectively.

first is that since the device is powered by a fixed flow of oxygen, driven through a fine needle at high pressure (typically 4 bar), it is often considered to be a 'flow generator' type of ventilator. Since flow generators deliver a constant flow regardless of the lung compliance and airways resistance, it is often considered that the Sanders injector might generate dangerously high airway pressures. However the Sanders injector is in fact a 'pressure generator' type of ventilator, and its maximum pressure can be predicted by knowledge of its geometry. Standard devices generate peak pressures of around 25 cmH$_2$O.

A second misconception is that the device operates to entrain air according the Venturi principle. The Venturi principle refers to the fact that the pressure in a fluid stream is lower in a narrow section compared to a broader section of pipe. However in the Sanders injector there is no constriction or dilatation, but simply an injection of gas at high velocity via a uniformly narrow needle injector. Entrainment of air is due to friction and shear forces between fast and slow airstreams as described below.

Consider a small injector of cross-sectional area a, placed inside a wider pipe (e.g., a bronchoscope, or the trachea itself) of cross-sectional area A, as shown in Figure 3.11.

Momentum rate

The driving gas is emitted at a high velocity (u_0) since it passes via a narrow 'needle'. In order to overcome the high resistance of this needle, the driving pressure needs to be high (say 4 bar).

At the point of injection, there will be considerable frictional forces between stream of oxygen and the surrounding air. These shear forces will force the surrounding air molecules to a higher velocity, whilst at the same time the sluggish air molecules will drag the once rapid oxygen molecules to a lower velocity. After a certain distance, the oxygen and air molecules will have a common velocity (u_2). At the tip of the injector, where the surrounding air is being dragged along and accelerated, air molecules are dragged and stretched apart which results in a drop in pressure (below atmospheric). This effect is buffered by the fact that air molecules can move in from outside, since $P_{atm} > P_1$.

Let us now consider the momentum of gas at various points in the device. The volume of gas which passes through a pipe per unit time is given by the product of the cross-sectional area and the velocity. So, considering the injector flow,

volume/unit time $= u_0.a$

The mass of gas is given by the volume multiplied by the density, therefore

mass/unit time $= \rho.u_0.a$

The momentum is given by the mass multiplied by the velocity, therefore

momentum/unit time $= \rho.u_0^2.a$

We can repeat this by also writing the momentum rates for the entrained air (u_1) and the oxygen/air mixture (u_2), as has been written in Figure 3.11. At the start of the entrainment process (i.e., at P_1) the sum of the momentum rates is $\rho u_0^2 a + \rho u_1^2 (A-a)$, and at the end of the process (i.e., at P_2) it is $\rho u_2^2 A$. Newton's second law dictates that the difference or *change* in the rates of momentum between these points is equal to the force applied. In our example, the force applied equals the pressure difference multiplied by the area. Hence

$$A(P_1 - P_2) = \rho u_2^2 A - \rho u0^2 a - \rho u_1^2 (A - a)$$

From this equation it can be appreciated that if P_2 rises, the velocity (and hence flow) of the gas mixture,

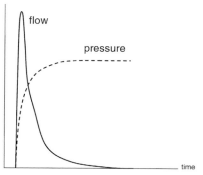

Figure 3.12. Flow and pressure profiles during inflation of the lung with a Sanders injector.

u_2, falls. So the output of the whole device is sensitive to 'back-pressure'. As the lung inflates, the back pressure rises to a degree determined by the lung compliance and airways resistance and so the flow output falls. It is possible to predict the back pressure at which flow output stops altogether (i.e., $u_2 = 0$). At this point no entrainment occurs and the driving oxygen simply flows backwards out of the airway. This so-called 'stalling pressure' represents the maximal inflation pressure which can be achieved. It is determined by the values a, A and u_0, i.e., by the dimensions of the device and the driving pressure. The airway pressure and flow profiles during inflation, which are typical of a 'pressure generator', are shown in Figure 3.12.

The above considerations apply to the use of a jet insufflator when used via a rigid bronchoscope or when applied directly into a patent airway or through the open vocal cords. These physical laws do not apply when a small bore needle is placed into a sealed system as might occur if the needle is placed via the cricothyroid membrane and the cords are closed, or upper airway obstructed. Under these circumstances jet ventilation, as defined above, does not occur. Here the device operates as a flow generator because the sole source of inflating gas is derived from the injector needle, and since this is supplied at high upstream pressure, its flow output is insensitive to downstream airway pressure (i.e., there is no back pressure effect). The flow output and the resultant airway pressure are not easy to predict or measure so great care must be exercised when operating in this way if airway and lung parenchymal trauma are to be avoided.

It could be argued that trans-cricothyroid 'jetting' should not be undertaken if the airway upstream is permanently obstructed since, as CO_2 would not be

effectively cleared, it would not offer any advantage over apnoeic oxygenation or gentle manual ventilation with the cricothyroid cannula.

Key points

- Flow tends to be turbulent in upper airway obstruction, so gas density is influential.
- The human upper airway has a 'collapsible' segment – the pharynx.
- Maintenance of pharyngeal airway patency is a complex neuromuscular phenomenon.
- Expiratory flow is less affected than inspiratory flow in upper airway obstruction; venting of gases through the upper airway is rarely a problem during trans-tracheal jet ventilation.
- In airway obstruction at the pharyngeal level, inspiratory flow may not be increased by increased inspiratory effort, but can be increased by positive pressure applied above the obstruction.

Further reading

Bartlett D Jr, St John WM. (1986). Influence of morphine on respiratory activities of phrenic and hypoglossal nerves in cats. *Respiration Physiology*, **64**, 289–294.

Bethune DW, Collis JM, Burbridge NJ, Forster DM. (1972). Bronchoscope injectors: A design for use with pipeline oxygen supplies. *Anaesthesia*, **27**, 81–83.

Eastwood PR, Szollosi I, Platt PR, Hillman DR. (2002). Collapsibility of the upper airway during anesthesia with isoflurane. *Anesthesiology*, **97**, 786–793.

Fogel R, Malhotra A, Shea S, Edwards J, White D. (2000). Reduced genioglossal activity with upper airway anesthesia in awake patients with OSA. *Journal of Applied Physiology*, **88**, 1346–1354.

Ho MH, Lee A, Karmakar MK, et al. (2003). Heliox vs air-oxygen mixtures for the treatment of patients with acute asthma. *Chest*, **123**, 882–890.

Malhotra A, Fogel R, Edwards J, Shea S, White D. (2000). Local mechanisms drive genioglossus activation in obstructive sleep apnea. *American Journal of Respiratory and Critical Care Medicine*, **161**, 1746–1749.

Mathru M, Esch O, Lang J, et al. (1996). Magnetic resonance imaging of the upper airway. Effects of propofol anesthesia and nasal continuous positive airway pressure in humans. *Anesthesiology*, **84**, 273–279.

Nandi PR, Charlesworth CH, Taylor SJ, Nunn JF, Dore CJ. (1991). Effect of general anaesthesia on the pharynx. *British Journal of Anaesthesia*, **66**, 157–162.

Sanders RD. (1967). Two ventilating attachments for bronchoscopes. *Delaware Medical Journal*, **39**, 170–176.

Airway reflexes

Jeremy A. Langton

Introduction

Knowledge of changes in upper airway reflex activity is of importance to anaesthetists. A clear airway allows safe ventilation of the lungs and oxygenation of the patient. It also provides a means by which the depth of inhalation anaesthesia can be rapidly altered. An increase in the sensitivity of airway reflexes during induction of anaesthesia increases the likelihood of laryngeal spasm and coughing. This may impair the smooth administration of inhalation anaesthesia and when severe may be life threatening. During recovery from anaesthesia the larynx plays a primary role in the protection of the lungs from aspiration of foreign material, an event which may predispose the patient to the development of post-operative chest infection, aspiration pneumonia and lung abscess.

Upper airway reflexes and receptors
Reflexes from the nose

The nasal mucosa receives sensory innervation from the trigeminal nerve (cranial nerve V) via branches of the anterior ethmoidal and maxillary nerves. There are not clearly structurally identified sensory end organs in the nose, however it is thought that non-myelinated nerve endings in the sub-epithelium mediate the nasal reflexes. Airborne chemical irritants cause discharges in the trigeminal nerves and these responses may be responsible for nasal reflexes such as sneezing and apnoea. Nasal irritation more commonly causes apnoea than a sneeze under experimental conditions. The apnoeic reflex is part of the complex diving response, caused by the physiological stimulus of water being applied to the face or into the nose. Apnoea can also be induced by odours or irritants and this response has been identified in all mammalian species studied. The apnoea is associated with cardiovascular changes and complete laryngeal closure which occurs as part of the diving response.

Chemical, mechanical stimuli and also mediators such as histamine can cause sneezing when applied to the nasal mucosa. Local application of capsaicin, which depletes substance P-containing nerves of their neuropeptide, can prevent the sneeze due to the inhaled irritants suggesting that non-myelinated nerves may be the receptors. Positive pressure applied to the nose and nasopharynx can stimulate breathing in man and experimental animals. In addition nasal irritation can cause bronchoconstriction or bronchodilation by two afferent pathways.

Anaesthetic vapours stimulate the nasal mucosa and elicit nasally mediated reflexes. Enflurane may produce the most marked influence on the breathing pattern. Following the start of insufflation of enflurane or isoflurane into the nose, there is a decrease in tidal volume with a prolongation in the expiratory time. Halothane has the least effect. Inhalation induction of anaesthesia using the volatile agents may be associated with breath-holding, coughing and laryngospasm. It is likely that these reflexes arise from stimulation of upper airway receptors. The nose is an important reflexogenic area, and stimulation of the nasal mucosa may cause some of the most frequently seen airway problems during anaesthesia.

Reflexes from the pharynx and nasopharynx

The nasopharynx is supplied by the maxillary nerve (V), and the glossopharyngeal (IX) nerve via the pharyngeal branch provides sensory innervation to the mucous membrane below the nasopharynx. Stimulation of the pharynx and nasopharynx may cause powerful reflexes including hypertension and diaphragmatic contraction.

Core Topics in Airway Management, Second Edition, ed. Ian Calder and Adrian Pearce. Published by Cambridge University Press.
© Cambridge University Press 2011.

Reflexes from the larynx

The innervation of the larynx is by the superior laryngeal nerve (X) and to a lesser extent by the recurrent laryngeal nerves (X). The internal branch of the superior laryngeal nerve contains afferent fibres from the cranial portion of the larynx. The recurrent laryngeal nerve provides afferent innervation to the subglottic area of the larynx. There are many nerve fibres which are thought to be sensory in almost all areas of the laryngeal mucosa and also in some deeper structures. There have been various types of nerve ending identified in and beneath the laryngeal mucosa, the most frequent type is of free nerve endings of myelinated and non-myelinated fibres in the mucosa and submucosa. The posterior supraglottic region has the highest density of free nerve endings, with the afferent fibres being transmitted via the superior laryngeal nerve. Some early work identified two types of receptor in the larynx: one a slowly adapting receptor and the second a rapidly adapting receptor thought to be especially sensitive to chemical stimulants.

Laryngeal afferent neurones with receptive fields in the epiglottis can be activated by a range of stimuli, including water, but mechanical stimuli are the most effective. The sensory units are thought to consist of free nerve endings that lie between the mucosal cells of the airway epithelium.

Laryngospasm

Laryngospasm is a common and potentially dangerous complication of general anaesthesia. It is defined as 'occlusion of the glottis by the action of the intrinsic laryngeal muscles' and is considered to be present when inflation of the lungs is hindered or made impossible by unwanted muscular action of the larynx.

Laryngeal spasm is essentially a protective reflex to prevent foreign material reaching lower down into the lungs. The laryngeal muscles are striated, the most important muscles involved in the production of laryngeal spasm being the lateral cricoarytenoid, thyroarytenoid (adductors of the glottis) and the cricothyroid (tensor of the vocal cords).

During laryngeal spasm in man, either the true vocal cords alone or the true and false cords become apposed in the midline and close the glottis. Rex stated that laryngeal spasm was the most frequent source of respiratory obstruction occurring during general anaesthesia. There are thought to be two initiators of laryngeal spasm during general anaesthesia. Direct irritation of the vocal cords may be caused by a sudden increase in concentration of irritant anaesthetic vapour or direct contact with blood or saliva, and second, traction on abdominal and pelvic viscera. There are many reports in the literature of the inhalation of irritant vapours producing laryngeal spasm, coughing and bronchospasm. Anaesthetic agents may sensitise the receptors, explaining why some inhaled and intravenous agents may easily precipitate laryngeal spasm.

This complication is not uncommon and may indeed be life threatening. In one large study of 156,064 general anaesthetics the overall incidence in all patient groups was 8.7/1000 patients. The incidence was high in children aged between 0 and 9 years, with a peak incidence of 27.6/1000 occurring in infants aged 1–3 months. Work in puppies demonstrated laryngeal adductor hyper-excitability in early life and a similar developmental neuronal imbalance may occur in humans, explaining the increased incidence in infants.

High risk patients are especially vulnerable to hypoxaemia, and therefore avoidance of factors contributing to laryngospasm is important. The incidence of laryngeal spasm is increased in patients with a history of asthma, and also in patients with a history of upper respiratory tract infection. In one study of anaesthesia in children with a history of recent upper respiratory tract infection (URTI) the incidence of laryngeal spasm was increased to 95.8/1000. Pre-existing conditions which are associated with an increased risk of developing laryngospasm may also predispose a patient to bronchospasm.

Factors affecting the sensitivity of upper airway reflexes

Using low inspired concentrations of ammonia vapour as an irritant chemical stimulus allows study of the upper airway in a repeatable and reliable manner. The lowest concentration of ammonia required to elicit a response is termed the threshold concentration (NH3TR). A low value of NH3TR indicates sensitive or reactive airways, whereas a higher NH3TR value represents a reduction in the sensitivity of upper airway reflexes and a depression of airway reflexes. This measure of airway sensitivity is used in several of the figures.

By measurement of the inspiratory flow pattern a measure of the sensitivity of the upper airway reflexes of a subject is made. Studying the sensitivity of upper airway reflexes in subjects suffering with, and recovering from, an URTI showed the sensitivity of airway reflexes was increased until day 15. This coincided with the presence of symptoms. Upper respiratory tract infections cause acute mucosal oedema followed by

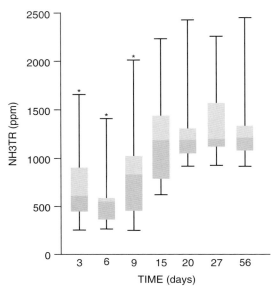

Figure 4.1. The effect of an URTI on upper airway reactivity. Ammonia threshold concentration (NH3TR) in volunteers with an upper respiratory tract infection (URTI) showing the median, interquartile range and the 10th and 90th percentiles **$P < 0.01$ (Wilcoxon). (Taken from Nandwani et al (1997).)

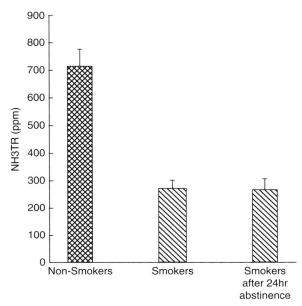

Figure 4.2. Mean (SEM) ammonia thresholds in 20 non-smokers and in 20 smokers before and after 24hr abstinence. ***$P =< 0.001$. (Taken from Erskine et al (1994).)

shedding of epithelial cells. Loss of airway epithelium can extend down to the basement membrane and may persist for up to 3 weeks. The mechanism for upper airway hyper-reactivity following viral infection may be due to increased exposure of intraepithelial sensory receptors to inhaled irritants. Bronchial reactivity to experimentally inhaled histamine is also increased during an URTI and persists for up to 7 weeks. The high incidence of laryngospasm during inhalation anaesthesia is likely to be due to a direct effect of irritant gases and vapours on the airways. In a cross-sectional study of complications of inhalation anaesthesia the overall incidence of laryngeal spasm was 12/1000 cases but patients receiving isoflurane had a much higher incidence of 29/1000 (see Figure 4.1).

Other factors, such as cigarette smoking are known to have an effect on the sensitivity of upper airway reflexes. Following abstinence from smoking this sensitivity is unaltered after 24 hours but the airway became less sensitive over the next 48 hours achieving a consistent change by day 10. It is known that chronic cigarette smokers develop dysplasia of the respiratory epithelium, which may disrupt the integrity of the respiratory epithelium. In addition smokers have depressed production of salivary epidermal growth factor which is known to stimulate epithelial proliferation. The

evidence for epithelial injury or inflammation causing increased airway sensitivity comes from work on the lower airway reflexes after damaging epithelium mechanically or chemically. Both ozone and acute smoke exposure have been shown to increase tracheal mucosal permeability with increased airway responsiveness. Nebulised lidocaine administered pre-operatively to a group of smokers, prior to induction of anaesthesia significantly improved the quality of induction of anaesthesia in smokers (see Figure 4.2).

Age is known to affect laryngeal reflexes, with the reactivity being thought to diminish with advancing age. Laryngeal reflexes in the elderly appear to be less active, both during induction of anaesthesia and in the recovery room, compared to a younger patient, suggesting that protection of the airway may be impaired in the elderly. A study of airway reflexes in different age groups found the sensitivity decreased by a factor of three between the third and ninth decade of life (see Figure 4.3).

Anaesthetic agents and laryngeal reflexes

Inhalation anaesthetic agents

The respiratory tract is hypersensitive to stimuli arising during light general anaesthesia. Rex examined

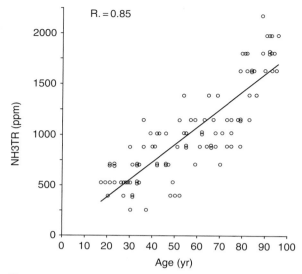

Figure 4.3. Correlation between age and ammonia threshold. Correlation coefficient +0.85. (Taken from Erskine et al (1993).)

the laryngeal responses induced by volatile anaesthetic agents and found that ether and halothane produced laryngeal spasm. Nishino investigated the effects of halothane, enflurane and isoflurane on receptors within the isolated upper airway of dogs and found that only halothane produced an inhibitory effect on receptor discharge. Other workers have reported the irritant effects of isoflurane during induction of anaesthesia. Desflurane is also known to have significant irritant effects on the airway during anaesthesia.

One comparison of the volatile agents found airway irritation most frequently with isoflurane, followed by enflurane, halothane and least frequently by sevoflurane. They concluded that sevoflurane did not elicit the cough reflex and was the least irritant of modern inhalation anaesthetics suggesting it was the preferential agent for inhalation induction of anaesthesia.

Intravenous anaesthetic agents

Thiopentone

Early work with thiopentone conducted in an animal model (cat), found that most of the animals would cough, sneeze or hiccup during thiopentone anaesthesia. Inspection of the glottis in these animals revealed hyperactive adducted vocal cords and lifting the epiglottis elicited complete closure of the glottis. The administration of large doses of atropine (3–5 mg kg^{-1}) would lead to relaxation of the vocal cords and it was concluded that the closure of the glottis following

intravenous barbiturates was probably mediated via the parasympathetic nervous system.

A number of later workers reported the occurrence of temporary closure of the glottis and the hyperactive state of the laryngeal reflex following induction of anaesthesia with thiopentone. Possible proposed mechanisms included (i) that peripheral afferent nerve endings are more sensitive to stimuli and (ii) increased sensitivity in the pathway between the afferent vagal nucleus of the solitary tract and the efferent vagal nucleus ambiguous.

Propofol

Since the introduction of propofol into anaesthetic practice more than 30 years ago, there have been several reports of a lack of excitatory upper airway effects associated with its use. De Grood noted that during induction of anaesthesia with propofol the vocal cords were abducted and tracheal intubation was possible using propofol alone. In contrast following thiopentone induction the vocal cords of >50% of subjects were closed. Another study used a fibrescope to measure the movements of the vocal cords on induction of anaesthesia with either thiopentone or propofol. With thiopentone the vocal cords often closed, whereas following induction with propofol the vocal cords remained abducted. This was thought to be due to a different action of these two agents on the sensitivity of airway reflexes. Other workers have reported that airway manipulation, insertion of airways and laryngeal mask insertion are more easily tolerated following induction of anaesthesia with propofol (see Figure 4.4).

Opioids

Fentanyl has been shown to depress airway reflex responses in a dose-related manner and has also been successfully used to reduce desflurane induced airway irritability. Remifentanil has been demonstrated to improve the intubating conditions in children during sevoflurane anaesthesia. There have also been many studies showing that remifentanil and alfentanil improve conditions for laryngeal mask insertion and during awake intubation.

Benzodiazepines

Benzodiazepines are widely used to produce short-term sedation and anxiolysis to facilitate endoscopy and minor surgical procedures. However it is known that these drugs produce depression of the sensitivity

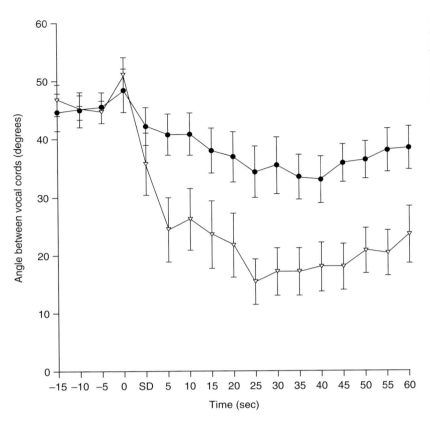

Figure 4.4. Angle between vocal cords after induction of anaesthesia with propofol or thiopentone (mean, SEM). Time 0 = start of the injection of thiopentone or propofol. SD = syringe drop. Circles: propofol; open triangle: thiopentone. (Taken from Barker et al (1992).)

of upper airway reflexes. This may impair the ability of the patient to protect their lower airway from aspiration. The effect of intravenous diazepam, midazolam and the benzodiazepine reversal agent flumazenil on the sensitivity of airway reflexes, assessed by the identification of reflex glottic closure in response to a threshold concentration of inhaled ammonia vapour, have been studied. Both diazepam (0.2 mg.kg^{-1}) and midazolam (0.07 mg.kg^{-1}) produced significant depression of the sensitivity of upper airway reflexes, maximal within 10 minutes of administration with baseline values regained within 60 minutes.

Flumazenil (300 micrograms) administered 10 minutes after midazolam resulted in significant reversal of the depression of airway reflexes. The same research group investigated the effect of oral diazepam and found significant depression of airway reflexes from 30 to 150 minutes following administration. Benzodiazepines also impair airway maintenance particularly by reducing the tonic contraction of genioglossus, muscle activity essential to keep the tongue away from the posterior pharyngeal wall.

Benzodiazepines should not be considered safe agents in airway obstruction.

Local anaesthetic agents

Local anaesthetic agents are often applied to the airway both to facilitate fibreoptic intubation in awake patients and also to reduce the reflex physiological effects of tracheal intubation and extubation. Raphael studied the effects of topical benzocaine and lidocaine applied to the airway. They investigated the effects of benzocaine lozenges, nebulised lidocaine and lidocaine applied directly on to the vocal cords. Benzocaine lozenges produced a significant effect within 10 minutes returning to normal within 25 minutes, whereas directly applied lidocaine produced a significant effect lasting 100 minutes. Nebulised lidocaine had an effect lasting 30 minutes (see Figure 4.5).

Local anaesthetic agents have also been used intravenously. Nishino investigated bolus administration of lidocaine 1.5 mg kg^{-1} intravenously on respiratory responses to airway irritation. Prior to the administration of lidocaine airway irritation caused not

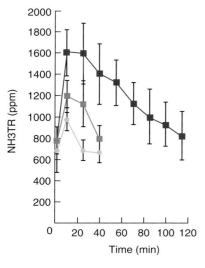

Figure 4.5. Effects of topical vocal cord lignocaine, nebulised lignocaine and oral benzocaine lozenges, on upper airway threshold response to ammonia stimulation (NH3TR) (mean, 95% CI). (Taken from Murphy et al (1994).)

only the cough reflex, but also other respiratory reflexes such as expiration, apnoea and spasmodic panting. Immediately following the administration of intravenous lidocaine (when plasma concentrations were >4.7 μg/ml), tracheal irritation elicited only brief apnoea, and other reflex responses were completely suppressed.

It should be noted that the initial application of local anaesthetic agents to the airway may be associated with laryngospasm. Several clinical reports describe loss of the airway immediately following topicalisation during preparation for awake intubation. This may a response to the initial stimulation of airway receptors by chemico-physical contact with the agent.

Airway patency

An important bony structure that determines the airway size is the mandible, to which muscle and soft tissue are attached. It can therefore act as a lever and tensor. There are more than 20 muscles surrounding the upper airway which constrict and dilate its lumen. For simplicity they can be lumped together as 'pharyngeal dilator muscles', but in reality these groups of muscles interact to determine the patency of the airway in a complex fashion which is not fully understood. The most widely studied of these muscles is genioglossus, which principally controls the position of the tongue and hyoid apparatus. Genioglossus has its origin at the symphysis menti and is inserted into the dorsum of the tongue and hyoid bone. Tonic contraction is required to keep the tongue forward and maintain airway patency. Genioglossus activity is diminished by anaesthesia and residual neuromuscular blockade.

It is thought unlikely that the pharynx is dilated by active dilatation on muscle groups within the pharyngeal wall, but rather paradoxically that these muscles actively *constrict*. Evidence for this is provided by the fact that the electromyographic (EMG) activity of these muscles *increases* as the pharynx dilates. It remains unclear whether the 'dilator' muscles act to dilate the airway, or whether the increase in muscle tone merely acts to stabilise the airway to withstand the collapsing forces present during inspiration.

Control of pharyngeal dilator activity

The activity of the pharyngeal dilator muscles is influenced by many factors, including arterial P_{O2} and P_{CO2}, airway P_{CO2}, arousal, hormones (progesterone/oestrogen), lung volume and intrapharyngeal negative pressure.

Local reflexes

The upper airway is richly supplied with receptors, including baroreceptors and chemoreceptors which play a role in modulating the baseline steady-state (i.e., tonic) EMG activity of pharyngeal dilators. Airway baroreceptors detect any fall in upper airway pressure and, possibly via a centrally mediated reflex, increase muscle tone to oppose the airway collapse which such a negative pressure would otherwise have produced. The tonic EMG activity is reduced if this reflex is blocked by application of local anaesthesia to the upper airway. Similarly, EMG activity is reduced when patients switch between breathing via the upper airway and breathing via a tracheostomy.

Phasic and central pharyngeal muscle activity

In addition to the background or 'tonic' activity, pharyngeal muscles also have 'phasic' activity, i.e., their EMG activity occurs in phase with tidal ventilation: increasing during inspiration, and diminishing in expiration. More interestingly, this activity can be shown to *precede* by a few milliseconds, the activation of the diaphragm (i.e., it occurs before airflow begins and before any local negative pressure sensors could be responsible for activating it), as if pre-activating the upper airway muscles in preparation for the impending negative pressure of inspiration. It is now thought that the pharyngeal dilators, in addition to the diaphragm, comprise the efferent output of the respiratory centre. Moreover, both hypoxic and hypercapnic drive to the respiratory centre, via stimulation of central and carotid body chemoreceptors, produce just as much of an increase in phasic efferent drive to the pharyngeal dilators as they do to the diaphragm. It is clear now that both *central* control of ventilation and control of airway patency are intimately linked.

Further reading

Barker P, Langton JA, Wilson IG, Smith G. (1992). Movements of the vocal cords on induction of anaesthesia with thiopentone or propofol. *British Journal of Anaesthesia*, **69**, 23–25.

Burstein CL, Rovenstine EA. (1938). Respiratory parasympathetic action of some shorter acting barbituric acid derivatives. *Journal of Pharmacology and Experimental Therapeutics*, **63**, 42–44.

Caranza R, Raphael JH, Nandwani N, Langton JA. (1997). Effect of nebulised lignocaine on the quality of induction of anaesthesia in cigarette smokers. *Anaesthesia*, **52**, 849–852.

De Grood PM, Van Egmond J, Van De Wetering M, Van Beem HB, Booij LH, Crul JF. (1985). Lack of effects of emulsified propofol (Diprivan) on vecuronium pharmacodynamics: Preliminary results in man. *Postgraduate Medical Journal*, **61**, 28–30.

Doi M, Ikeda K. (1993). Airway irritation produced by volatile anaesthetics during brief inhalation: Comparison of halothane, enflurane, isoflurane and sevoflurane. *Canadian Journal of Anaesthesia*, **40**, 122–126.

Empey DW, Laitinen LA, Jacobs L, Gold WM, Nadel JA. (1976). Mechanisms of bronchial hyperreactivity in normal subjects after upper respiratory tract infection. *American Review of Respiratory Disease*, **113**, 131–139.

Erskine RJ, Murphy PJ, Langton JA. (1994). Sensitivity of upper airway reflexes in cigarette smokers: Effect of abstinence. *British Journal of Anaesthesia*, **73**, 298–302.

Erskine RJ, Murphy PJ, Langton JA, Smith G. (1993). Effect of age on the sensitivity of upper airway reflexes. *British Journal of Anaesthesia*, **70**, 574–575.

Golden JA, Nadel JA, Boushey HA. (1978). Bronchial hyperreactivity in healthy subjects after exposure to ozone. *American Review of Respiratory Disease*, **118**, 287–294.

Groves ND, Rees JL, Rosen M. (1987). Effects of benzodiazepines on laryngeal reflexes. *Anaesthesia*, **42**, 808–814.

Harrison GA. (1962). The influence of different anaesthetic agents on the response to respiratory tract irritation. *British Journal of Anaesthesia*, **34**, 804–811.

Herbstreit F, Peters J, Eikermann M. (2009). Impaired upper airway integrity by residual neuromuscular blockade. *Anesthesiology*, **110**, 1253–1260.

Hoglund NJ, Michaelsson M. (1950). A method for determining the cough threshold with some preliminary experiments on the effects of codeine. *Acta Physiologica Scandinavica*, **21**, 168–173.

Langton JA, Murphy PJ, Barker P, Key A, Smith G. (1993). Measurement of the sensitivity of upper airway reflexes. *British Journal of Anaesthesia*, **70**, 126–130.

Lee J, Oh Y, Kim C. (2006). Fentanyl reduces desflurane induced airway irritability following thiopentone administration in children. *Acta Anaesthesiologica Scandinavica*, **50**, 1161–1164.

Lew JK, Spence AA, Elton RA. (1991). Cross sectional study of complications of inhalational anaesthesia in 16,995 patients. *Anaesthesia*, **46**, 810–815.

Murphy PJ, Erskine R, Langton JA. (1994). The effect of intravenously administered diazepam, midazolam and flumazenil on the sensitivity of upper airway reflexes. *Anaesthesia*, **49**, 105–110.

Nandwani N, Raphael J, Langton JA. (1997). Effect of an upper respiratory tract infection on upper airway reactivity. *British Journal of Anaesthesia*, **78**, 352–355.

Nishino T. (2000). Physiological and pathophysiological implications of upper airway reflexes in humans. *Japanese Journal of Physiology*, **50**, 3–14.

Nishino T, Anderson JW, Sant'Ambrogio G. (1993). Effects of halothane, enflurane, and isoflurane on laryngeal receptors in dogs. *Respiratory Physiology*, **91**, 247–260.

Nishino T, Hiraga K, Sugimari K. (1990). Effects if intravenous lignocaine on airway reflexes elicited by irritation of the tracheal mucosa in humans anaesthetised with enflurane. *British Journal of Anaesthesia*, **64**, 682–687.

Nishino T, Tanaka A, Ishikawa T, Hiraga K. (1991). Respiratory, laryngeal and tracheal responses to nasal isufflation of volatile anaesthetics in anesthetised humans. *Anesthesiology*, **75**, 441–444.

Olsson GL, Hallen B. (1984). Laryngospasm during anaesthesia. A computer aided incidence study in 136,929 patients. *Acta Anaesthesiologica Scandinavica*, **28**, 567–575.

Pontoppidan H, Beecher HK. (1960). Progressive loss of protective reflexes in the airway with the advance of age. *Journal of the American Medical Association*, **174**, 2209–2213.

Raphael JH, Stanley GD, Langton JA. (1996). Effects of topical benzocaine and lignocaine on upper airway reflex sensitivity. *Anaesthesia*, **51**, 114–118.

Rex MAE. (1966). Stimulation of laryngospasm in the cat by volatile anaesthetics. *British Journal of Anaesthesia*, **38**, 569–571.

Rex MAE. (1970). A review of the structural and functional basis of laryngospasm and discussion of the nerve pathways involved in the reflex and its clinical significance in man and animals. *British Journal of Anaesthesia*, **42**, 891–899.

Sasaki CT. (1979). Development of laryngeal function: Etiological significance in the sudden infant death syndrome. *Laryngoscope*, **89**, 1964–1982.

Tagaito Y, Isono S, Nishino T. (1998). Upper airway reflexes during a combination of propofol and fentanyl anaesthesia. *Anesthesiology*, **88**, 1459–1466.

Verghese ST, Hannallah RS, Brennan M. (2008). The effect of intranasal administration of remifentanil on intubating conditions and airway response after sevoflurane induction of anaesthesia in children. *Anesthesia and Analgesia*, **107**, 1176–1181.

Widdicombe JG. (1981). Nervous receptors in the respiratory tract and lungs. In: Hornbein TF (Ed.), *Regulation of Breathing*. **Vol. 1**. New York: Dekker. pp. 429–472.

Chapter 5

Decontamination of airway equipment

Adrian Pearce

The medical devices used to manage the airway come into contact with mucous membranes and there is a risk of cross-infection if they are reused. There is now extensive guidance on the appropriate policies to be followed to prevent cross-infection. The organisms responsible are mainly viruses, bacteria, spores and yeasts but concern has also been expressed about the risk of transmission of spongiform encephalopathies.

Transmissable spongiform encephalopathies (TSE)

Human TSEs are rare degenerative neurological disorders and include Creutzfeldt-Jakob disease (CJD), kuru and fatal familial insomnia. CJD is the commonest (prevalence ~ 1/million people) and occurs worldwide in a sporadic (90%) and familial form (10%). There have been a few hundred cases of iatrogenic CJD transmitted by contaminated medical devices, extracted pituitary hormones or implantation of contaminated cornea or dural grafts. A variant form (vCJD) first appeared in the UK in 1994 related to the ingestion of beef infected with bovine spongiform encephalopathy. Patients with vCJD are younger at presentation (mean 29 yr) than with sporadic CJD (65 yr) and usually show sensory and psychiatric symptoms. In February 2010 there have been 169 deaths in the UK from vCJD (peaking in year 2000) with 25 in France. Lymphoid tissue such as the tonsil is deemed of medium infectivity for vCJD.

The infective agent for TSE transmission is an abnormal prion protein. The conversion of the normal cellular prion protein (PrP^c) into the abnormal form (PrP^{sc}) involves a conformational change such that the α-helical content diminishes and the β-pleated sheet increases. No prion-specific nucleic acid is involved in disease transmission, and abnormal prion-protein

infectivity is not controlled by standard decontamination procedures of standard autoclaving or cold-chemical sterilisation.

NICE guidance has been issued on the prevention of iatrogenic CJD through surgical instruments in contact with the high-risk tissues of the outer layer of the brain, optic nerve and retina. Reusable equipment should never be used in patients known or suspected of having CJD unless the equipment is to be destroyed after use. In the case of flexible fibre-scopes, dedicated endoscopes may be obtained from the National CJD Surveillance Unit in Edinburgh or there may be a local policy. The tonsillar bed has been identified as a high-risk area and in routine practice tracheal tubes, supraglottic and oral airways should be discarded after use in this procedure. A previous recommendation that a disposable laryngoscope blade should always be used for tonsillectomy has been modified by the latest Working Party of the Association of Anaesthetists of Great Britain and Ireland (AAGBI) which suggests that the risk is so low that a reusable one may be used but only if it is considered superior in clinical performance to a disposable blade. There are currently no known cases of TSE transmission via reused airway equipment.

Definitions

Decontamination is the combination of processes, including cleaning, disinfection and/or sterilisation, used to render a reusable medical device safe for further use.

Disinfection means the elimination of all vegetative pathogenic organisms such as bacteria and viruses.

Sterilisation indicates the elimination of all pathogens including spores. For a terminally sterilised

Core Topics in Airway Management, Second Edition, ed. Ian Calder and Adrian Pearce. Published by Cambridge University Press.
© Cambridge University Press 2011.

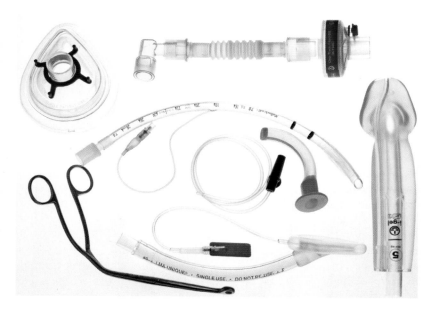

Figure 5.1. Most airway equipment is single use.

medical device to be labelled sterile, the theoretical probability of there being a viable microorganism present on the device should be equal to or less than 1×10^{-6}.

UK legal framework

In January 2009 the Health Act (2006) was superseded by the Health and Social Care Act (2008) which contains a Code of Practice for the NHS with regard to prevention and control of healthcare-associated infections. With effect from 1 April 2009 the Care Quality Commission (CQC) is the regulatory body with authority to take any actions necessary to protect patients. There are nine specific criteria in the latest Hygiene Code detailing the standards required within a hospital and unannounced visits are part of the inspection process. All Trusts should have Infection Control Committees and Teams which are responsible for preparing infection control policies to conform to all national and international standards and recommendations. Health Technical Memorandum HTM 01–01 series covers the essential information and is currently under revision.

A guideline on infection control within anaesthesia was published by the AAGBI in 2008 and provides valuable advice. There are three possible options for airway equipment – single use equipment, steam sterilisation or cold chemical sterilisation.

Single use, disposable

Single use equipment eliminates the risk of cross-infection between patients through the airway device and is the preferred option. The term is used for both equipment used only once (e.g., a suction catheter) and equipment reused within a patient event such as a laryngoscope or yankauer suction. It has the additional benefits;

- Sterile (often by γ irradiation) and packed ready for use
- Does not require the laborious process of in-hospital cleaning and sterilisation
- No structural deterioration through use or repeated sterilisation.

It has become standard for tracheal tubes, oral and nasopharyngeal airways, catheter mounts, breathing filters/humidifiers, plastic facemasks, introducers, stylets, airway exchange catheters and suction apparatus (Figure 5.1). Some metal laryngoscope blades and Magill forceps are produced so cheaply now that they too are labelled single use. It is easy to envisage that all breathing systems, laryngoscope blades, laryngeal masks and facemasks will become single use in future, and the advances here are limited by cost or supply pressures and concerns about the comparable clinical performance of single use versus reusable airway devices. Packaging should not be removed until the point of use to ensure infection control, accurate identification of component, traceability in the case of manufacturer's recall or hazard notice and safety. Plastic equipment should always be checked before use in case of manufacturing fault – one of the causes of failed ventilation is a blocked catheter mount or tube.

Items marked for single use only may not be reused without compromising the Trust Clinical Negligence Scheme or exposing patients to the risk of cross-infection. Various disposable sheaths have been developed which fit over rigid and flexible fibrescopes, but they are not popular and tend to decrease the transmitted light intensity. Some of the new indirect laryngoscopes use a plastic disposable blade. Whilst the part of the device in the mouth is discarded after single use, the rest of the instrument may become contaminated by handling with soiled gloves. A high incidence of bacterial contamination of laryngoscope handles has been found despite low-level disinfection.

The disadvantages of single use equipment are mainly the problems of ordering, storage and disposal of large volumes of stock. These problems are partly within the hospital but there is also an ecological cost dealing with mass produced disposable plastic components. Another concern with single use equipment is whether it behaves comparably with a reusable version. This has been evident in the early single use introducers in comparison with the original 'gum-elastic bougie'. Another notable example was with the use of single use surgical instruments for tonsillectomy. The equipment was not of the same standard or design as the reusable instruments and there was a rise in the incidence of post-tonsillectomy bleeding.

Heat sterilisation

Sufficient heat will destroy viruses, bacteria and spores but may damage thermally sensitive equipment such as flexible fibrescopes. Repeated cycles of heat sterilisation will produce loss of transmitted light in rigid laryngoscope bundles. It remains the mainstay for surgical equipment (too expensive for single use status) but is commonly used currently for reusable laryngeal masks (classic, Proseal and intubating) (Figure 5.2), laryngoscope blades and handles without batteries, black rubber facemasks, rubber or silicone catheter mounts and some types of Magill forceps. While dry-heat may be used, it is more common to use saturated steam under pressure. The thermal

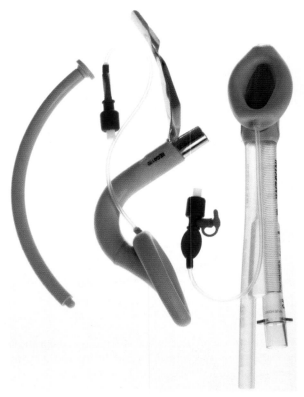

Figure 5.2. Reusable Proseal and intubating laryngeal masks should be autoclaved.

energy of steam is many times higher than dry air at the same temperature.

The process starts with instrument cleaning to remove all blood, tissue or body fluids from the instrument. Studies from surgical instruments which are ready for use have shown that many are still contaminated with blood or tissue from previous patients. This is extremely worrying when one considers that prions are not destroyed by the temperatures reached in normal autoclaving. Apparently clean reusable anaesthetic equipment such as laryngeal masks and laryngoscope blades can be contaminated with a deposit which stains red with erythrosin, the dye which indicates the presence of plaque – a proteinaceous aggregate which rapidly develops on anything placed in the mouth (Figure 5.3). Manual cleaning, external and internal, with a scrubbing brush, warm water and detergent can be very effective but is time consuming and has no quality standard – some people are more diligent scrubbers! Immersion in a enzymatic detergent with an agitated wash or

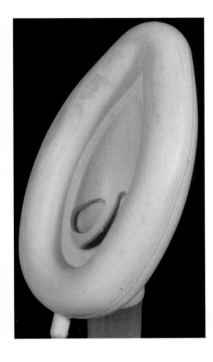

Figure 5.3. Pink staining proteinaceous material on 'clean' reusable laryngeal mask.

Table 5.1. Properties of an ideal cold chemical sterilising agent

Cheap

Long shelf-life

Sterilant rather than disinfectant

Short stand time (~5 minutes) to achieve sterilisation

No adverse effects on fibrescope or disinfection equipment

Non-toxic to healthcare workers

No special requirement for disposal of used solution

ultrasonic cleaning cycle will have a better quality standard. Air should be evacuated from all cuffs and pilot balloons.

Porous-load sterilisers (autoclaves) use vacuum assistance to remove air from the chamber prior to steam ingress and are suitable for all airway devices including those with lumens (e.g., laryngeal masks). The stages of the operating cycle are air evacuation, sterilising and post-vacuum or drying. A typical cycle incorporates a temperature of 134–138°C held for 12 minutes. Simple bench-top sterilisers without vacuum assistance are unsuitable for wrapped loads or devices with lumens. Regular functional testing of the steriliser is required. This is aided by chemical process indicators which may be distributed within the test load and demonstrate a change of colour when exposed to heat. The chemical indicators may be autoclave tape, test tubes containing chemical indicator or sterilisation bags. Reusable laryngeal masks can be autoclaved 40 times and the special reusable tubes for the ILMA 10 times before they should be discarded.

Cold chemical sterilisation

Cold chemical sterilisation is appropriate for devices which are not single use and are thermally sensitive. Intubating fibrescopes are now the only commonly used airway equipment sterilised in this manner. Until recently the standard agent was 2% activated glutaraldehyde and, after cleaning with detergent, the fibrescope was fully immersed for 10–20 minutes. This immersion time was considered suitable for vegetative organisms but was ineffective against spores so that these immersion times allowed disinfection but not sterilisation. Glutaraldehyde vaporises easily and is toxic, irritant and allergenic. The Control of Substances Hazardous to Health (COSHH) Regulations 1988 limits occupational atmospheric exposure to 0.05 ppm.

Developments in cold sterilising chemicals have concentrated on killing all organisms (sterilisation), reducing the stand-time to no more than 5–10 minutes, making the agents non-toxic to healthcare professionals, patients and to the fibrescopes themselves. The characteristics of the ideal cold chemical sterilising agent are shown in Table 5.1. Newer substances include:

- Peracetic acid (NuCidex, Gigasept, Perasafe)
- Ortho-phthalaldehyde (Cidex-OPA)
- Super-oxidised water (Sterilox)
- Chlorine dioxide (Tristel).

Immediately after use the fibrescope should be decontaminated by thorough manual washing/scrubbing of the external surface and working channel in a low-foaming, enzymatic detergent solution to remove blood, mucus and biofilm (Figure 5.4). Biofilm bacteria are firmly attached to one another by exopolysaccharide making them difficult to remove. Any suction valves should be removed and disassembled for cleaning and the working channel cleaned with an appropriate single use channel cleaning brush. The stage of cleaning is essential because disinfectants do not penetrate mucus or biofilm.

39

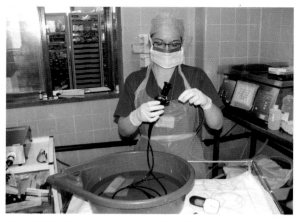

Figure 5.4. Detergent cleaning and brushing the working channel of a fibrescope.

The scope is rinsed with water to remove the detergent and taken to an automated disinfector which generally starts with a detergent cycle and rinse (including irrigation of the working channel), followed by a stand-time of appropriate length in the disinfectant or sterilant. A final rinse with sterile or filtered water renders the fibrescope ready for reuse. Automated processes are superior to manual cleaning because they are more open to quality control. A label indicating satisfactory cleaning should be attached to the patient's notes along with a record of the fibrescope identity, and a patient register should be maintained for each fibrescope. This allows tracking of the clinical use of a fibrescope.

Irrigation of the working channel with isopropyl alcohol is recommended before the scope is stored in a dry environment, without the suction valve in place and with the insertion tube hanging down to let the working channel dry out. If fibrescopes are stored in non-sterile cupboards it is recommended they undergo another automated sterilisation cycle before use, if the interval between disinfection and elective clinical use is more than a few hours. Ultraviolet cabinets are available which maintain sterility of a sterilised fibrescope for 72 hours. If the fibrescope is packed as for a surgical instrument it will remain sterile until the pack is open.

Ethylene oxide

Ethylene oxide (C_2H_4O, MW 44) is a flammable, colourless gas at temperatures above $11\,^{\circ}C$. It is normally mixed with 85% carbon dioxide for storage and

the cylinder has red and yellow shoulder rings to notify explosive and poisonous contents. It possesses good sterilant properties but has a number of serious disadvantages. The gas is flammable and toxic causing eye pain, sore throat, dizziness, nausea, headache, convulsions and death in high concentrations. It is also carcinogenic. It may be used for thermally sensitive equipment such as an intubating fibrescope. However the cycle time for gassing and degassing is several days and stock levels must take account of this.

Key points

- Cross-infection may occur through reusable airway devices.
- Airway equipment should be single use disposable when possible.
- Reusable equipment should be heat sterilised if possible.
- Porous-load autoclaves are required for equipment with lumens.
- Chemical disinfection is required for fibrescopes.
- Automated disinfectors should be used for fibrescopes.
- Abnormal prion proteins are not destroyed by standard autoclave or chemical disinfection cycles.

Further reading

Association of Anaesthetists of Great Britain and Ireland (2008). Infection control in anaesthesia. *Anaesthesia*, **63**, 1027–1036.

Bannon L, Brimacombe J, Nixon T, Keller C. (2005). Repeat autoclaving does not remove protein deposits from the classic laryngeal mask airway. *European Journal of Anaesthesiology*, **22**, 515–517.

Barnett M, Rios M. (2009). Preventing hospital-acquired infections from reprocessed multiple-use medical devices. *Journal Clinical Engineering*, **34**, 139–141.

Blunt MC, Burchett KR. (2003). Variant Creutzfeldt–Jakob disease and disposable anaesthetic equipment – balancing the risks. *British Journal of Anaesthesia*, **90**, 1–3.

British Society of Gastroenterology. (2008). *Guidelines for Decontamination of Equipment for Gastrointestinal Endoscopy.* Available at: www.bsg.org.uk.

Bucx MJ, Dankert J, Beenhakker MM, Harrison TE. (2001). Decontamination of laryngoscopes in the Netherlands. *British Journal of Anaesthesia*, **86**, 99–102.

Call TR, Auerbach FJ, Riddell SW, Kiska DL, Thongrod SC, Tham SW. (2009). Nosocomial contamination of laryngoscope handles: Challenging current guidelines. *Anesthesia Analgesia*, **109**, 479–483.

Dettenkofer M, Block C. (2005). Hospital disinfection: Efficacy and safety issues. *Current Opinion in Infectious Diseases*, **18**, 320–325.

Miller DM, Youkhana I, Karunaratne WU, Pearce A. (2001). Presence of protein deposits on 'cleaned' reusable anaesthetic equipment. *Anaesthesia*, **56**, 1069–1072.

National Institute for Health and Clinical Excellence. (2006). *Patient safety and reduction of risk of transmission of Creutzfeld-Jakob disease (CJD) via interventional procedures*. Available at: www.nice.org.uk/IPG196.

Rowley E, Dingwall R. (2007). The use of single-use devices in anaesthesia: Balancing the risks to patient safety. *Anaesthesia*, **62**, 569–574.

Seoane-Vazquez E, Rodriguez-Monguio R. (2008). Endoscopy-related infection: Relic of the past? *Current Opinion in Infectious Diseases*, **21**, 362–366.

Weber DJ, Rutala WA. (2002). Managing the risk of nosocomial transmission of prion diseases. *Current Opinion in Infectious Diseases*, **15**, 421–425.

Clinical

Basic principles of airway management

Ian Calder and Adrian Pearce

Serious airway problems are not common, which makes rigorous, ethical, research into whether one treatment is better than another almost impossible. Hanley and Lippman-Hand pointed out in their classic publication 'If nothing goes wrong, is everything all right?', that it is unwise to claim that a technique is safe, or safer than an alternative, until a great many successful interventions have been achieved.

Complete agreement about fairly basic matters, such as whether cricoid pressure is worthwhile, or the proper use of neuro-muscular blocking drugs (NMBD), is lacking. Nevertheless, almost everybody agrees about some things (Box 6.1).

Planning airway management

A process that might help to ensure safe management of the airway was suggested by the American Society of Anesthesiologists (ASA) in 1993. It remains a sensible approach.

Evaluation of the airway

Evaluation of the airway seeks to establish which airway device will provide the appropriate level of airway protection and maintenance for the proposed treatment, and whether there will be any difficulty. All patients managed by an anaesthetist should have an airway evaluation because even those undergoing surgery under sedation, local or regional anaesthesia may require conversion to general anaesthesia or resuscitation. Predicting airway difficulty is covered in detail in Chapter 7. Predicting difficulty may lead to postponement of surgery, undertaking surgery under local or regional anaesthesia, assembling additional help or equipment, planning ways of managing the airway and allows discussion with the patient about possible

---

Box 6.1 Airway management – basic principles

1. **Preparation is paramount:** this includes ensuring that the correct staff and equipment are assembled.
2. A suitably trained assistant increases safety.
3. Pre-oxygenation gives valuable extra time for establishment of a patent airway.
4. Difficulty is more likely when the procedure is part of emergency management.
5. Have a self-inflating bag and suction available at all times.
6. Good monitoring equipment reduces the frequency of serious complications.
7. The airway should be expected to become less patent as the conscious level declines.
8. Aspiration of material into the lungs becomes a possibility when the conscious level declines.
9. If difficulty with an airway is possible, consideration should be given to regional or local anaesthesia.
10. If the airway is likely to be uncontrollable with facemask, supraglottic device or by laryngoscopic introduction of a tracheal tube after induction, then a tracheal airway should be established before induction: the problem here is the definition of 'likely' – see Chapter 7.

Box 6.2 Steps in airway management (ASA)

Evaluation of the airway
Preparation for difficulty
Airway strategy at the start of 'anaesthesia'
Airway strategy at the end of 'anaesthesia'
Follow-up

---

options. Evaluation is an imperfect process so that patients regarded as normal may not be, and patients predicted to be difficult may not be.

Preparation for difficulty

Practitioners have to make plans based on their perception of the degree or nature of the difficulty expected. A plan requires at least thought, time, personnel, drugs and equipment. We need to be sure that we have access to the drugs and equipment we will need to implement alternative plans when difficulty occurs unexpectedly. The equipment for routine airway management should be on a trolley in every anaesthetic area but the anaesthetist has the duty of checking that all equipment is ready before starting each patient. More specialised equipment used only in difficult circumstances is commonly kept on a difficult airway trolley. Suggestions for the contents of standard and difficult airway equipment trolleys are given on the Difficult Airway Society (DAS) website www.das.uk.com. If difficulty is predicted there is time to get help from another practitioner. Two people's thoughts about the way to manage a certain problem will be more wide-ranging than one person's and there is much benefit in open discussion. Arbous et al have confirmed that the presence of two trained practitioners improves outcome. The plan will involve the whole team looking after the patient.

Airway strategy

A strategy is a combination of plans and is generally described as formulating a primary or initial Plan A and back-up Plan B, C or more. It is essentially a 'what if' exercise. This process has to be followed for both induction and emergence from anaesthesia (see Chapter 17). Airway difficulty is not predicted in a proportion of cases, so that practitioners need to develop a template that they will implement when time, assistance and equipment are restricted. If face-mask anaesthesia is Plan A and this proves unsatisfactory, Plan B is often to insert a laryngeal mask. If Plan A is insertion of a laryngeal mask and this proves to be unsatisfactory, Plan B is usually tracheal intubation. If tracheal intubation is required in Plan A and this fails, it is possible to make a decision that the operation can, after all, be undertaken with a laryngeal mask (see Chapter 20). Generally, however if tracheal intubation is considered to be the correct level of airway maintenance and protection it may be considered desirable for Plan B also, in which case equipment for alternative methods of intubation should be available (See Chapter 19). In extreme, but fortunately rare, cases establishment of cardio-pulmonary bypass (femoro–femoro) *before* induction of anaesthesia is required.

Algorithms and flow-charts

One of the ways of producing some structure to the way in which we think about managing normal and difficult airways is by algorithm or flow-chart. In order to be useful, it is probable that difficult airway flow-charts should use only a range of core skills which are in the training syllabus, that the flow-chart addresses a well-defined common airway scenario and that the chart contains information about the individual steps. Flow-charts, appropriate to the UK, describing routine or default intubation strategy, failed rapid sequence induction and failed ventilation were produced by the Difficult Airway Society in 2004 and are available as a published article and also on the DAS website (www.das.uk.com).

Routine or default intubation strategy

One of the DAS flow-charts (Figure 6.1) covers the commonest clinical scenario which gives rise to problems, that of unanticipated difficult intubation in an elective surgical patient. The prevalence of failure to intubate by direct laryngoscopy aided by a bougie, by a trained anaesthetist, is probably only about 1:500–2000 in general surgical patients in whom no problem is predicted. This means that an 'average' anaesthetist will fail to intubate in a general surgical patient no more than once every 3 to 5 years. One of the problems is that managing failed direct laryngoscopy is not commonly practised in patients.

The flow-chart is applicable, therefore, to most patients undergoing tracheal intubation under general anaesthesia in an operating theatre environment. The primary Plan A of this situation is oxygenation by facemask ventilation around intubation attempts, intubation is attempted by optimal direct laryngoscopy with the possibility of using an alternative laryngoscope or blade and laryngeal reflexes are abolished by neuro-muscular blocking drugs (NMBDs). If facemask ventilation proves impossible after the induction of general anaesthesia and NMBD administration, Plan B for failed ventilation is activated – an ascending sequence of oral airway, two handed facemask ventilation, laryngeal mask insertion and emergency cricothyrotomy.

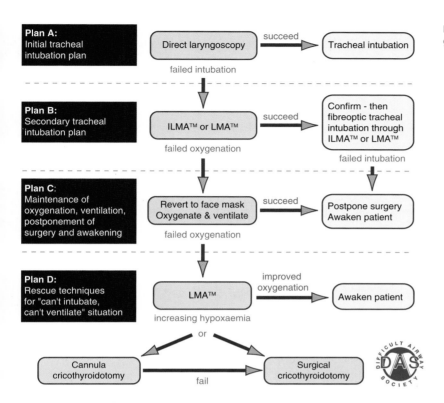

Figure 6.1. Difficult Airway Society guideline for unanticipated difficulty.

Figure 6.2 shows Plan B of the DAS guideline for failed tracheal intubation by direct laryngoscopy. It recommends insertion of a laryngeal mask or intubating laryngeal mask, stabilisation of oxygenation and anaesthesia before attempting to intubate through the supraglottic airway. The emphasis must be that repeated fruitless attempts at direct laryngoscopy should not be made as this can cause the conversion of a patient from being possible to ventilate by face-mask to being impossible to ventilate, the 'can't ventilate, can't intubate' (CVCI) situation.

Within the guideline for unanticipated difficult direct laryngoscopy is Plan C in which intubation through the supraglottic airway has also failed. In an elective patient oxygenation and anaesthesia should be maintained with the supraglottic airway until the patient can be woken. Surgery is postponed and the airway managed in another way at a later date. It is worth remembering when having life-threatening difficulty in airway management in elective patients that the option that is likely to be preferred *by the patient* is waking up to come back another time. Sugammadex may make it easier to make the decision

to antagonise residual neuromuscular blockade and activate wake-up.

One deficiency of current guidelines is that they have not offered advice about what should be done if a patient becomes impossible to mask ventilate after induction, before a NMBD has been given. The anaesthetist must decide whether to await spontaneous awakening or give further medication to allow tracheal intubation (see below – 'squirt, puff, squirt').

Follow-up

When difficulty with airway management has been encountered detailed notes should be made, which describe the problem(s) and their management. Perforation of the pharyngeal mucosa can lead to deep cervical infection or mediastinitis (see Chapter 11) and surveillance must be instituted. The patient needs to be reviewed so that any other morbidity can be found and treated, with an explanation to the patient of what problem was encountered. The patient should be encouraged to remember that difficulty was encountered and to tell the next anaesthetist. A letter

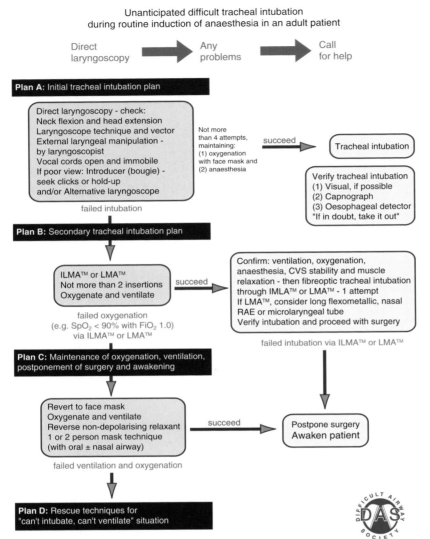

Figure 6.2. Plan B of the DAS guideline.

Unanticipated difficult tracheal intubation
during routine induction of anaesthesia in an adult patient

Difficult Airway Society Guidelines Flow-chart 2004 (use with DAS guidelines paper)

to the patient, copied to the GP, hospital notes and to a department register should repeat the oral explanation. It is easiest to use a form for this and one is available on the DAS website (www.das.uk.com) used with permission from the authors who described it in 2003. If the problem is serious or life-threatening, will recur with future anaesthetics and is not obvious from external examination the patient should be encouraged to join Medic Alert and wear a bracelet inscribed with 'Difficult Intubation' or 'Difficult Airway'.

The aftermath of an airway disaster will be a harrowing period, and colleagues should offer support. Recommendations for supporting a colleague are contained within the free booklet 'Catastrophes in Anaesthetic Practice – dealing with the aftermath' from the AAGBI (www.aagbi.org). A certain way to make a terrible situation worse is for those involved to be less than completely open and honest about events. When a complication occurs we should try to avoid outcome or hindsight bias, where unhappy outcomes attract criticism of a technique, which would have been deemed acceptable had the outcome been good. Hindsight bias is the tendency, knowing the outcome, to predict with false certainty that particular outcome from a series of judgements or actions.

Some contentious topics

Sedation

Sedation makes treatments such as endoscopies, tracheal intubation, dental treatment and minor surgical procedures more tolerable.

What level of consciousness denotes sedation rather than anaesthesia is not universally agreed. Sedation is defined in the UK by communication – the patient must be capable of understanding and reacting to verbal or hand signal communications. However it is not always easy to maintain a steady level of sedation and we (the authors) acknowledge that periods of time during our attempts at sedation could be described as anaesthesia. Deeper levels of sedation are recognized in the USA, described as 'Monitored Anesthesia Care' (MAC). The difference between MAC and anaesthesia is hard to discern. 'Deep' sedation can have unexpected consequences, such as facial burns due to added oxygen and diathermy during facial surgery. Sedation can be a very appropriate and valuable aid to treatment, but there is a danger of it being used as an alternative to anaesthesia for reasons of economy, or indeed profit.

It can be difficult to decide whether it is more appropriate to attempt sedation or insist on establishing a reliable airway, but one will rarely regret a secure airway. An analogy between safety at depressed levels of consciousness and safety in a submarine is often made, where safety is greatest when at adequate but not excessive depth, because most of the dangers are encountered near the surface. Death and brain damage due to obstructed airways have been reported during sedation. There is probably a perception amongst the public, and even the medical population, that sedation is inherently safer than anaesthesia but this belief is unjustified, largely because the airway is not controlled.

Poor access to the airway, unfavourable patient characteristics both physical and mental, doubts about the duration and extent of the procedure or the operator's capabilities and the likelihood of complications, such as bleeding, all militate for the establishment of a reliable airway.

The place of neuro-muscular blocking drugs (NMBDs) in airway management

NMBDs are powerful drugs, indubitably dangerous in untrained hands. When the authors were beginning their training, it was common practice to give curare or pancuronium *before* the thiopentone, because thiopentone was less airway friendly than propofol and it was believed airway control (both mask ventilation and tracheal intubation) was hastened by early neuromuscular blockade. At some point the pendulum has swung away from this approach, and in 2008 Schmidt et al. from an American hospital reported that residents performing emergency tracheal intubations outside theatre used a NMBD on only 17% of occasions.

It has been suggested that anaesthetists should try not to advance to a position from which they cannot retreat and giving an NMBD has been, until recently, a largely irrevocable step. If an NMBD has not been given to a patient who cannot be ventilated there is a chance that the patient will restore their own ventilation, whereas there is much less chance if a NMBD has been given, so that a policy of not using relaxants, unless necessary, is attractive. However it is not certain that avoiding NMBDs is in patients' interests. Mask ventilation is generally easier when relaxation has been established, and it has been found that intubation without NMBDs is associated with more traumatic complications and an increased failure rate. It could be that a majority of patients would be disadvantaged.

An important facet of this problem is the matter of experience. Authors on both sides of the Atlantic have suggested that inexperienced practitioners should use NMBDs with caution. And yet the evidence shows that NMBDs make both mask ventilation and tracheal intubation easier, which should benefit the less experienced more than the expert. Will more patients die or be damaged if trainees are inhibited from, or encouraged in, the use of NMBDs? In our opinion trainees should be made aware of the fact that airway control is more successful when blockade has been induced, but should be well informed about the problems that are associated with their use – see Table 6.1.

NMBDs make a vital contribution to patient safety; it is worth recalling what anaesthetic practice must have been like without them (Box 6.3)

47

Table 6.1. NMBDs and airway management: pros and cons

For	Against
Allow rapid control of the airway	Spontaneous breathing will not return until effect of relaxant ceases
Make face-mask ventilation easier and more successful	Increase risk of awareness
Increase success rate for direct laryngoscopy intubation	Anaphylaxis
Reduce trauma caused by laryngoscopy and intubation	Inadequate reversal and/or side effects of reversal drugs
Reliably abolish unwanted reflex activity such as breath-holding and laryngospasm	Serious complications in some neurological, muscle, renal conditions, particularly with suxamethonium
Increase cardiovascular stability during airway management	Intubation without relaxant (e.g., propofol/alfentanil) can decrease list turnover time – but whether an 'intubating' dose of opioid allows an earlier return of breathing than an equivalent dose of suxamethonium is not known.

Box 6.3

Dr John Snow's Casebook
  'Administered chloroform to Mr Brewster – there was rigidity – and then the breathing became very stridulous, and he became livid in the face'
  Saturday 15th August 1857.

'Squirt, puff, squirt' (Steve Yentis)

Over the past 20 years a practice of confirming that mask ventilation is possible before a NMBD is given has come to be regarded as safe practice, although when patients are believed to be at risk of aspiration it seems to be widely accepted that relaxation should be immediate and complete, without preliminary testing for the ability to facemask ventilate. The origin of the 'squirt, puff, squirt' tactic is obscure, but the idea is that if mask ventilation proves impossible the patient

---

Box 6.4 Mrs Bromiley

Mr Martin Bromiley, a professional pilot, has released a report on his wife's death, in the hope that the anaesthetic community will follow the example of the aviation industry and learn lessons. http://www. chfg.org/resources/07_qrt04/Anonymous_Report_ Verdict_and_Corrected_Timeline_Oct_07.pdf).

The anaesthetist appears to have encountered muscle rigidity after induction, possibly due to remifentanil, which prevented facemask ventilation or LMA insertion. A NMBD was not given for seven or more minutes, by which time the SpO_2 may have been less than 40%. Suxamethonium was given and there were then several failed intubation attempts before ventilation was established via an ILMA. In hindsight, since an ILMA was successful after muscle relaxation had occurred, it seems possible that an LMA or mask ventilation would have been successful had the muscle rigidity been treated with a NMBD at the outset. The authors do not know whether a NMBD was not given because the anaesthetist was obeying the 'squirt, puff, squirt' doctrine.

---

can be awoken. Calder and Yentis have questioned the validity of the concept on several grounds.

1. It has no evidence base.
2. In the majority of cases anaesthetists do not find it expedient to wake the patient. Kheterpal et al reported on 77 cases of failed mask ventilation in 53 041 attempts. Two of the patients were awoken but 73 were given a NMBD and their tracheas were intubated. Two patients had crico thyrotomy. Why anaesthetists do not wake up patients when they find they cannot facemask ventilate is not known. It is likely that the onset of desaturation means that some action *has* to be taken.
3. There is a possibility that anaesthetists might administer too little induction agent, especially in patients that they think might be difficult to mask ventilate, resulting in a false positive failure.
4. Anaesthetists might fail to administer a NMBD when it is indicated, as in cases of opiate-induced muscle stiffness or laryngospasm. Opiates can cause muscle rigidity ('wooden chest'), and Bennet et al showed that opiate rigidity caused vocal cord closure, which was only relieved by neuromuscular paralysis (see Box 6.4).
5. Most experienced practitioners believe that neuromuscular blockade makes mask ventilation easier in the overwhelming majority of cases. Szabo et al

have shown that mask ventilation is more successful if rocuronium is given at induction.

6. Anaesthetists are more likely to use suxamethonium (65 out of 73 cases in Kheterpal's study) if they are trying to induce relaxation after failed mask ventilation. Suxamethonium has some serious side-effects (see Chapter 18), amongst which is an increase in oxygen consumption due to fasciculation. It may be that the introduction of sugammadex, which effectively reverses the effect of 1.2 mg/kg of rocuronium after 2 minutes (16 mg), will alter practice.

7. Finally, retreat to spontaneous ventilation is often not a real option for patients with impaired consciousness, circulatory or respiratory failure, gross sepsis, airway obstruction, or when the intervention is part of resuscitation.

Should squirt, puff, squirt be abandoned?

We will be surprised if this practice ceases. Broomhead et al have pointed out that there are other examples of humans wishing to acquire evidence, which they would rather have than not have, even when they accept that their ultimate behaviour will not be altered by the knowledge.

Instructors who advise trainees to adopt the practice should include a discussion of what is to be done when impossible mask ventilation is encountered. A decision must be taken whether to attempt to await recovery, perhaps in the face of desaturation, or to 'do something'. The evidence indicates, that in the majority of cases the administration of a NMBD will assist the practitioner and result in a favourable outcome. There has been a gap in airway management algorithms, in that they have not made clear what a practitioner who encounters failed mask-ventilation should do. However El-Orbany and Woehlck have recently suggested an algorithm to be considered if difficult mask ventilation (DMV) is encountered – see Figure 6.3. This algorithm includes NMBDs in the first list of options to be considered if DMV is encountered.

In our view it would not be in the patient's interests if a surgical airway or cricothyroid cannula was inserted without trying the effect of a NMBD, if ventilation is difficult after induction.

NMBDs and the difficult airway

This is a very difficult subject to discuss dispassionately. We are the product of our own experience and,

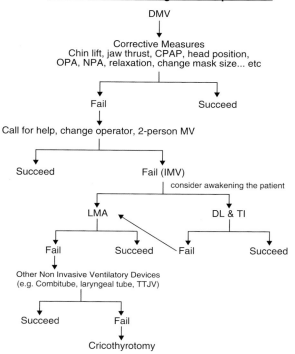

Figure 6.3. An algorithm for difficult mask ventilation. (Reproduced with permission from El-Orbany and Woehlck (2009).)

in particular, our early training. Really difficult airways are unusual enough to prevent controlled trials.

In the authors' opinion it is not sensible to suggest that NMBDs cannot be used if difficulty with the airway is expected. The test is whether we are prepared *to induce general anaesthesia*. Once we induce anaesthesia we may prefer not use a NMBD, but we should accept that we may have to – for instance an NMBD might be required if a patient known to be a Grade IV laryngoscopy develops laryngospasm. Patel et al's work with patients with stridor (see below) has shown that NMBDs and positive pressure can be useful when the airway is critically obstructed.

The obstructing airway – are there techniques and drugs we should and should not use?

The classic causes of acute airway obstruction include haematomas or tissue swelling after thyroid or anterior cervical spine or carotid surgery, trauma, or pharyngeal and laryngeal infections. We suspect that there is no real consensus about the best policy to be followed in such cases, although most would agree that it is best to:

1. Open the wound to relieve tissue tension (see Chapter 26). The wound should probably always be opened before induction.
2. Assemble staff and equipment suitable for surgical tracheotomy or cricothyroidotomy.
3. Avoid nitrous oxide because of its high density, which will impede gas flow, if flow is turbulent.

Should spontaneous breathing be preserved and intravenous agents avoided?

The decision-making process involved in managing an obstructing airway is easiest if obstruction is complete. When faced with a completely obstructed airway, we know that anything we do is unlikely to be criticised, as long as we get on and do what can be done, which will generally be an attempt at laryngoscopy, insertion of a bougie and intubation, followed by insertion of a supraglottic airway device (SAD) if intubation fails and surgical or needle cricothyrotomy if the SAD fails.

However when the obstruction is incomplete, practitioners are burdened with the anxiety that their induction may result in complete failure to ventilate and a potentially fatal outcome.

The prospect of finding oneself unable to ventilate a patient makes the idea of preserving spontaneous breathing until it is possible to show that either tracheal intubation can be performed, or that one can ventilate with a mask or SAD, an attractive one.

Nevertheless there are logical inconsistencies in the concept of inducing anaesthesia via an obstructing airway. First, induction will be prolonged or even impossible. Second, physical principles dictate that negative pressure tends to aggravate upper airway obstruction (see Chapter 2). The group led by Patel at the Royal National ENT Hospital in London have shown that patients with stridor due to laryngotracheal stenosis experience better gas flow rates after intravenous induction, paralysis and ventilation via a Laryngeal Mask Airway, than they can achieve when awake (see Chapter 25). The phenomenon of obstructive sleep apnoea being relieved by CPAP is another example of the inherent problems of negative pressure being ameliorated by positive pressure.

However many practitioners with experience of obstructed airways recommend a spontaneous breathing technique, and if a level of anaesthesia can be achieved that allows intubation then all is well, but if the airway becomes completely obstructed when the laryngeal reflexes are still active it may be necessary to administer intravenous agents (propofol is widely regarded as the most appropriate agent), or a NMBD. Hari and Nirvala reported a case of retropharyngeal abscess, in which the airway became completely obstructed during inhalational induction, but was relieved by intravenous propofol, and Neff et al reported a case of Ludwig's angina where laryngospasm developed during inhalational induction when the abscess burst, and suxamethonium was used to allow intubation. Combes et al reported four cases of incipient airway obstruction successfully intubated with a rapid-sequence technique and direct laryngoscopic insertion of a gum-elastic bougie.

'*Awake*' *intubation and the obstructed airway:* commonly performed with a flexible fibreoptic laryngoscope, but this can also be accomplished with direct laryngoscopy. Awake intubation has been used successfully in many cases, notably in cases of Ludwig's angina, and can often be the best option. However fibreoptic intubation is unlikely to succeed when the airway is totally obstructed and it must be remembered that topical application of lidocaine to the airway can produce temporary partial or complete glottic closure (see Chapter 26).

Conclusion: it should be accepted that there is no universally applicable technique in these desperate situations. Practitioners should recognise the danger of deterioration in airway patency after induction, or fibreoptic intervention, try to assemble the best team and equipment that time allows and then be prepared to utilise whatever drugs and equipment seem likely to help. Direct laryngoscopy has succeeded after fibreoptic laryngoscopy has failed and a gum-elastic bougie is a vital item.

'Human factors'

'No passion so effectually robs the mind of all its powers of acting and reasoning as fear'   (Edmund Burke 1757)

In the period between the publication of the first and second edition of this book, medicine has followed the aviation industry in recognising that excellence of equipment provision and utilisation is important, but not the whole story. Humans make errors, which in retrospect can seem distressingly obvious. Those

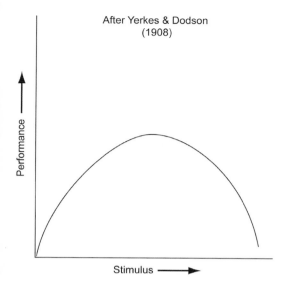

Figure 6.4. The relationship between stimulus and performance. A certain amount of stimulus is helpful but performance can deteriorate dreadfully if the situation overwhelms the practitioner's abilities and/or experience.

involved in airway management need to appreciate that in critical situations there will not be time for detailed, analytical decision making, and be wary of fixating on issues or techniques that are not contributing to success. They must make allowance for the phenomenon of stress making their own or their assistants' actions less effectual, and realise that communication between members of the team can be crucial. Team-working is much more formalised in the aviation industry with use of standard operating procedures (SOP) covering many of the more likely (but still rare) serious problems. Some airway management SOPs are evident in pre-hospital care. There is no doubt that SOPs make team-working more effective since each person knows their role, and practical theatre-based airway management team-working courses have now started to appear (Figure 6.4).

Interested parties and individuals (notably the relatives of injured patients) have pressed for study of these human factors and Non-Technical Skills (NOTECHS). The website of the Clinical Human Factors Group may be found at www.chfg.org, and this description of human factors is taken from there.

'*Human factors are all the things that make us different from logical, completely predictable machines. How we think and relate to other people, equipment and our environment. It is about how we perform in our roles and how we can optimise that performance to* improve safety and efficiency. In simple terms it's the things that affect our personal performance.*'

The Difficult Airway Society and the Royal College of Anaesthetists have performed a year long audit of serious airway problems (those that have resulted in death or brain damage or unexpected admission to intensive care – NAP4), which is now complete. The results are expected in 2011. This audit will hopefully help to elucidate the contribution of patient, equipment, human or other factors.

Key points

- Suction apparatus and a self-inflating bag to allow inflation of the patient's lungs in the event of anaesthetic machine failure must always be present.
- Expect and prepare for difficulty, assemble and check the function of the appropriate equipment drugs and staff before induction.
- Know what you will do if your starting plan fails.
- Ask for help at an early stage.
- Follow-up the patient.
- Be aware of the possibility of error in crisis situations.

Further reading

Academy of Medical Royal Colleges. (2001). *Implementing and Ensuring Safe Sedation Practice for Healthcare Procedures in Adults*. London: Royal College of Anaesthetists. Available at: http://www.rcoa.ac.uk/docs/safesedationpractice.pdf.

Arbous MS, Meursing AE, van Kleef JW, et al. (2005). Impact of anesthesia management characteristics on severe morbidity and mortality. *Anesthesiology*, **102**, 257–268.

Belmont MJ, Wax MK, DeSouza FN. (1998). The difficult airway: Cardiopulmonary bypass – the ultimate solution. *Head Neck*, **20**, 266–269.

Bennett JA, Abrams IT, Van Riper DF, Horrow JC. (1997). Difficult or impossible ventilation after sufentanil-induced anesthesia is caused primarily by vocal cord closure. *Anesthesiology*, **87**, 1070–1074.

Benumof JL, Dagg R, Benumof R. (1997). Critical hemoglobin desaturation will occur before return to an unparalyzed state following 1 mg/kg intravenous succinylcholine. *Anesthesiology*, **87**, 979–982.

Bhananker SM, Posner KL, Cheney FW, et al. (2006). Injury and liability associated with monitored anesthesia care: A closed claims analysis. *Anesthesiology*, **104**, 228–234.

Broomhead R, Marks RJ, Ayton P. (2010). Confirmation of the ability to ventilate by facemask before administration of neuromuscular blocker: A non-instrumental piece of information? *British Journal of Anaesthesia*, **104**, 313–317.

Bromiley M. (2008). Have you ever made a mistake? *Royal College of Anaesthetists' Bulletin*, **48**, 2442–2445.

Calder I, Yentis SM. (2008). Could 'safe practice' be compromising safe practice? Should anaesthetists have to demonstrate that face mask ventilation is possible before giving a neuromuscular blocker? *Anaesthesia*, **63**, 113–115.

Calder I, Yentis S, Patel A. (2009). Muscle relaxants and airway management. *Anesthesiology*, **111**, 216–217.

Caplan RA, Posner KL, Cheney FW. (1991). Effect of outcome on physician judgement of appropriateness of care. *Journal of the American Medical Association*, **265**, 1957–1960.

Combes X, Andriamifidy L, Dufresne E, et al. (2007). Comparison of two induction regimens using or not using muscle relaxant: Impact on postoperative upper airway discomfort. *British Journal of Anaesthesia*, **99**, 276–281.

Combes X, Dumerat M, Dhonneur G. (2004). Emergency gum elastic bougie-assisted tracheal intubation in four patients with upper airway distortion. *Canadian Journal of Anaesthesia*, **51**, 1022–1024.

Conacher ID, Curran E. (2004). Local anaesthesia and sedation for rigid bronchoscopy for emergency relief of central airway obstruction. *Anaesthesia*, **59**, 290–292.

Davis DP, Ochs M, Hoyt DB, Bailey D, Marshall LK, Rosen P. (2003). Paramedic-administered neuromuscular blockade improves prehospital intubation success in severely head-injured patients. *Journal of Trauma*, **55**, 713–719.

De Boer HD, Driesen JJ, Marcus MA, et al. (2007). Reversal of rocuronium-induced (1.2 mg/kg) profound neuromuscular block by sugammadex: A multicenter, dose-finding and safety study. *Anesthesiology*, **107**, 239–244.

El-Orbany M, Woehlck HJ. (2009). Difficult mask ventilation. *Anesthesia and Analgesia*, **109**, 1870–1880.

Hanley JA, Lippman-Hand A. (1983). If nothing goes wrong, is everything all right? Interpreting zero numerators. *Journal of the American Medical Association*, **249**, 1743–1745.

Hari MS, Nirvala KD. (2003). Retropharyngeal abscess presenting with acute airway obstruction. *Anaesthesia*, **58**, 712–713.

Henderson JJ, Popat MT, Latto IP, Pearce AC. (2004). Difficult Airway Society guidelines for management of the unanticipated difficult intubation. *Anaesthesia*, **59**, 675–694.

Kheterpal S, Martin L, Shanks AM, Tremper KK. (2009). Prediction and outcomes of impossible mask ventilation. A review of 50,000 anesthetics. *Anesthesiology*, **110**, 891–897.

King KP. (2002). Where is the line between deep sedation and general anesthesia? *American Journal of Gastroenterology*, **97**, 2485–2486.

Lundstrøm LH, Møller AM, Rosenstock C, et al. (2009). Avoidance of neuromuscular blocking agents may increase the risk of difficult tracheal intubation: A cohort study of 103812 consecutive adult patients recorded in the Danish Anaesthesia Database. *British Journal of Anaesthesia*, **103**, 283–290.

Mencke T, Echternach M, Kleinschmidt S, et al. (2003). Laryngeal morbidity and quality of tracheal intubation. A randomized controlled trial. *Anesthesiology*, **98**, 1049–1056.

Mort TC. (2007). Complications of emergency tracheal intubation: Immediate airway-related consequences: part II. *Journal of Intensive Care Medicine*, **22**, 208–215.

Neff SP, Merry AF, Anderson B. (1999). Airway management in Ludwig's angina. *Anaesthesia and Intensive Care*, **27**, 659–661.

Nouraei SA, Giussani DA, Howard DJ, Sandhu GS, Ferguson C, Patel A. (2008). Physiological comparison of spontaneous and positive-pressure ventilation in laryngotracheal stenosis. *British Journal of Anaesthesia*, **101**, 419–423.

Schmidt UH, Kumwilaisak K, Bittner E, George E, Hess D. (2008). Effects of supervision by attending anesthesiologists on complications of emergency tracheal intubation. *Anesthesiology*, **109**, 973–977.

Shakespeare WA, Lanier WL, Perkins WJ, Pasternak JJ. (2010). Airway management in patients who develop neck haematomas after carotid endarterectomy. *Anesthesia and Analgesia*, **110**, 588–593.

Shaw IC, Welchew EA, Harrison BJ, Michael S. (1997). Complete airway obstruction during awake fibreoptic intubation. *Anaesthesia*, **52**, 582–585.

Szabo TA, Reves JG, Spinale FG, Ezri T, Warters RD. (2008). Neuromuscular blockade facilitates mask ventilation. *Anesthesiology*, **109**, A184.

Yentis SM. (2010). Of humans, factors, failings and fixations. *Anaesthesia*, **65**, 1–3.

Difficult airways: causation and identification

Ian Calder

What is a 'difficult airway'?

Humans cannot survive for long unless oxygen is absorbed and carbon dioxide excreted. These essentials require that the airway must be at least partially patent. A difficult airway is therefore one in which the standard airway maintenance manoeuvres (head tilt, jaw thrust, recovery position, facemask, supraglottic airway (SGA), tracheal tube, tracheostomy) are hard or impossible to implement. However an airway that is difficult to maintain using one method may be easily controlled with another (a patient who is difficult to mask ventilate may be easy to intubate or vice versa), so that the broad term 'difficult airway' needs to be qualified when applied to patients.

Causes of difficulty

Non-patient factors

- **Operator and assistant:** the skill and experience level of the operator can affect the degree of difficulty reported.
- **Equipment and location:** even the most skilled operator may be ineffectual if deprived of appropriate equipment and drugs, or placed in an unfamiliar or challenging environment (see Chapter 29).
- **Drug issues:** the depth of anaesthesia, or lack of it, may affect the operator's control of the airway. In general, the airway is easiest to control at a depth of anaesthesia that obtunds the airway reflexes. Adequate neuro-muscular blockade tends to allow effective and atraumatic control of the airway, but the matter is not without controversy (see Chapters 6 and 19). Opioid drugs can cause muscular rigidity, possibly as a result of central

stimulation of mu_1 receptors. This can cause laryngeal closure. Suxamethonium can cause masseter spasm, which may be without sequelae, but can herald malignant hyperpyrexia.

Patient factors

- **Unwanted reflex activities** – excess salivation, breath-holding, and laryngospasm provide the most frequent problems. (see Chapter 4)
- **Stiffness, deformity, or swelling** – of the joints and tissues of the cranio-cervical junction (CCJ), temporo-mandibular joint (TMJ), face, mouth, pharynx, cervical spine, glottis or trachea cause difficulty. It is tedious to list all the described causes; 'pathological sieves' can be applied, such as congenital or acquired, traumatic, neoplastic, inflammatory, endocrine and iatrogenic, or 'in the lumen', 'in the wall', 'outside the wall' (Table 7.1). Increasing age is associated with difficulty because the range of motion of the CCJ, cervical spine and TMJ decreases with age. An increasingly recognised cause of airway obstruction is angio-oedema associated with angiotensin-converting enzyme inhibiting drugs.
- **Background factors** – include heart or lung disease, or other conditions which may increase the likelihood of hypoxaemia or circulatory collapse. Constraints and stress may be imposed on the anaesthetist by factors such as impossible venous access, aspiration risk, and uncooperative patients. Obesity is a good example of a condition, in which any problem with airway control is compounded by poor venous access and rapid desaturation (Figure 7.1). There is a higher

Core Topics in Airway Management, Second Edition, ed. Ian Calder and Adrian Pearce. Published by Cambridge University Press.
© Cambridge University Press 2011.

Table 7.1. Some classic causes of airway difficulty

- Pierre Robin
- Treacher-Collins
- Klippel-Feil
- Rheumatoid arthritis
- Ankylosing spondylitis
- Facial/cervical trauma including burns
- Head and neck irradiation
- Acromegaly
- Epiglottitis
- Tumours
- Foreign bodies
- Ludwig's angina
- Anterior cervical swelling or haematoma
- Cervical fixator devices
- Lingual tonsil
- Angio-oedema in patients taking ACE inhibitors

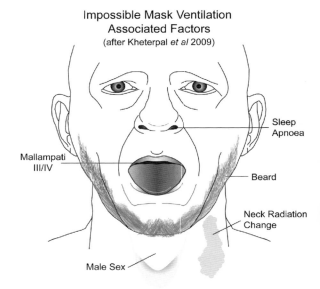

Impossible Mask Ventilation
Associated Factors
(after Kheterpal *et al* 2009)

Sleep Apnoea

Mallampati III/IV

Beard

Neck Radiation Change

Male Sex

Figure 7.2. Factors found to be associated with impossible facemask ventilation (IMV) by Kheterpal et al. The predictive value of these factors is poor, as IMV occurred in less than 1% of the cases of all the factors, even the most strongly associated factor (neck radiation changes – 3 out of 320 cases).

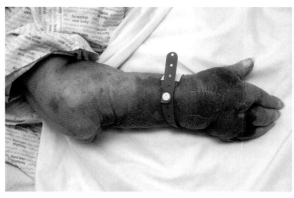

Figure 7.1. Poor venous access due to rheumatoid arthritis. Difficult venous access can be a background factor in airway difficulty.

incidence of difficult intubation in emergency cases, particularly if the patient is not in the operating theatre environment.

Types of difficulty

Difficult mask ventilation – facial pathology may make facemask fit difficult to achieve. Edentulous patients are a common problem; many practitioners prefer to allow patients to keep their dentures in, which helps with mask anaesthesia, but it is vital to ensure that they do not become dislodged and impacted in the pharynx or oesophagus (many dentures are radiolucent, so a missing denture may not be detected by radiography).

It is hard to elucidate the incidence of difficult mask ventilation as it is a subjective experience. Objective criteria such as expired carbon dioxide are of limited value as it is a common experience to be able to mask ventilate without detecting expired carbon dioxide. A four-grade classification has been proposed by Kheterpal et al (Figure 7.2).

Grade 1. Ventilated by mask

Grade 2. Ventilated by mask with oral airway/adjuvant

Grade 3. Difficult ventilation (inadequate, unstable or requiring two providers)

Grade 4. Unable to ventilate

Kheterpal et al encountered 77 grade 4 patients in 53 041 attempts (0.15%). A further 2.2% of the patients were grade 3.

Difficult direct laryngoscopy – the outdated term 'anterior larynx' is still sometimes used, but has no value. The four-point score proposed by Cormack and Lehane is the most widely used method of

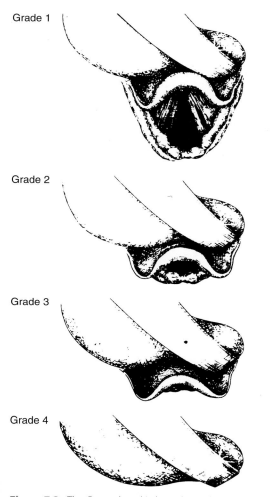

Grade 1

Grade 2

Grade 3

Grade 4

Figure 7.3. The Cormack and Lehane Score. (Reprinted with permission from Williams KN, Carli F, Cormack RS. *Br J Anaesth* 1991; 66:38–44.)

Table 7.2. The Danish Anaesthesia Database tracheal intubation score (difficult intubation is defined as a score of >1)

Score	Definition
1.	Intubated by direct laryngoscopy by the first anaesthetist and in two attempts maximally
2.	Intubated by direct laryngoscopy by the first anaesthetist but with more than two attempts or intubated by a supervising anaesthetist after one or more failed attempts
3.	Intubated by a method other than direct laryngoscopy
4.	Intubation failed after multiple attempts, no tracheal tube inserted.

recording laryngeal visibility (Figure 7.3). Grade 3 (epiglottis only) occurs in about 2–5% of general surgical patients. Grade 4 (no laryngeal structure visible) is rare. In practice, the most important distinction is between those patients whose laryngeal visibility allows the insertion of a bougie at direct laryngoscopy and those in whom this is not possible. Cook suggested a modification of the Cormack score to describe this distinction; patients in whom direct laryngoscopy revealed the epiglottis but did not allow insertion of a bougie are described as 3b. Grade 4 and 3b patients are thus the 'difficult' ones.

Difficult intubation – the term difficult intubation is often inaccurately, but perhaps practically, used synonymously with difficult direct laryngoscopy. The advent of video-laryngoscopy has made the division more relevant, since it is not unusual to obtain a good view of the larynx but have difficulty with intubation. Various intubation difficulty scores have been suggested, which seek to include data such as the number of attempts and operators, and the time required. The score used in the Danish Anaesthesia Database seems practical (Table 7.2).

Can't ventilate, can't intubate (CVCI) – this term is generally used to denote failure of facemask ventilation and tracheal intubation. It is extremely rare to encounter CVCI in a patient who does not have any obvious airway abnormalities, and has been properly anaesthetised. The most important avoidable causes of CVCI are inadequate anaesthesia or muscle relaxation, and difficulty with facemask ventilation arising after repeated failed attempts at intubation. Kheterpal et al have shown that impossible facemask ventilation does not mean impossible intubation. Of the 77 impossible facemask ventilation patients in their study, 73 were intubated (after muscle relaxants had been given).

Difficult tracheotomy/ostomy – is mostly due to cervical spine flexion deformity, soft tissue swelling or tumour, or burns including radiotherapy.

Predicting difficulty – striking a balance between identifying true positives and generating false positives

Nearly all the patients whose lives are at risk at induction are so obviously abnormal, that decisions can be made 'from the end of the bed' (Figures 7.4, 7.5).

55

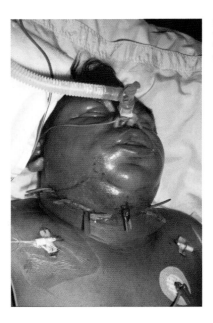

Figure 7.4. Gross tissue swelling due to infection after dental extraction.

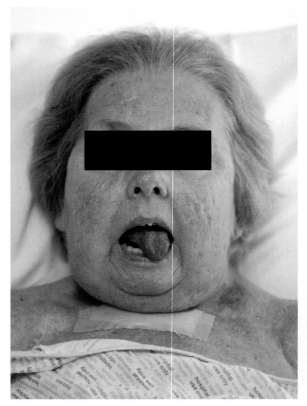

Figure 7.5. Rheumatoid arthritis involving the cervical spine and temporomandibular joint.

Conversely, it is hard to identify the few relatively normal-looking patients who are seriously difficult to manage. Our attempts to do so are accompanied by the creation of numerous false positives and failure to identify some of the true positives. Two consequences flow from this – first, *unexpected difficulty* with an airway is an unwelcome but inevitable facet of anaesthetic practice, and second, our efforts to identify these patients produce *large numbers of false positive predictions*, which tends to make the process fall into disrepute.

Wilson pointed out that it is more important for an anaesthetist to be trained to expect and be capable of coping with unexpected difficulty, than to perform numerous airway examinations. On the other hand, a basic airway assessment must always be performed so that problems that do not render the patient particularly abnormal-looking (severe limitation of mouth-opening, for instance) are not missed.

One sometimes hears or reads statements such as 'anaesthetists should not use techniques liable to cause apnoea when difficulty with the airway is predicted'. This needs qualification, because what constitutes a 'prediction' of difficulty is an uncertain issue. Bedside prediction of airway difficulty in apparently normal patients is of limited value. The following material may help to explain the problems.

Sensitivity and specificity

These concepts are important and useful. It is not at all difficult to become confused but it is well worth making the effort to understand them.

Sensitivity is positivity in disease. If we applied a test to 100 diseased people and the test is positive in 50 of them, then the sensitivity of the test is 50%. The rate at which this test acquires true positives is 50%, but it misses half the true positives and these are false negatives.

Specificity is negativity in health. If we applied a test to 100 healthy people and the test managed to remain negative in 90 of them, then the specificity of the test is 90%. In 10 healthy people the test failed to remain negative and declared them to be falsely positive, so that the test has a false positive rate of 100–90 = 10%. So if the prevalence of true positives in the population being tested is low, any test that is not highly specific, and can remain negative when the disease is

Table 7.3. Some values of likelihood ratios from Shiga et al 2005

Test	Sensitivity	Specificity	Likelihood ratio
Mallampati	49	86	3.7
TMD[*]	20	94	3.4
SMD[*]	62	82	5.7
Mouth opening	22	97	4.0
Wilson Risk Sum	46	89	5.8
Mall + TMD	36	87	9.9

[*]Thyro-mental distance, Sterno-mental distance

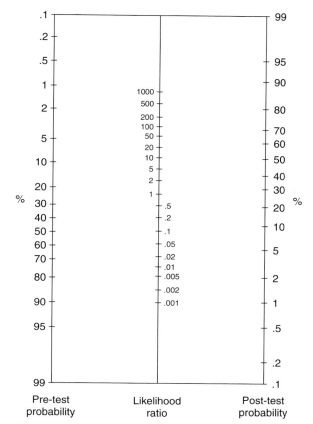

Figure 7.6. Fagan's nomogram. Post-test probability can be determined by drawing a line from the pre-test probability through the likelihood ratio. (Reprinted with permission from Sacket DL et al. (1991) *Clinical Epidemiology: A Basic Science for Clinical Medicine*, 2nd ed. Boston/Toronto: Little Brown and Company.)

not present, might generate as many or more false positives as true positives. The fact that tests that are highly sensitive tend to be unspecific is an inconvenient fact of life, which makes our attempts to plot a safe and sensible course difficult. In other words, a test which identifies most of the true positives is likely to generate a lot of false positives at the same time.

Likelihood ratios. We must accept that any test will generate false positives as well as identify true positives. What matters is the ratio between true positive acquisition and false positive declaration. This ratio is known as the likelihood ratio, and is the true positive rate divided by the false positive rate (sensitivity/1 − specificity) (Table 7.3). Tests with likelihood ratios over 10 are regarded as powerful discriminators. The likelihood ratio is the ratio of the probability of the specific test result in people who have the disease to the probability in people who do not, or roughly, the number of times more likely it is that a patient with a positive test result actually has the disease. Negative likelihood ratios can also be calculated, but are of limited value in this context, since we already know that nearly all normal-looking patients will not be difficult.

Post-test probability. With a knowledge of the sensitivity and specificity of a test we can use the likelihood ratio to estimate the post-test probability, or positive predictive value (the proportion of positive tests that are correct). The pre-test probability (p_1), is the estimated or known prevalence of the problem in the population being tested. Strictly speaking we should use the pre-test odds in the calculation when calculating the post-test probability (p_2), but a

nomogram described by Fagan is available which allows the use of probabilities without conversion to odds [pre-test odds can be calculated as odds $= p_1 / (1 − p_1)$]. A line is drawn from the pre-test probability through the likelihood ratio to give the post-test probability, or positive predictive value (Figure 7.6).

It can be seen that when the pre-test probability is low, tests must have a high likelihood ratio to generate worthwhile post-test probabilities. The predictive value of tests such as the Mallampati or thyro-mental distance is low, and not suitable for screening a low prevalence population. Greater significance can be attached to a positive result in a higher prevalence population, such as rheumatoid arthritis affecting the cervical spine.

Combining tests. If two or more tests are found to be positive the predictive value increases. Shiga et al

57

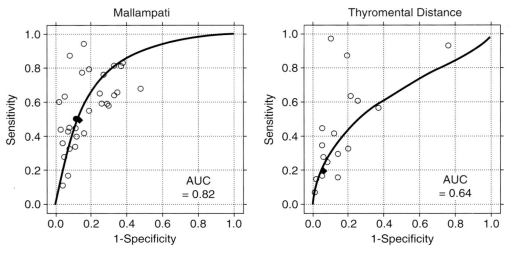

Figure 7.7. Receiver operating characteristic (ROC) curves for studies of the Mallampati and thyro-mental distance. Each open circle represents the results of a study. The diamonds represent pooled point estimates of sensitivity and specificity. The area under the curve is greater for the Mallampati, suggesting that it has greater discriminatory power than the thyro-mental distance test. (Reproduced with permission from Shiga et al (2005).)

found that the likelihood ratio of the combination of the Mallampati and the thyro-mental distance nearly reached 10. An objection to combination is that the sensitivity inevitably decreases, so that there is an increase in false-negative results. However this is not really a problem in practice since we instinctively adopt a 'Bayesian' approach. That is, when we find one piece of data, we seek another and add the probabilities (Thomas Bayes, English vicar and mathematician, 1702–61).

Receiver operating characteristic (ROC) curves. If the true positive rate is plotted against the false positive rate (sensitivity against 1 − specificity) for a series of sensitivities and specificities obtained from multiple studies, or different threshold values (such as different values of thyro-mental distance) one can construct a curve. Theoretically a 45-degree bisector from bottom left to top right (an area under the curve [AUC] of 0.5) represents a value that could be obtained by guessing. The principal value of ROC curves is in comparing one test against another. AUCs of greater than 0.7 are taken to have clinical significance (Figure 7.7).

Predicting difficulty in practice

When possible, a history, examination, and special investigations approach is appropriate (it may not be possible in emergency situations when patients are obtunded or unable to cooperate) (Figure 7.8).

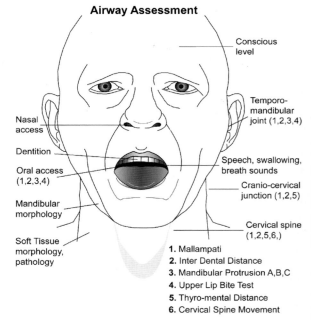

Figure 7.8. Areas of interest in airway assessment and relevant examinations.

History: a history of difficulty or of a disease associated with difficulty must be of interest. However Lundstrøm et al found that a history of difficult or failed intubation gave likelihood ratios of about 6 and 22 for prediction of subsequent difficult

Table 7.4. Symptomatology (and signs) of impending airway obstruction

Symptom/signs	Note
Sudden waking at night with feeling of obstruction	Said to be characteristic of glottic obstruction
Feeling of 'not being able to breathe'	An obvious, but sometimes undervalued symptom
Wanting to sit up	A constant feature
Difficulty in speaking and swallowing	Ultimately dysphagia will result in drooling
Stridor	May not occur in supraglottic obstruction; can be misdiagnosed as asthma in subglottic obstruction
SpO_2	If the FiO_2 is high SpO_2 may be preserved until obstruction is complete

intubation, which suggests that a history of failure should be taken very seriously but a history of difficulty may not be a good predictor of subsequent difficulty.

Symptoms: one of the principal difficulties in predicting airway problems under anaesthesia is that in most unexpected cases there are no symptoms. The symptoms associated with obstructed sleep apnoea (OSA) syndrome should be sought in suspected cases. Anaesthetists should be aware of the symptomatology (and signs) of impending airway obstruction (Table 7.4).

Examination: the first consideration is whether a seal can be obtained with a facemask. If this is impossible then apnoea could be disastrous if an LMA or tracheal intubation fails. A history of snoring or OSA, beards, obesity, age greater than 55 years, poor Mallampati grade, thyro-mental distance less than 6 cm, poor mandibular protrusion, and radiotherapy scars are all associated with difficult facemask ventilation, but these factors, even in combination, have poor predictive value. If there is serious doubt about the practicality of facemask ventilation because of a poor seal or inability to maintain the airway, then awake intubation must be considered.

The presence of large quantities of blood, pus or mucus is significant because fibreoptic endoscopy will be impeded.

Specific areas of examination

Conscious level: This is a basic piece of data that may influence management profoundly. This element of the examination includes items such as intoxication, age, language barriers, educational and emotional immaturity.

Dental health: This should be examined and patients warned of possible damage to loose, restored or diseased teeth. It is vital that one can be certain about whether the patient has the same number of teeth at the end of the anaesthetic as she/he had at induction. Dental prostheses can be displaced and may be difficult to find, as most are radiolucent.

Mouth opening: The lower 95% confidence limit of inter-dental distance is 3.7 cm in young people. Assessment is generally by 'eye', but measurement should be performed when restriction is detected. Fingerbreadths have been used as a unit, but are inaccurate. Few studies have examined inter-dental distance as a factor, and there is little information to allow us to determine an acceptable minimum distance. LMA insertion is likely to be difficult if inter-dental distance is less than 2 cm, so this could be about the minimum acceptable.

Mandibular protrusion is a vital part of normal mouth opening (and airway management) and should be assessed by asking the patient to place the lower incisors in front of the upper incisors. An ABC classification has been used but a modification known as the Upper Lip Bite Test (ULBT) may be easier to perform. The patient is asked to cover the upper lip with their bottom incisors. Eberhardt et al found that the ULBT had a likelihood ratio of 3.7. Nasal access becomes very important if oral access is poor.

Mallampati: The original three grades of oro-pharyngeal visibility were increased to four by Sansoom and Young, who hoped that there would be a correlation with the four grades of laryngeal visibility at direct laryngoscopy. There is no basis for this concept, and there is no need for more than two grades: 1 ('not bad') and 2 ('bad'). The Mallampati has serious inter-observer variability and poor sensitivity and specificity, but is the best test yet devised.

Cranio-cervical extension: Cranio-cervical extension is a vital part of airway management for basic airway management and direct laryngoscopy, but unfortunately there is no reliable method of assessment. One reason for this is that poor movement at the CCJ can be compensated for at lower inter-vertebral levels, so that the total cervical range of movement appears reasonably normal. One often only detects cranio-cervical junction (CCJ) stiffness at the moment when one tries to extend the head on the neck for direct laryngoscopy. Curiously, the Mallampati examination may be the best method of assessing poor cranio-cervical movement because restricted cranio-cervical extension causes poor mouth opening. There is a characteristic appearance during mouth opening in patients with restricted cervical movement – the chin seems to disappear into the neck and folds appear in the submental soft tissue (see Figure 7.5). The best predictive results ever obtained with the Mallampati were in a study of patients with cervical spine disease. Readers practicing in salubrious areas may find the 'Champagne Sign' useful – patients with stiff necks find drinking from a champagne flute difficult (see Chapter 1).

Thyro-mental and sterno-mental distances: The suggested cut offs are 6 cm and 12 cm. These values are compromises aimed at maximising sensitivity without losing too much specificity. Unfortunately the positive predictive values reported have been worse than the Mallampati. A drawback of these tests as bedside methods is that they require a measurement of length. Fingerbreadths are not accurate and a further source of inaccuracy is that the exact points of measurement are not entirely clear.

Special investigations

'Quick look' laryngoscopy: This can be undertaken under topical anaesthesia in patients being considered for awake intubation. If an adequate view is obtained with a direct or video-laryngoscope general anaesthesia can be induced.

Ultrasound: This can be used to determine the position of the trachea before percutaneous tracheostomy (see Chapter 28). It has also been claimed that estimation of the quantity of cervical fat can predict difficult laryngoscopy.

Radiology: In selected patients it can be very useful to examine cervical spine radiographs, CT or MRI scans (to assess CCJ mobility or major deformity – see Chapter 26). Abnormalities of the cranio-cervical junction are more often associated with difficult laryngoscopy than lesions below C3. The patency of the airway can be assessed by CT or MRI scans (see Chapter 25).

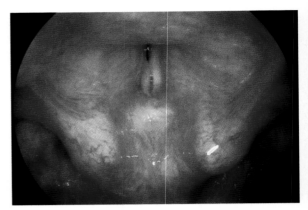

Figure 7.9. Glottic stenosis due to rheumatoid arthritis. Crico-arytenoid joint involvement leads to fixation of the vocal cords. Intubation trauma can cause obstruction after extubation. (Reproduced with permission from Benjamin B. (1998) *Endolaryngeal Surgery.* London: Martin Dunitz.)

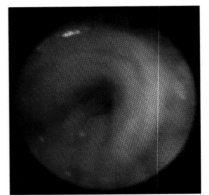

Figure 7.10. Glottic stenosis due to acromegaly. Intubation trauma can cause obstruction after extubation.

Predicting airway problems after anaesthesia

The possibility of airway difficulty after anaesthesia must also be considered. Sleep apnoea patients in particular may well be at greater risk in the postoperative period than at induction, whilst some types of surgery are notorious for engendering airway difficulty post-operatively; facio-maxillary and anterior cervical surgery are examples. The trauma caused by tracheal intubation may aggravate laryngeal and tracheal stenosis, resulting in obstruction after extubation. Rheumatoid and acromegalic disease of the larynx are particularly prone to post-extubation obstruction, so that the smallest possible size of tracheal tube should be used (Figures 7.9, 7.10).

Table 7.5 Indications for consideration of intra-operative tracheostomy

- Major head and neck surgery (such as free flap graft)
- High cervical or base of skull surgery involving maxillotomy or mandibular and tongue splits
- Pre-existing severe high cervical myelopathy or cranial nerve palsies
- Laryngeal or pharyngeal trauma

In some patients an intra-operative tracheostomy is the sensible option (Table 7.5)

Serious morbidity and mortality and prediction of airway difficulty

Unexpected difficulty with facemask ventilation or direct laryngoscopy is a feature of life for anaesthetists. Anaesthetists must keep in mind that mortality associated with airway management is most often due to loss of airway after repeated attempts at intubation, infection after perforation of the pharyngeal mucosa and oesophageal intubation (see Chapter 11). A minimum examination of dental health, inter-dental distance and mandibular protrusion should be routine. It would be unconscionable to find that a patient had an interdental distance of only 1 cm after induction.

Documentation and communication

Difficulty should be documented and disseminated to the patient and their medical advisors. The patient should be given a document containing a brief summary of the problems and solutions. Medic-Alert bracelets are a particularly attractive option for relatively normal-looking patients with severe problems. A suitable document is available from the Difficult Airway Society website (www.das.uk.com).

Key points

- No special training or aptitude is required to recognise most patients with seriously difficult airways.
- It is difficult to identify the rare, relatively normal-looking patients who present important degrees of difficulty during anaesthesia.
- Nevertheless, a basic assessment of dental health, oro-pharyngeal visibility, mandibular protrusion and cranio-cervical flexibility should always be made.

- Anaesthetists should expect and be capable of dealing with unpredicted airway difficulties.
- Serious upper-airway obstruction can be present without stridor or desaturation.
- In some cases predictable airway difficulty can be caused by the surgery or the sequelae of tracheal intubation.
- Mortality and serious morbidity as a result of unexpected difficulty with airway management is avoidable in many cases, by avoiding multiple fruitless attempts to intubate, being alert to the risks of oesophageal intubation and perforation of the mucosa.

Further reading

Baker PA, Depuydt A, Thompson JM. (2009). Thyromental distance measurement – fingers don't rule. *Anaesthesia*, **64**, 878–882.

Calder I, Picard J, Chapman M, O'Sullivan C, Crockard A. (2003). Mouth opening – a new angle. *Anesthesiology*, **99**, 799–801.

Conlon NP, Sullivan RP, Herbison PG, et al. (2007). The effect of leaving dentures in place on bag-mask ventilation at induction of general anesthesia. *Anesthesia and Analgesia*, **105**, 370–373.

Cook TM. (2000). A new practical classification of laryngeal view. *Anaesthesia*, **55**, 274–279.

Deeks JJ, Altman DG. (2004). Diagnostic tests: 4. Likelihood ratios. *British Medical Journal*, **329**, 168–169.

Eberhart LH, Arndt C, Cierpka T, et al. (2005). The reliability and validity of the upper lip bite test compared with the Mallampati classification to predict difficult laryngoscopy: An external prospective evaluation. *Anesthesia and Analgesia*, **101**, 284–289.

El-Orbany M, Woehlck HJ. (2009). Difficult mask ventilation. *Anesthesia and Analgesia*, **109**, 1870–1880.

Hanley JA, McNeil BJ. (1982). The meaning and use of the area under a receiver operating characteristic (ROC) curve. *Radiology*, **143**, 29–36.

Jones PM, Harle CC. (2006). Avoiding awake intubation by performing awake GlideScope laryngoscopy in the preoperative holding area. *Canadian Journal of Anesthesia*, **53**, 1264–1265.

Kheterpal S, Martin L, Shanks AM, Tremper KK. (2009). Prediction and outcomes of impossible mask ventilation. A review of 50,000 anesthetics. *Anesthesiology*, **110**, 891–897.

Lau E, Kulkarni V, Roberts GK, Brock-Utne J. (2009). 'Where are my teeth' A case of unnoticed ingestion of a dislodged partial denture. *Anesthesia and Analgesia*, **109**, 836–838.

Lee A, Fan TY, Gin T, Karmakar MJ, Ngan Kee WD. (2006). A systematic review (meta-analysis) of the accuracy of the Mallampati tests to predict the difficult airway. *Anesthesia and Analgesia*, **102**, 1867–1878.

Lundstrøm LH, Møller AM, Rosenstock C, et al. (2009). A documented previous difficult tracheal intubation as a prognostic test for a subsequent difficult tracheal intubation in adults. *Anaesthesia*, **64**, 1081–1088.

Lundstrøm LH, Møller AM, Rosenstock C, et al. (2009). Avoidance of neuromuscular blocking agents may increase the risk of difficult tracheal intubation: A cohort study of 103812 consecutive adult patients recorded in the Danish Anaesthesia Database. *British Journal of Anaesthesia*, **103**, 283–290.

Lundstrøm LH, Møller AM, Rosenstock C, Astrup G, Wettersley J. (2009). High body mass index is a weak predictor for difficult and failed tracheal intubation: A cohort study of 91,332 consecutive patients scheduled for direct laryngoscopy registered in the Danish Anesthesia Database. *Anesthesiology*, **110**, 266–274.

Mort TC. (2007). Complications of emergency tracheal intubation: Immediate airway-related consequences: part II. *Journal of Intensive Care Medicine*, **22**, 208–215.

Nouraei SA, Giussani DA, Howard DJ, Sandhu GS, Ferguson C, Patel A. (2008). Physiological comparison of spontaneous and positive-pressure ventilation in laryngotracheal stenosis. *British Journal of Anaesthesia*, **101**, 419–423.

Ovassapian A, Glassenberg R, Randel GI, et al. (2002). The unexpected difficult airway and lingual tonsil hyperplasia. *Anesthesiology*, **97**, 124–132.

Parmet JL, Colonna-Romano P, Horrow IC, et al. (1998). The laryngeal mask airway reliably provides rescue ventilation in cases of unanticipated difficult tracheal intubation along with difficult mask ventilation. *Anesthesia and Analgesia*, **87**, 661–665.

Pemberton P, Calder I, O'Sullivan C, Crockard HA. (2002). The Champagne Angle. *Anaesthesia*, **57**, 402–403.

Segebarth PB, Limbird TJ. (2007). Perioperative acute upper airway obstruction secondary to severe rheumatoid arthritis. *Journal of Arthroplasty*, **22**, 916–919.

Shiga T, Wajima Z, Inoue T, Sakamoto A. (2005). Predicting difficult intubation in apparently normal patients: A meta-analysis of bedside screening test performance. *Anesthesiology*, **103**, 429–437.

Tham EJ, Gildersleve CD, Sanders LD, Mapleson WW, Vaughan RS. (1992). Effects of posture, phonation, and observer on Mallampati classification. *British Journal of Anaesthesia*, **68**, 32–38.

Thompson T, Frable MA. (1993). Drug-induced, life threatening angioedema revisited. *Laryngoscope*, **103**, 10–12.

Tse JC, Rimm EB, Hussain A. (1995). Predicting difficult endotracheal intubation in surgical patients scheduled for general anesthesia: A prospective blind study. *Anesthesia and Analgesia*, **81**, 254–258.

Urakami Y, Takennaka I, Nakamura M, et al. (2002). The reliability of the Bellhouse test for evaluating extension capacity of the occipitoatlantoaxial complex. *Anesthesia and Analgesia*, **95**, 1437–1341.

Wilson ME. (1993). Predicting difficult intubation. *British Journal of Anaesthesia*, **71**, 333–334.

Yentis SM. (2002). Predicting difficult intubation – worthwhile exercise or pointless ritual? *Anaesthesia*, **57**, 105–109.

Yentis SM. (2006). Predicting trouble in airway management. *Anesthesiology*, **105**, 871–872.

Chapter 8

Obstructive sleep apnoea and anaesthesia

Peter J.H. Venn

Worldwide, obstructive sleep apnoea (OSA) is the most common medical disorder affecting sleep, afflicting about 3–4% of the middle aged population of the UK, of whom about 70% are male. The full range of sleep disorders has been classified by the American Academy of Sleep Medicine (Table 8.1). The high prevalence of OSA means that anaesthetists are frequently involved with such patients presenting either for surgery as part of treatment for the condition itself, or for unrelated surgery. This chapter deals with the pathophysiology of the condition and its presenting features, investigations and treatment. It concludes with management during the peri-operative period. Sleep apnoea in children is also considered briefly.

Definition and presentation of OSA

OSA is defined as a repetitive obstruction of the upper airway during sleep causing hypoxaemia with arterial oxygen desaturation, which leads to a reduced quality of sleep. When this results in excessive daytime sleepiness (EDS) the condition is often referred to as sleep apnoea syndrome. There is almost always a history of snoring that has worsened over the preceding few years, often causing patients to sleep separately from their partners. The obstruction to the airway may arise from a number of discrete anatomical causes that are listed in Table 8.2, but in the absence of abnormal anatomy, it is relaxation of the pharyngeal constrictor muscles during sleep that allows collapse of the airway. There is evidence that these muscles are hypertonic during wakefulness, and that fatigue may become unmasked during sleep, leading to excessive relaxation. Physical associations with obstructive sleep apnoea include being male, a collar size of 17 inches or greater, a large tongue and often some degree of retrognathia. The association with a high

body mass index means that most of these patients will fall into the category of potentially difficult intubations as classified in the anaesthetic literature. The incidence of the condition rises with age, some studies citing a prevalence of greater than 30% in elderly populations of between 65 and 95 years of age. Medical associations include hypothyroidism, acromegaly and glycogen storage diseases, whilst congenital causes include Down's syndrome, Pierre Robin sequence and other facial anomalies.

To meet the criteria for diagnosis, apnoea from complete obstruction of the airway should occur repeatedly during sleep for more than 10 seconds in the presence of continued movement of the diaphragm, leading to a reduction of greater than 4% in arterial oxygen saturation (SaO_2) from the baseline. Cessation of diaphragm movement resulting in absence of ventilation is called central sleep apnoea and, whilst not uncommon and usually indicative of circulatory conditions, is not the subject of this article. Cessation of breathing due to a combination of central and obstructive apnoeas is termed complex sleep apnoea. Furthermore, obesity hypoventilation syndrome may produce a sustained fall in oxygen saturation during sleep, often with superimposed further falls due to airway obstruction.

Typically in obstructive sleep apnoea, airway obstruction occurs at the level of the pharynx, hypopharynx or both, for between 30 seconds and 1 minute (and occasionally considerably longer), during which time attempted inspiration becomes increasingly vigorous as arterial oxygen desaturation progresses, finally leading to a partial arousal from sleep and sudden reopening of the airway. This causes an explosive intake of breath usually accompanied by some movement of the body or twitching of the limbs indicating sleep disruption or fragmentation.

Core Topics in Airway Management, Second Edition, ed. Ian Calder and Adrian Pearce. Published by Cambridge University Press.
© Cambridge University Press 2011.

Table 8.1. Classification outline of sleep disorders published by the American Academy of Sleep Medicine

1. **Dyssomnias**

    A. Intrinsic sleep disorders

    B. Extrinsic sleep disorders

    C. Circadian rhythm sleep disorders

2. **Parasomnias**

    A. Arousal disorders

    B. Sleep–wake transition disorders

    C. Parasomnias usually associated with REM sleep

    D. Other parasomnias

3. **Medical/psychiatric sleep disorders**

    A. Associated with mental disorders

    B. Associated with neurological disorders

    C. Associated with other medical disorders

1A. Intrinsic sleep disorders

1. Psychophysiological insomnia

2. Sleep state misperception

3. Idiopathic insomnia

4. Narcolepsy

5. Recurrent hypersomnia

6. Idiopathic hypersomnia

7. Post-traumatic hypersomnia

8. Obstructive sleep apnoea syndrome

9. Central sleep apnoea syndrome

10. Central alveolar hypoventilation syndrome

11. Periodic limb movement disorder

12. Restless legs syndrome

Table 8.2. Anatomical and physiological reasons for the development of sleep disordered breathing

1. Macroglossia and a wide tongue base

2. Retrognathia

3. Tumours of the upper airway

4. Craniofacial disorders

5. Neuromuscular disorders

6. Tonsillar hypertrophy

7. Neck girth of 17 inches or more

The resulting fragmented and poor quality sleep leads to a lack of refreshment on awakening with excessive daytime sleepiness (EDS) as measured by the Epworth Sleepiness Scale (Figure 8.1). Epworth scores above 8 out of the maximum 24 possible are regarded as above normal, and a score of greater than 12 impacts upon social and family life as well as daytime performance – particularly vehicle driving ability. Sufferers are consequently a potential danger to themselves, and to others who may be dependent upon their judgement. Drivers of large goods vehicles are predisposed to the condition partly as a result of their typical lifestyle.

Although complete and repeated apnoea represents the worst case scenario, some individuals experience only partial degrees of upper airway obstruction that do not lead to overt arterial oxygen desaturation. Sleep arousals may still occur, probably due to the increased upper airway resistance still causing a rise in diaphragmatic work. The resulting reduction in tidal volume due to partial upper airway obstruction is called hypopnoea, and often results in EDS in the absence of actual OSA.

Recurrent night time hypoxaemia can lead to several cardiovascular complications, including arterial and pulmonary hypertension, cor pulmonale, an increased incidence of heart disease and cerebrovascular events. There is unequivocal evidence that treating OSA reduces raised arterial blood pressure. Furthermore, there is mounting evidence of an association with the development of type II adult onset diabetes and metabolic syndrome. Metabolic syndrome has been defined by the World Health Organization (WHO) according to the criteria in Table 8.3, and is estimated to increase the risk of major cardiovascular events six fold. This has been referred to recently as Syndrome X, and appears to be due to the development of insulin resistance.

Electro-encephalography (EEG) shows evidence of cortical or sub-cortical arousal from sleep due to a combination of arterial oxygen desaturation combined with increased inspiratory effort and diaphragmatic work. Hyperventilation follows re-establishment of the airway for a short time, but as sleep deepens again, airway obstruction returns causing the cycle to restart. The worst cases may have up to 60 of these cycles per hour (apnoea index) giving 400–500 episodes in a sleep period of 8 hours, with each dip in oxygen saturation as low as 60%.

THE EPWORTH SLEEPINESS SCALE

How likely are you to fall asleep or doze in the situations described in the boxes below, in contrast to just feeling tired?

Use the following scale to choose the most appropriate number for each situation.

Not at all	Score 0
Slight chance	Score 1
Moderate chance	Score 2
High chance	Score 3

ACTIVITY	SCORE
Sitting and reading	
Watching TV	
Sitting inactive in a public place, (e.g., in a theatre or meeting)	
Sitting quietly after lunch without alcohol	
Sitting in a car as a passenger for an hour without a break	
Lying down to rest in the afternoon when circumstances permit	
Talking to someone	
In a car, whilst stopped for a few minutes in traffic	

Figure 8.1. The Epworth Sleepiness Scale, used to assess the amount of daytime dysfunction due to fragmented sleep at night. This is the most widely used scoring system in the world at the present time, although other scoring systems are becoming popular.

Clinical presentation

History

The symptoms of snoring, apnoea and EDS often lead to consultations with ENT surgeons, but other medical symptoms may precipitate alternative presentations to chest physicians, neurologists or cardiologists. Furthermore, daytime sleepiness can mimic clinical depression and lead to psychiatric referral.

Although the clinical presentation varies and diagnosis requires an index of suspicion, the typical patient is male, with weight gain over adulthood leading to a current body mass index (BMI) of 30 kg m^{-2} or more, and an increase in collar size of 1.5 inches to around 17 inches during adulthood (Figure 8.2). There is a history of increasingly intrusive snoring in all positions during sleep, with reports of sleep apnoea and daytime sleepiness. A full medical history should include details of the presenting complaint, as well as enquiry about nocturia, loss of libido, nightmares and sudden awakening in the night with fear or palpitations, all of which are associated. Gastro-oesophageal reflux is common in this group and also leads to sudden awakening during sleep with choking and dyspnoea. A detailed cardiovascular history including the end-organ consequences of hypertension should be sought, as well as prescribed and non-prescribed drugs, tobacco and alcohol consumption. More often than not, patients are already taking antihypertensive drugs, and increasing numbers are on hypocholesterolaemics and aspirin. Unfortunately some patients still present on night sedatives, their morning lack of refreshment being attributed to insomnia. Benzodiazepines and more modern alternatives such as zaleplon, zolpidem and zopiclone (so called Z-drugs) tend to worsen pharyngeal relaxation, and exacerbate the situation. A commonly associated feature is poor subjective ability to breathe through the nose, and previous nasal surgery may already have been carried out, or become necessary as part of the ongoing management of the condition.

Table 8.3. The criteria for diagnosis of metabolic syndrome as laid down by the World Health Organisation (1999)

The presence of either diabetes mellitus, or impaired glucose tolerance, impaired fasting glucose and insulin resistance are necessary, together with two or more of the following:	
Criterion	**Value**
Body weight	W/H ratio > 0.9 in males
Raised waist/hip ratio	W/H ratio > 0.85 in females
	Central obesity and increased intra-abdominal fat
Body mass index	> 30 kg/m²
High density lipoprotein (HDL)	< 1.7 mmol/litre
Low density-lipoprotein (LDL)	> 0.9 mmol/litre
Arterial Blood Pressure	> 140/90 mmHg
Micro-albuminuria	Urine albumin excretion > 20 mg/min
Inflammatory state	Elevated C-reactive protein

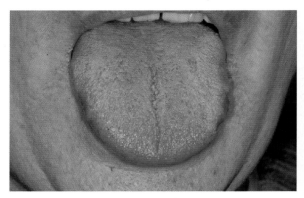

Figure 8.3. The typical appearance of the tongue in a patient with obstructive sleep apnoea. Notice the 'crenulations' (indentations) on the lateral borders of the tongue made by the teeth, and the Mallampati score of 4.

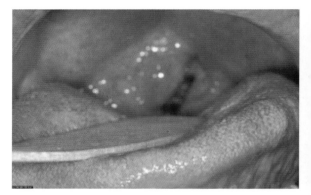

Figure 8.4. The restricted pharyngeal volume with redundant mucosal folds often seen in association with obstructive sleep apnoea.

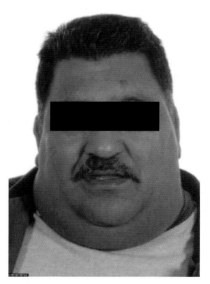

Figure 8.2. The typical facial features of a patient with obstructive sleep apnoea. Notice the width of the neck.

Physical examination

A full examination of the upper airway should be undertaken, with attention to the collar size, Mallampati score, dental occlusion and pharyngeal volume.

Tonsillar hypertrophy should be recorded because this may be the underlying problem, and usually is so in children presenting with OSA. The facial profile should be studied to detect degrees of mandibular retrognathia. The tongue may have crenulations – small indentations on the lateral borders made by the teeth. These indicate that it is being squeezed inwards and backwards into the pharyngeal space when the mouth is closed (Figure 8.3). The pharyngeal volume is often very reduced with redundant mucosal folds limiting the lateral diameter (Figure 8.4). The patient should be asked to sublux the jaw forwards to measure the amount of movement, because good degrees of movement of greater than 5 millimetres may allow treatment with intra-oral mandibular advancement devices, rather than continuous positive airway pressure devices.

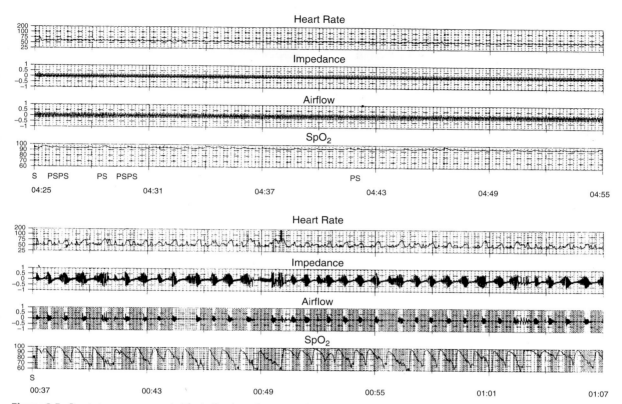

Figure 8.5. Respiratory traces recorded for half an hour from two subjects whilst asleep. The four channels show from top to bottom; heart rate, chest movement, airflow and arterial oxygen saturation. The top trace is taken during unobstructed quiet sleep and shows a steady heart rate with normal respiration and levels of oxygen saturation. The lower trace shows obstructive sleep apnoea with cyclical dips in oxygen saturation due to regular cessation of airflow with consequent rises and falls in heart rate as each partial arousal from sleep occurs.

Investigations

Investigations include blood tests to exclude other causes of EDS such as hypothyroidism, anaemia and narcolepsy (which is associated with HLA DQB1*0602 typing), but the diagnosis is readily confirmed by carrying out a sleep study called a polysomnogram (PSG). Full polysomnography is complicated, and includes monitoring of the chest movement, airflow dynamics, heart rate and blood pressure, arterial oxygen saturation, EEG and electro-oculogram (EOG), together with a pre-tibial electromyogram (EMG) to detect limb movements, all during sleep. EEG monitoring is used to assess the stage of sleep (Stage I, II, III, IV non-REM, or REM sleep) and is a valuable tool in the diagnosis of complex sleep disorders. However at least in the UK, comparatively few sleep laboratories have this facility, and cardio-respiratory monitoring alone is usually carried out, this being adequate to diagnose OSA.

Video-telemetry using an infrared camera for night time recording combined with sound is a very useful supplement. Comparisons of a normal respiratory PSG with one from a patient with florid OSA are shown in Figure 8.5.

Treatment of OSA

The gold standard of treatment for OSA is to submit the patient to nasal continuous positive airway pressure (nCPAP) whilst asleep. CPAP devices are now in common usage worldwide, and a wide choice of products is available. CPAP is applied to the airway through a nasal mask (Figure 8.6) and works by applying positive airway pressure to the pharynx throughout the breathing cycle to overcome the obstructive forces due to pharyngeal collapse. CPAP is best commenced in hospital for 1 night under supervision whilst the correct level of airway pressure

67

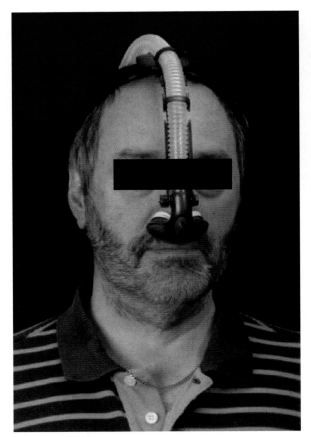

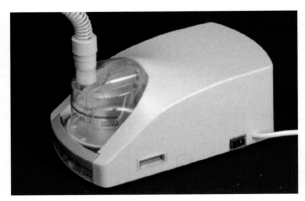

Figure 8.7. The Fisher Pakel CPAP device with an inbuilt heated water bath for humidification of inspired air.

Figure 8.6. Application of nCPAP to the airway using nasal prongs and harness. The minimal amount of hardware attached to the patient's face increases the acceptability of the device.

measured in centimetres of H_2O is set for the individual. However there are now automated devices available which sense the airflow of each inspiration and adjust the pressure accordingly to overcome any obstruction (auto-titration). Whilst the pressure energy should be high enough to overcome the pharyngeal collapse causing the obstruction, it should not be so high as to reach the lower airway and raise the functional residual capacity, because there is evidence that this in itself disrupts sleep. Pressure requirements range from as low as 5 cmH$_2$O to as high as 15–20 cmH$_2$O depending upon the severity of the obstruction.

Many studies have been carried out to evaluate and predict the compliance to treatment of patients who use CPAP at home. Clearly, non-compliance brings no benefit or relief from symptoms, but every laboratory has its group of such patients. Good compliance predictors include self-referral due to EDS (as opposed to referral under pressure from partners or family because of snoring), a patent nasal airway and, most importantly, relief of daytime sleepiness on CPAP with an improved quality of life. Despite treating OSA adequately with CPAP, about 10% of patients remain excessively sleepy by day, and the reason for this has recently been debated but remains unclear. The level of compliance is recorded in hours of usage by a meter built into the device, and at least 4 hours of use per night is necessary for a reduction in EDS as evaluated by pre- and post-treatment Epworth Scores.

There are no serious side effects of CPAP treatment, but minor untoward effects may decrease compliance and benefit. Of these, inflammation of the nasal mucosa from the pressurised airflow often leads to symptoms of rhinitis and nasal blockage that can be troublesome, and is sometimes a reason for failure to comply with treatment. Nasal blockage usually causes the user to mouth breathe with loss of the required pharyngeal pressure, airflow entering through the nose but escaping through the mouth. These patients awaken with sore and dry throats that may be distressing. Nasal blockage can be treated with topical steroid sprays, but responds well to humidification of the pressurised airflow, the humidifier usually being an integral part of the machine design (Figure 8.7). Where the nasal airway persistently blocks despite simple measures, a full facemask covering the nose and mouth can be tried, with resort to nasal surgery if all else fails. Occasionally, other complaints about CPAP include noise emission from the device disturbing the sleep of the partner or patient, discomfort from the mask, the development of pressure sores on the nasal bridge, or feelings of claustrophobia.

Whilst the most noticeable effect of CPAP is to reduce daytime sleepiness, physiological benefits also occur. Hypertensive patients treated with CPAP show a beneficial reduction in both systolic and diastolic blood pressure, the effect of which appears to increase with time. The strong association of asthma with OSA also benefits, as does nocturia, the reduction of which improves sleep quality in itself. With time, patients become very adept in managing their CPAP therapy, putting it on, adjusting it and going to sleep within only a few minutes.

As previously stated, some patients can be treated for mild OSA with mandibular advancement devices (MAD), which posture the mandible forwards, pulling the tongue away from the posterior pharyngeal wall through traction on the geniohyoid and genioglossus muscles. Mandibular advancement depends upon a partial dislocation of the temporomandibular joint. Patients who benefit most from this treatment tend to be mandibular retrognathic, with a class II dental malocclusion where the bottom incisors lie behind the top incisors when the mouth is closed. They have snoring predominantly from behind the tongue that may cause varying degrees of upper airway obstruction during sleep, even in the absence of true OSA. However the disadvantage of both CPAP and MADs is that they must be used every night to be effective and, therefore, many patients prefer to seek a permanent surgical solution. This has led to the development of a number of operations, resulting in varying degrees of success.

Recently, radio frequency coagulation of the palate (somnoplasty) and ablation of the base of the tongue have been used with some success in the treatment of palatal snoring, as have soft palate implants to stiffen the tissues. Since 2005, the National Institute of Clinical Excellence (NICE) in the UK has reviewed these procedures but do not recommend them for routine clinical use at the time of writing, although they note some benefit. However many consider them preferable to the unpleasant operation of uvulopalatopharyngoplasty (UPPP), where the soft palate is surgically removed completely. In the author's opinion, there is no place for UPPP in the modern management of sleep apnoea, although laser assisted palatoplasty is still carried out on the unwary, and many patients with OSA present to sleep clinics having undergone such surgery previously. Its use has declined due to poor results and the long-term serious complication of velopharyngeal incompetence.

The most recent surgical development in the treatment of OSA is bimaxillary osteotomy in selected patients. Where an MAD proves effective, either moving the mandible forwards alone using a sagittal split osteotomy, or in combination with the upper jaw using a Le Fort I osteotomy, can produce a permanent cure for the condition. This may be a protracted process, necessitating up to 2 years of orthodontic treatment before surgery, so producing a normal dental occlusion post-operatively. The production of a clearer nasal airway is often an additional benefit.

Finally, the increased numbers of morbidly obese patients have produced a working relationship between sleep centres and those undertaking bariatric surgery. Both gastric banding, and the more complicated operation of gastric bypass, can lead to profound levels of weight loss with a beneficial reduction in metabolic and physiological risk.

In conclusion, because there is now a broad range of options, both surgical and non-surgical, careful assessment is required before advising on a suitable treatment for patients with OSA.

Obstructive sleep apnoea and anaesthesia

Pre-operative assessment

The most serious risk for patients with OSA undergoing surgery is loss of the airway caused by the use of anaesthetic, sedative and opioid drugs, combined with the increased risk of anaesthesia from clinical obesity and hypertension. The high prevalence of OSA means that anaesthetists will meet it frequently. Most sufferers remain undiagnosed, and reliance cannot therefore be put on the patient to volunteer information about their symptoms. Patients may present for surgery as part of the overall management of their sleep apnoea, most often on the nasal airway, palate, tongue, tonsils or mandible, where there is the added complication of shared airway anaesthesia. However the undiagnosed and unrecognised patient presenting for unrelated surgery poses the greatest risk, and where there is a suspicion of sleep apnoea, elective surgery should be postponed until the patient has been fully investigated and treated.

Planning for surgery should start well before the day of admission, because special investigations may be needed as part of the peri-operative workup. Previous anaesthetic records grading ease of direct

69

laryngoscopy and intubation are invaluable if available. All patients using CPAP at home should be instructed to bring their device with them on the day of admission for use during their hospital stay, and the staff looking after them on the ward and in the recovery room should be familiar with the concept of CPAP, and its use.

The anaesthetic assessment of the airway should begin routinely by enquiring about a history of snoring or apnoea during sleep. Most patients will be aware of the disharmony in the bedroom due to their condition, even if no medical help has previously been sought. A concurrent history of daytime sleepiness suggests some degree of airway obstruction during sleep that may well be transposed to anaesthesia. Enquiry about cardio-respiratory symptoms is mandatory to evaluate right and left ventricular function, and the presence of cor pulmonale, together with the consequences of end organ dysfunction. Examination and prediction of the difficult airway has been extensively documented in the anaesthetic literature, and a detailed analysis will not be given here. However the degree of mouth opening, Mallampati score and thyro-mental distance should be recorded, together with a Wilson summation score. Patients requiring shirt collars of greater than 17 inches should be assumed to have sleep apnoea unless proved otherwise.

A frank discussion with the patient is necessary about the increased risk of general anaesthesia, and should include a detailed explanation of the anaesthetic technique deemed appropriate. The high association with clinical obesity and acid reflux may affect the planning of the anaesthetic.

Premedication with sedatives and opioids should be avoided, or used with extreme caution if deemed absolutely necessary. Constant vigilance is required once these drugs have been administered, and monitoring of the arterial oxygen saturation should be considered.

Anaesthetic technique

This group of patients present a formidable challenge to the anaesthetist in terms of intubation, extubation, and post-operative analgesia. Of interest is a retrospective study that concludes that, whilst morbid obesity in itself is not a predictor of difficult direct larygoscopy, a history of OSA is so, with Cormack grade III and IV views in 90% of OSA patients studied.

No global rules can be applied to the choice of anaesthetic technique, and each patient should be considered according to their individual needs. However induction under full monitoring is required and, whatever means is used to secure the airway, most agree that tracheal intubation is preferable to use of the laryngeal mask airway. Regard should be given to possible regurgitation of stomach acid during induction. A full range of aids for difficult intubation should be ready, and attendant staff should be familiar with the use of such equipment.

Some authors advocate awake fibreoptic intubation under topical anaesthesia for all patients with OSA, although obtunded airway reflexes after local anaesthesia to the upper airway have been reported to cause increased levels of obstruction in the post-operative period. Whatever technique is chosen for induction and intubation, the attention and skill of all staff is of paramount importance. At least two plans should be made to maintain the airway in the event of failure of the first.

Extubation should be predicted to be 'stormy' and not be undertaken until the patient is awake. Intra-operative use of local anaesthesia for pain relief will allow sparing administration of opioid drugs, and regional techniques using infusions are useful adjuncts in the post-operative period, especially where catheters can be placed with great accuracy using ultra-sound guidance.

Although avoidance of sedative and opioid drugs during the peri-operative period is the recommended practice, sedatives and opioids have been used freely in conjunction with CPAP therapy without complication in the post-operative period.

Post-operative management

The patient's CPAP device should be sent to the recovery room during surgery and made ready for use immediately on emergence from anaesthesia. Under no circumstances should the patient be left unattended or without cardiorespiratory monitoring until fully awake, and even then consideration should be given to the enterohepatic circulation of any sedative or opiate drugs. Up to 20% of patients require major medical intervention including re-intubation in the immediate post-operative period. Nursing staff should be familiar with such complications and ready to maintain a difficult airway if needed and, obviously, the anaesthetist should be available immediately.

Subsequent management in an intensive care or high dependency unit should be considered for any major surgical intervention, especially vascular surgery, where significant oxygen desaturation has been recorded during the first two post-operative nights, possibly due to rebound levels of REM sleep following anaesthesia. One recommendation is for nocturnal oxygen post-operatively and for at least one more night after opioid therapy has stopped.

Sleep apnoea in children

Obstructive sleep apnoea in children is a specialised area, but most often presents on ENT operating lists for correction of adenoidal or tonsillar hypertrophy. It is appropriate to enquire of the parents about a history of snoring, and the child's breathing quality during sleep. A diminished ventilatory response to CO_2 has been recorded in these patients, and they require trained paediatric staff in the recovery room. Although children are less amenable than adults, they can be successfully managed with CPAP in specialised centres, Great Ormond Street Hospital for Sick Children in London claiming success in up to 86% of children of various ages with OSA not relieved by adenotonsillectomy.

Rarer associations with OSA in children include congenital conditions such as the mucopolysacharridoses, Down's syndrome and hypothyroidism. Conditions of craniofacial deformity are also seen, Pierre Robin sequence, Treacher-Collins syndrome and Goldenhars syndrome representing more common examples. Such cases require treatment in specialized centres with multidisciplinary planning and should not be managed outside an appropriate environment.

Key points

- OSA is a common condition, often unrecognised.
- OSA recognised at pre-operative evaluation needs proper assessment before elective surgery.
- Airway management may be more difficult both intra- and post-operatively.
- OSA increases post-operative morbidity and mortality.
- Established therapy, such as nasal CPAP, should be continued in the post-operative period.
- Opioid therapy presents particular problems and patients require cardiorespiratory monitoring.
- Supplemental oxygen is required for 1 night longer than opioid therapy.

Further reading

Benumof JL. (2002). Obstructive sleep apnea in the adult obese patient: Implications for airway management. *Anesthesiology Clinics of North America.* **20**, 789–811.

Bolden N, Smith CE, Auckley D. (2009). Avoiding adverse outcomes in patients with obstructive sleep apnea (OSA): Development and implementation of a perioperative OSA protocol. *Journal of Clinical Anesthesia,* **21**, 286–293.

Brown KA. (2009). Intermittent hypoxia and the practice of anesthesia. *Anesthesiology,* **110**, 922–927.

Brown KA, Morin I, Hickey C, Manoukian JJ, Nixon GM, Brouillett RT. (2003). Urgent adenotonsillectomy: An analysis of risk factors associated with postoperative respiratory morbidity. *Anesthesiology,* **99**, 586–595.

Candiotti K, Sharma S, Shankar R. (2009). Obesity, obstructive sleep apnoea, and diabetes mellitus: Anaesthetic implications. *British Journal of Anaesthesia,* **103**(Suppl 1), 123–130.

Chung F, Elsaid H. (2009). Screening for obstructive sleep apnea before surgery: Why is it important? *Current Opinion in Anaesthesiology,* **22**, 405–411.

Chung SA, Yuan H, Chung F. (2008). A systemic review of obstructive sleep apnea and its implications for anesthesiologists. *Anesthesia and Analgesia,* **107**, 1543–1563.

den Herder C, Schmeck J, Appelboom DJ, de Vries N. (2004). Risks of general anaesthesia in people with obstructive sleep apnoea. *British Medical Journal,* **329**, 955–959.

Eastwood PR, Szollosi I, Platt PR, Hillman DR. (2002). Comparison of upper airway collapse during general anaesthesia and sleep. *Lancet,* **359**(9313), 1207–1209.

Ezri T, Medalion B, Weisenberg M, Szmuk P, Warters RD, Charuzi I. (2003). Increased body mass index per se is not a predictor of difficult laryngoscopy. *Canadian Journal of Anaesthesia,* **50**, 179–183.

Gross JB, Bachenberg KL, Benumof JL, et al. (2006). Practice guidelines for the perioperative management of patients with obstructive sleep apnea: A report by the American Society of Anesthesiologists Task Force on Perioperative Management of patients with obstructive sleep apnea. *Anesthesiology,* **104**, 1081–1093.

International Diabetes Federation. *Worldwide Definition of Metabolic Syndrome.* Available at: www.idf.org/metabolic_syndrome.

Isono S. (2009). Obstructive sleep apnea of obese adults: Pathophysiology and perioperative airway management. *Anesthesiology,* **110**, 908–921.

Liao P, Yegneswaran B, Vairavanathan S, Zilberman P, Chung F. (2009). Postoperative complications in patients with obstructive sleep apnea: A retrospective matched cohort study. *Canadian Journal of Anaesthesia,* **56**, 819–828.

Lim J, McKean M. (2003). Adenotonsillectomy for obstructive sleep apnoea in children. *Cochrane Database of Systematic Reviews*, (1), CD003136.

Logan AG, Tkacova R, Perlikowski SM, et al. (2003). Refractory hypertension and sleep apnoea: Effect of CPAP on blood pressure and baroreceptor reflex. *The European Respiratory Journal*, 21, 241–247.

Massa F, Gonsalez S, Laverty A, Wallis C, Lane R. (2002). The use of nasal continuous positive airway pressure to treat obstructive sleep apnoea. *Archives of Disease in Childhood*, 87, 438–443.

National Institute for Health and Clinical Excellence. *Radiofrequency Ablation of the Soft Palate for Snoring*. NICE Interventional Procedural Guideline 124. Available at: www.nice.org.uk.

National Institute for Health and Clinical Excellence. *Continuous Positive Airway Pressure for the Treatment of Obstructive Sleep Apnoea/Hypopnoea Syndrome*. NICE technology appraisal guidance 139. Available at: www.nice.org.uk.

Ramachandran SK, Josephs LA. (2009). A meta-analysis of clinical screening tests for obstructive sleep apnea. *Anesthesiology,* **110**, 928–939.

Schwengel DA, Sterni LM, Tunkel DE, Heitmiller ES. (2009). Perioperative management of children with obstructive sleep apnea. *Anesthesia and Analgesia,* **109**, 60–75.

Strauss SG, Lynn AM, Bratton SL, Nespeca MK. (1999). Ventilatory response to CO_2 in children with obstructive sleep apnea from adenotonsillar hypertrophy. *Anesthesia and Analgesia,* **89**, 328–332.

Facemasks and supraglottic airway devices

Tim Cook

Fundamentals

Nothing is more fundamental to the practice of general anaesthesia than the maintenance of a clear upper airway.

Almost every general anaesthetic requires maintenance of the airway with a facemask after induction and more than 60% of anaesthetics in some countries involve use of a supraglottic airway during maintenance of anaesthesia.

Basic airway care

General anaesthesia almost invariably causes loss of airway reflexes and respiratory arrest (apnoea). As it is usually performed in the supine position airway obstruction is almost inevitable. Unless this is relieved rapidly hypoxia is inevitable. Due to the shape of the oxygen haemoglobin dissociation curve hypoxia is often delayed after the induction of anaesthesia. However when hypoxia becomes evident (SpO_2 85%) life-threatening hypoxia (SpO_2 <50%) will develop in 20–40 seconds if the airway is not established and maintained by the anaesthetist. The speed and severity of hypoxia is increased in those with abnormal airway anatomy (e.g., congenital morphology, tumours, trauma), decreased oxygen reserves (e.g., pregnancy, obesity, children, lung pathology), increased oxygen consumption (e.g., pregnancy, sepsis, burns) or circulatory insufficiency.

Mechanism of obstruction

After the induction of anaesthesia respiratory drive is usually depressed or absent. Normal airway muscular tone is profoundly reduced. Airway reflexes are either reduced or completely abolished. The patient is usually lying supine. In these circumstances there is a natural tendency for the mouth to close, the jaw to recess and the soft tissues fall backwards under gravity. In particular the tongue falls back until it occludes the oro/hypopharynx. Epiglottic occlusion and loss of tone in the larynx also contribute. The soft palate may obstruct the nasal airway. All these factors contribute to an increased likelihood of airway obstruction with increasing depth of anaesthesia. Obstruction below the nasopharynx blocks the common path of both the nasal and oral airway. It is the submandibular soft tissue structures (tongue and epiglottis) that are the principal causes of airway obstruction. The tongue is attached to the inner surface of the mandible and movement of the mandible is transmitted to the tongue. Reversing or preventing airway obstruction is achieved by manoeuvres that draw the mandible forward and increase submandibular space.

Much can be achieved by patient positioning and simple airway manipulations. In some cases, however, these procedures are inadequate and airway control requires use of airway adjuncts

Anaesthesia (and sedation) that may alter airway tone and lead to airway obstruction should only be undertaken by those appropriately trained, in an appropriate area with trained assistance, recommended monitoring in place and resuscitation equipment available. Minimum monitoring for anaesthesia has been defined by the AAGBI and should include measurement of delivered oxygen, blood pressure, pulse oximetry and capnography. Administration of high flow oxygen to all patients prior to induction of anaesthesia increases oxygen reserves in the lungs. It reduces the incidence of hypoxia and increases the margin of safety of anaesthetic induction. After induction all patients require the airway to be cleared

Core Topics in Airway Management, Second Edition, ed. Ian Calder and Adrian Pearce. Published by Cambridge University Press.
© Cambridge University Press 2011.

and maintained. Establishing a patent airway involves reversing those factors that have led to airway obstruction.

Anaesthesia facemasks

After induction of anaesthesia oxygenation and ventilation are maintained with facemask ventilation. A clear airway is achieved with the use of a combination of head and neck positioning and airway clearing manoeuvres (i.e., chin lift and jaw thrust) (Figure 9.1).

Anaesthesia facemasks are designed to fit the variable contours of the patient's face and provide a low pressure seal to enable leak-free ventilation during both spontaneous and controlled ventilation.

Facemask anaesthesia may be suitable for airway maintenance for short anaesthetic procedures. However this technique requires constant hand contact by the anaesthetist and is not suitable for surgery close to the head or neck. The anaesthetist may be freed by use of a harness securing the mask in place, but these are mainly of historical interest. Prolonged use of a tight fitting mask or harness may (rarely) lead to injury to branches of the trigeminal or facial nerves (particularly intraorbital and trochlear nerves).

Standard facemasks are plastic or rubber cones designed to fit over the nose and mouth. A 22 mm connector allows attachment to an anaesthetic breathing circuit and an air-filled edge allows a gas-tight seal to be made with the face. Anaesthetic masks come in a variety of sizes to fit infant to large adult. While masks have historically been made of antistatic rubber, with the discontinuation of highly flammable anaesthetic agents this material is redundant. Most are now made of clear plastic, which affords patient comfort and allows patient colour and secretions to be observed by the anaesthetist. Observing condensation of exhaled humidified gas can be a useful respiratory monitor. Specialised masks exist for anaesthetising using the nose only (nasal masks – see Chapter 24). In paediatric practice the dead space of conventional mask becomes significant and masks such as the Baker-Rendell-Soucek mask are designed to overcome this problem.

To allow ventilation the mask may be attached to a ventilating bag. This is usually a self-inflating bag in non-anaesthetic practice, and the reservoir bag of the anaesthetic circuit filled with anaesthetic gases during anaesthetic practice.

Many anaesthesia facemasks are delivered with a multipronged o-ring around the collar of the

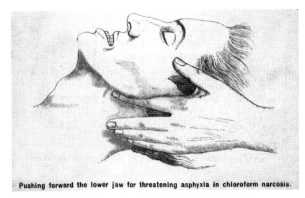

Pushing forward the lower jaw for threatening asphyxia in chloroform narcosis.

Figure 9.1. Jaw thrust. (From Esmarch F. (1877) by kind permission of The Royal Society of Medicine.)

connector. This ring is designed to enable attachment of a harness that keeps the mask in place and allows hands-free airway maintenance. With the advent of supraglottic airways this technique is largely redundant. The o-rings interfere with comfortable mask holding and should generally be removed before use.

There are many manufacturers of anaesthesia facemasks and design and quality varies between products. Mask ventilation is a fundamental skill of anaesthesia and when intubation and other techniques have failed it may be a life-saving technique. Therefore there should be no compromise on quality.

Bag and mask ventilation requires several things to be achieved by the anaesthetist: 1) maintenance of a patent airway 2) an effective seal between mask and the face 3) effective and smooth ventilation by compression of the bag (reservoir). This is a fundamental skill but one that is neither easy, nor well performed routinely. In many patients achieving a seal may prove difficult and this is particularly so in elderly patients with no teeth, in whom the mid-face has a tendency to collapse. An oral airway adjunct may be required.

One person technique: an experienced anaesthetist may use one hand to lift the bony part of the jaw and effect a seal with the mask while the second hand squeezes the bag to achieve ventilation. The thumb and index finger press the mask to the face, while the middle and ring fingers pull the mandible into the mask and the little finger is hooked under the angle of the jaw lifting anteriorly. Even in the most experienced hands this technique may fail and a two person technique may be needed.

Two person technique: particularly useful for individuals with small hands, for large patients and those with small chin and a beard (a popular combination!). One person clears the airway with two handed jaw thrust while the second squeezes the bag. Three fingers of both hands are used to apply jaw thrust and lift the mandible into the facemask while the thumb and index finger apply downward pressure on the mask to achieve an effective seal. The overall direction of application of force should lead to chin lift and upper cervical extension. Excessive force downwards will lead to flexion of the upper cervical spine and worsen airway obstruction.

Whatever technique is used poor airway seal leads to gas leak and ineffective ventilation. Poor airway clearance and use of excessive volumes or pressure during assisted ventilation leads to gas preferentially entering the oesophagus, rather than the larynx, with gastric distension and increased risk of regurgitation. Attention to the 'feel' of the airway, as well as inspection of chest wall movement, reservoir bag filling, and capnography will indicate success or otherwise. High inflation pressures without chest movement indicate airway obstruction. Loss of gas from the system (inability to keep the reservoir bag full) indicates gas leaking from the mask because the seal is inadequate. Using high fresh gas flow when mask ventilation is difficult will improve success. What constitutes difficult mask ventilation is by no means easy to describe or quantify, see Chapter 7.

Airway adjuncts

Maintenance of the patient's airway may be facilitated by use of an oropharyngeal or nasopharyngeal airway. In both cases the adjunct passes through the route of the natural airway to lie in the pharynx thereby overcoming airway collapse/obstruction.

Guedel (oropharyngeal) airway

The Guedel airway was first described in 1933 and is a hollow partially flattened plastic tube formed in the shape of the superior surface of the tongue. It acts both to open the mouth and to lift the tongue from the hypopharynx, so clearing the airway. The tip should lie in the oropharynx. There are up to seven sizes and size is approximated by measuring from the midline (incisors) to the angle of the jaw. Adult sizes are 90–110 mm in length (Size 3–5). In adults the airway is inserted upside-down (convexity downwards) until the soft palate is reached and it is then rotated 180 degrees and advanced into place. This technique

minimises the risk of inadvertently forcing the tongue backwards during insertion. In children, placement under direct vision, using a tongue depressor or laryngoscope blade is preferred and this is equally suitable for adults. Insertion of a Guedel of the wrong size or in light planes of anaesthesia may lead to airway obstruction, laryngospasm or regurgitation. The Guedel is designed for single use and costs less than £0.50.

Size	Length (mm)
00	40–45
0	50–55
1	75
2	80
3	90
4	100
5	110

Nasopharyngeal airway

A nasopharyngeal airway is designed to be passed along the floor of the nose, behind the soft palate to position its tip in the oropharynx. It is used infrequently during general anaesthesia but may be useful in sedated or obtunded patients. Specifically designed airways or cut-down tracheal tubes are both appropriate. Diameter is selected as approximately 1 mm smaller than the appropriate tracheal tube. The nasal airway should not cause blanching of the nostril when inserted, and a size greater than 7.0 mm is not necessary. The length of the airway may be estimated from the tip of the nose to the tragus of the ear and is about 3 cm longer than an oral airway.

The lubricated airway is inserted into the nostril then advanced parallel to the roof of the mouth below the inferior turbinate. Insertion is stimulating, but once the device is inserted it is well tolerated and may be left in place until the patient is fully awake. The principal complication of the use of a nasal airway is bleeding (which may be profuse), though sub-mucosal placement is also possible. A proximal flange prevents loss of the airway into the nasal cavity but in softer devices a safety pin may also be needed. Nasal airways should not be used in the presence of base of skull fractures or severe bleeding diatheses. Nasal airways are designed for single use and cost £2–3.

Supraglottic Airway Devices (SADs)

The term supraglottic airway device (SAD) describes a group of airway devices designed to establish and maintain a clear airway during anaesthesia. SADs have several roles including anaesthesia, airway rescue after failed intubation or out of hospital, use during cardiopulmonary resuscitation and as conduits to assist (difficult) tracheal intubation. Some prefer the term extraglottic airway device (EAD), but SAD is more widely accepted and is used here.

Prior to 1998 almost all general anaesthesia was conducted with facemask or tracheal tube. The classic laryngeal mask airway (cLMA) was introduced in 1988 and rapidly transformed the way in which anaesthesia is practiced through much of the world. Since that time, and particularly in the past 5 years there has been an explosion of new SADs designed to compete with the cLMA. These devices vary considerably in the degree to which they have been evaluated before and since marketing. Several devices have been modified several times since introduction so interpretation of literature on device performance must be made with great care to ensure the device reported on is the device currently produced. There are currently too few comparative trials between devices to determine the clinical role (if any) for individual devices. The ProSeal LMA (PLMA) and Laryngeal Tube (LT) are the most extensively investigated of the newer SADs. The LMA Supreme and i-gel are also supported by an increasing body of evidence.

The majority of SADs are designed to lie with their tip at the origin of the oesophagus, effectively 'plugging' the oesophagus. A seal around the larynx is then achieved by a more proximal cuff, which acts to elevate the base of the tongue and lift the epiglottis and seal the oropharynx. Some cuffs encircle the laryngeal inlet while others simply lie above it. All airways that are inserted beyond the epiglottis (all SADs except the COPA) may lead to down-folding of the epiglottis and airway obstruction. One of the design challenges of these devices is to allow placement of the distal portion of the device behind the cricoid cartilage without displacing the epiglottis during insertion.

Efficacy, safety and new SADs

As indicated above, SADs may have a number of roles, and different designs and performance characteristics may be required for each role. In anaesthesia the cLMA was originally used almost exclusively for brief, peripheral operations, performed in slim patients, usually breathing spontaneously. The popularity of the cLMA has led to an evolution in practice such that SADs have become increasingly used for longer, more complex operations. Changes in patient morphology have led to an increase in their use in obese patients. An increase in laparoscopic surgery has led to use of SADs for intra-abdominal surgery, whether laparoscopic or open. Use during controlled ventilation has also become commonplace.

All these expansions of use offer potential benefit to patients but also raise questions of efficacy and safety. During spontaneous ventilating anaesthesia the cLMA provides a clear airway and enables hands-free anaesthesia in more than 95% of uses. The *efficacy* of the cLMA for controlled ventilation diminishes rapidly as lung resistance increases (i.e., obesity, laparoscopy etc.) and both hypoventilation and gastric distension increase. This raises concerns over the *safety* of its use in these situations.

In the past decade more than 40 new SADs have been introduced. The majority are simply attempts to copy and compete with the cLMA: of interest to purchasers and managers. Of more interest to the anaesthetist are those designed to improve SAD performance (efficacy and safety) and thereby increase the clinical utility of such devices.

Many studies comparing different SADs are inadequately powered to determine even efficacy. None address the issue of safety directly, and this needs a different approach.

Efficacy depends on a number of factors including ease of insertion, manipulations required to maintain a clear airway throughout anaesthesia and tolerance during emergence. Efficacy during controlled ventilation requires the ventilation orifice of the SAD to sit over the larynx and that the SAD seals well with the laryngopharynx (*pharyngeal seal*).

Safety reflects the risk of complications occurring at all stages of anaesthesia and afterwards. Prevention of aspiration requires a good quality seal with the pharynx and oesophagus (*oesophageal seal*) to 1) prevent gas leaking into the oesophagus and stomach and 2) prevent regurgitant matter passing from the oesophagus into the airway. A functioning drain tube will enable regurgitant matter to bypass the larynx and be vented outside: both protecting the airway and giving an early indication of the presence of regurgitation.

Recent studies have shown that the extent of oesophageal seal varies considerably between different

SADs. Those with a drain tube will effectively vent regurgitant fluid if the drain tube is not occluded.

First and second generation SADs

There are several classifications of SADs with most based on device anatomy and positioning. They add little to the practical understanding of SAD use.

This author simply divides SADs into first and second generation SADs. First generation SADs (e.g., cLMA) are simply airway tubes, with no specific design features to improve safety (or ventilation efficacy). Second generation SADs in contrast have specific design features to make them safer (and often more effective for controlled ventilation).

First generation SADs

These include the following:

- Classic LMA
- Flexible LMA
- All LMs
- CobraPLA

Classic LMA (cLMA)

The cLMA was designed by Dr Archie Brain in the United Kingdom in the early 1980s and introduced to anaesthetic practice in 1988. It has been used in approximately 200 million anaesthetics globally. There are over 2500 studies published on the device. Consequently the cLMA must be considered the gold standard for SADs.

The cLMA consists of a transparent silicone tube with a small oval-shaped silicone mask at the distal end. The mask has an anterior cuff, with pilot balloon and its posterior surface is reinforced to prevent folding. Across the distal end of the airway tube are two flexible bars that prevent the tongue impeding insertion and the epiglottis causing obstruction after placement. Correctly placed the mask lies with the airway orifice facing anteriorly, the tip at the origin of the oesophagus and the cuff encircling the laryngeal inlet. The lateral cuff lies against the pyriform fossa and the upper cuff the base of the tongue. The mask is held in a stable position by the hypopharyngeal constrictor muscles laterally and cricopharyngeus inferiorly. Inflation of the mask cuff produces a low pressure seal around the larynx.

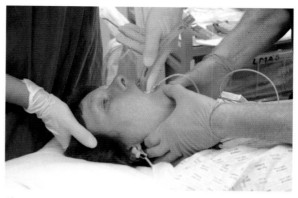

Figure 9.2. cLMA insertion technique.

The cLMA is designed for use up to 40 times. Standard masks are not MRI compatible due to metal in the pilot tube valve. MRI compatible masks are available with a metal-free valve and are colour coded with a yellow pilot balloon.

There are eight sizes of cLMA available (1, 1½, 2, 2½, 3, 4, 5, 6) for use from neonates to large adults. Size selection is according to patient weight (Table 9.1). Using a larger size cLMA for a given patient is likely to result in an improved laryngeal seal. As a 'rule of thumb' in Western populations a size 4 is used for adult women and a size 5 for adult men. In Asian populations one size smaller may be appropriate.

The cLMA performs optimally during spontaneous ventilation, but it is also widely used for controlled ventilation. It is an alternative both to anaesthesia with facemask or tracheal tube. Its introduction has transformed the routine practice of anaesthesia and facemask anaesthesia is now rarely practiced. However the cLMA is not suitable for all cases and good case selection is the key to successful use. Most importantly the cLMA should not be regarded as providing protection against aspiration of regurgitated gastric contents and so is contraindicated for patients who are not starved or who may have a full stomach. The cLMA seals with the pharynx to a pressure of 16–24 cmH$_2$O and to higher pressures with the oesophagus, 40–50 cmH$_2$O, but has no drain tube. The cLMA does provide good protection from pharyngeal secretions above the cuff and is suitable for nasal and dental surgery.

Contraindications include: risk of aspiration (often difficult to define), morbid obesity, reduced lung compliance such that airway pressure >20 cmH$_2$O

Table 9.1. Characteristics of cLMAs

Size	Patient group	Weight range (kg)	Maximum cuff volume (ml)	Length of airway tube (mm)	Maximum size of TT
1	Neonate	<5	4	108	3.5
1.5	Infant	5–10	7	135	4.5
2	Child	10–20	10	140	5.0
2.5	Child	20–30	14	170	6.0
3	Child/small adult	30–50	20	200	6.5
4	Adult	50–70	30	205	6.5
5	Adult	70–	40	230	7.0
6	Large adult	>100	45	–	–

Length of airway tube: from connector to grille.
Maximum size of tracheal tube: based on an uncuffed, well lubricated, Portex blue line tracheal tube, without forcing.

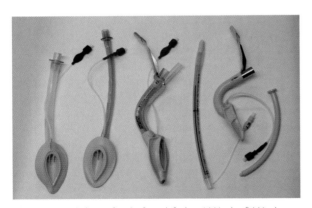

Figure 9.3. The LMA family: from left the cLMA, the fLMA, the PLMA and the ILMA.

is required, major oral or pharyngo-laryngeal pathology.

Insertion is best performed with the patient in the 'sniffing position'. The cLMA should be visually inspected, free from foreign bodies and the mask completely deflated. Failure of a cLMA to maintain complete deflation indicates a cuff leak. Full deflation may be assisted by using the manufacturer's cuff shaper.

The smaller the leading edge of the device is, the less likely it is to catch on the tongue or epiglottis during insertion, both of which may impair placement. Full deflation allows the cLMA to slide behind the cricoid cartilage. The posterior of the mask should be well lubricated. The airway is held like a pen, with the index finger placed at the anterior junction of the airway tube and mask. The mouth is opened, the mask inserted and its posterior aspect pressed onto the hard palate. The index finger is then advanced towards the occiput, which causes the cLMA to pass along the roof of the mouth and then the posterior pharynx. The device is advanced in a single smooth movement until it is felt to stop, on reaching the cricopharyngeus muscle. During insertion the non-intubating hand holds the head to prevent flexion of the head. Chin lift or jaw thrust applied by an assistant may ease insertion. Once fully inserted the tube should be held while the intubating finger is withdrawn (Figure 9.2).

The cuff should be inflated before attaching the anaesthetic circuit. When correctly inserted the black line on the posterior of the cLMA will remain in the midline and during cuff inflation the device rises out of the mouth some 1–2 cm while the anterior neck fills. The manufacturer indicates volumes of air that may be inserted into the mask. These are *maximum* volumes and a volume of half the maximum is often sufficient. Alternatively the cuff may be inflated with a manometer in which case a pressure of 60–70 cmH$_2$O is recommended. Most of the airway seal is achieved with the first 10 ml of air inserted into the cuff and is achieved with cuff pressure of below 30 cmH$_2$O. High intracuff pressure maintained for a long period may cause pharyngeal and laryngeal mucosal or nerve damage. Inflation to manufacturer's maximum volumes routinely leads to intracuff pressure >120 cmH$_2$O. If nitrous oxide is used during anaesthesia this will diffuse into the cuff and lead to increases in volume and pressure particularly in the first 30 minutes of anaesthesia. Injuries to the lingual (particularly when large masks are used), hypoglossal and recurrent laryngeal nerves have been infrequently reported. These are likely to be minimised by meticulous insertion, positioning and maintaining intracuff pressure below 70 cmH$_2$O.

Once the cLMA is inserted ease of manual ventilation should be assessed. Adequate ventilation should be achieved with no audible gas leak at a pressure below 20 cmH$_2$O. If this cannot be achieved consideration should be given to use of an alternative size of cLMA or a different airway. Airway noise or poor filling of the reservoir bag (impaired expiration) may indicate poor placement and should lead to further investigation or repositioning of the airway.

The cLMA should be secured by tape or tie to reduce the likelihood of extrusion or displacement. Use of a bite block (rolled gauze placed between the molar teeth) is recommended until the cLMA is removed. This is particularly important during emergence.

Misplacement may occur due to rotation, the tip of the device bending backwards, folding of the epiglottis or insertion of the tip of the device into the glottis. Careful technique reduces all these misplacements. Insertion of the tip of the device into the laryngeal inlet may mimic laryngospasm with high airway pressures, slow expiration and wheeze. The presence of the cLMA tip behind the larynx may occasionally shorten the vocal cords leading to partial extrathoracic airway obstruction during spontaneous ventilation and paradoxical cord movement during controlled ventilation. If the origin of the oesophagus lies within the bowl of the cLMA the use of controlled ventilation may lead to gastric distension. This misplacement may occur in up to 15% of cases and may not be clinically apparent.

At the end of surgery, where controlled ventilation has been used the transition to spontaneous ventilation is usually seamless. The cLMA is tolerated until very light planes of anaesthesia. The cLMA should be left in place during transfer to the recovery unit. Maintenance of the patient in the supine position is recommended. Oxygen is administered by T-piece, Venturi or T-bag. Of these the T-bag is preferred as it is economical, provides a high oxygen concentration with as little as 2 litre/min gas flow and provides an auditory and visual indicator of breathing as well as allowing controlled ventilation if required.

Though not all studies support this, the consensus and recommendations are that removal of the bite block and cLMA should not be attempted until the patient regains consciousness and airway reflexes return. It is recommended to deflate the cuff at the time of removal, however removal without cuff deflation is usually well tolerated and without complications. Airway suction is not necessary or desirable unless secretions are excessive as pharyngeal secretions are removed with the airway. The cLMA may be removed with the patient supine or on their side. Where there is no reason to turn the patient on the side before waking this is generally unnecessary for airway management. The evidence on timing of removal of the cLMA in children is less clear and some clinicians prefer to remove the cLMA in infants and small children before emergence.

After use the cLMA should be rapidly and thoroughly cleaned before being sterilised by autoclave (up to 137°C for 3 minutes with the cuff fully deflated) and stored in sterile packaging thereafter.

Predictors of difficult laryngoscopy/tracheal intubation do not correlate with ease or difficulty with cLMA placement, though markedly reduced mouth opening will also impede cLMA placement. In patients who are edentulous with loss of alveolar bone, it may prove difficult to achieve a stable airway with the cLMA.

The depth of anaesthesia required for cLMA insertion is greater than that needed for insertion of a Guedel airway, but less than for several other SADs. Prior to insertion there should be no eyelash reflex and no response to jaw thrust. Propofol is the ideal anaesthetic induction agent for insertion as it profoundly reduces airway reflexes (in contrast to thiopentone) and addition of a rapidly acting opioid and intravenous lignocaine reduce both the required dose of induction agent and improve insertion conditions. Neuromuscular blocking drugs are not needed. The cLMA may also be inserted with topical anaesthesia of the airway or bilateral supraglottic nerve blocks. Insertion causes minimal haemodynamic response.

The flow resistance of the cLMA is approximately 1/6th of the resistance of a tracheal tube of appropriate size, however as the cLMA lies outside the larynx it is more appropriate to compare the resistance of the whole airway. During use of the cLMA airway resistance (tube plus laryngeal resistance) is similar to that of a conventional tracheal tube (size 4 cLMA versus 7.5–8.5 mm internal diameter tracheal tube). Correct positioning of the cLMA contributes to reduced resistance and a downfolded epiglottis, rotation of the cLMA or mechanical shortening of the vocal cords may increase laryngeal and therefore overall resistance.

Movement of head and neck does little to alter cLMA position over the larynx. However head and neck flexion or rotation both lead to an increase in laryngeal seal pressure and intracuff pressure. Head and neck extension has the opposite effects.

When first introduced into anaesthetic practice in 1988 the cLMA was greeted with a degree of scepticism. Where used, this was almost exclusively for elective patients undergoing minor peripheral surgery while breathing spontaneously. The cLMA was avoided in all overweight patients and controlled ventilation. While this conservative approach was entirely appropriate, since then there has been a gradual but inexorable widening of the applications and reduction in the contraindications to cLMA use. Whether the more laissez-faire approach to use of the device is appropriate is not known, but the effect on routine anaesthesia care that the cLMA has had is remarkable, as is its safety record. In 1993 a large study showed 30% of all surgical cases performed with a cLMA. In 2002 this figure had risen to 65% with almost half of these patients receiving controlled ventilation.

The incidence of airway-related critical incidents was 0.16% during spontaneous ventilation and 0.14% during controlled ventilation. The incidence of aspiration in carefully selected elective patients is variously estimated as 1 in 5–11 000. The accuracy of these figures is unclear but is of a similar order to reported incidences of aspiration during tracheal tube anaesthesia (1 in 2–4000).

Meta-analysis has been used to compare cLMA anaesthesia with tracheal tube or facemask anaesthesia. Advantages over the facemask include improved oxygenation and less hand fatigue. Advantages over tracheal intubation include improved haemodynamic stability, reduced anaesthetic requirements during maintenance, improved emergence (better oxygenation and less cough) and reduced sore throats in adults. The cLMA lessens laryngeal morbidity compared to tracheal intubation with reduced mechanical and neurological vocal cord dysfunction. The use of the cLMA for controlled ventilation remains controversial. The main concern is the issue of airway protection from regurgitated gastric contents and the possibility of gastric distension during controlled ventilation. Detractors point to several factors; while the cLMA has been shown to modestly reduce lower oesophageal sphincter pressure, much more importantly as peak airway pressure increases, the risk and extent of gastro-oesophageal insufflation increases. However when oropharyngeal leak occurs during controlled ventilation with the cLMA the leak is into (and out of) the mouth in approximately 95% of cases. Cadaver work shows the cLMA does provide some protection from oesophageal fluid when compared to the unprotected airway. Large series have reported use of controlled ventilation in 44–95% of cases with no increase in aspiration or airway-related critical incidents. Proven aspiration with the cLMA remains infrequent and there are few reports of long-term sequelae after aspiration during cLMA use. When the cLMA is used for controlled ventilation, case selection and correct positioning are both critical. Imperfect position should not be accepted. Airway pressures should be kept to a minimum and pressures above 20 cmH_2O should be avoided altogether. Recently the PLMA has been introduced and wherever controlled ventilation is required this is a more suitable device than the cLMA.

Use of the cLMA for laparoscopic surgery is also controversial. The use of controlled ventilation, raised intra-abdominal pressure and the lithotomy position all theoretically increase aspiration risk. Several small trials support the use of the cLMA for gynaecological laparoscopy and suggest controlled ventilation with muscle relaxation or spontaneous ventilation are both acceptable. Proof of safety is absent but series of up to 1500 cases with no cases of aspiration are reported.

Another useful role for the cLMA is to maintain the airway after tracheal extubation. Tracheal extubation can be associated with undesirable haemodynamic and respiratory complications and in particular coughing and oxygen desaturation (see Chapter 17). These are reduced during emergence with a cLMA in place. The cLMA may be inserted posterior to the tracheal tube, using the tracheal tube as a guide prior to its removal. This technique is used widely in some centres at the end of neurosurgical cases but might be considered appropriate for all extubations.

The breadth of cases that the cLMA has been used for is enormous. There are reports of the use of the cLMA for elective laparotomy, abdominal aortic aneurysm surgery, caesarean section, neurosurgery, all extubations and cardiac surgery. In intensive care medicine the cLMA has been used for brief periods of controlled ventilation in selected cases, as a bridge to extubation following neurosurgery, as an aid for weaning from mechanical ventilation and during percutaneous dilational tracheostomy. However successful use does not indicate safety or even efficacy. 'Can do' does not equate to 'should do'!

In addition to its role during the maintenance of anaesthesia the cLMA is a useful device for accessing the trachea and for management of difficult airways. In 75–90% of cases the larynx is visible from the bowl of the cLMA. This allows access to the trachea either with a small tracheal tube, a bougie or exchange catheter. This has led to the use of the cLMA as a conduit (dedicated airway) during blind attempts at tracheal intubation, elective fibreoptic intubation and for bronchoscopy. Techniques using a fibrescope, allowing the procedure to be performed under direct vision, are preferable, as blind access to the trachea via the cLMA is unreliable. In the emergency setting after failed intubation the cLMA may be used as a rescue device. After failed tracheal intubation the priority is oxygenation and the cLMA is usually effective in establishing the airway. In this context several points should be noted. 1) The tip of the cLMA seats behind the cricoid cartilage so placement is impaired in the presence of cricoid pressure. If cricoid pressure is applied it should be reduced or removed to allow cLMA placement. Once placed cricoid pressure may be reapplied but may interfere with effective ventilation. 2) The cLMA does not reliably protect against aspiration and where this risk is high a more secure airway may be needed. 3) In patients with difficult airways controlled ventilation via the cLMA may be difficult; in particular if high airway pressures are required there may be considerable airway leak. The cLMA is included in almost all national guidelines as a rescue device for management of failed tracheal intubation.

Outside of use during anaesthesia the cLMA has an important role during cardiopulmonary resuscitation. After instruction relative novices are able to achieve a clear airway and provide controlled ventilation in a high proportion of cases. Ventilation is achieved by unskilled personnel with the cLMA with greater success than either a facemask or a tracheal tube. The cLMA is one of the airway devices recommended for airway control during CPR by ILCOR (international liaison committee on resuscitation).

In these circumstances the risk of pulmonary aspiration must not be forgotten. However aspiration in these circumstances is probably less if the airway is maintained with a cLMA than with the facemask.

The cLMA costs approximately £90 and is reusable 40 times.

Flexible (reinforced) LMA (fLMA)

The flexible or reinforced LMA is identical to the cLMA except for the airway tube, which is made of soft silicone with spiral wire reinforcement. This means that the airway tube is more flexible and does not kink when bent. This allows the proximal end of the fLMA to be moved in any direction as necessary and this is useful when surgery is close to the face. The fLMA is particularly suitable for head and neck, dental, ophthalmic and ENT surgery. The wire in the airway tube makes the fLMA unsuitable for use in the MRI scanner.

The fLMA is available in sizes 2–5. A single use fLMA is available in sizes 2.5–5.

The fLMA airway tube is longer and narrower than the cLMA with a consequent increase in airway resistance. Resistance is similar to an equivalent size tracheal tube. So when laryngeal resistance is added, the overall airway resistance with a fLMA is somewhat higher than for a tracheal tube. This translates to an increase in work of breathing during spontaneous ventilation but the increase is rarely clinically important. The narrower airway tube also makes the fLMA less suitable than the cLMA for exchange techniques if access to the trachea is needed.

Insertion technique is identical to the cLMA but requires considerably greater attention to detail to prevent axial rotation. Poor technique may lead to a 'backwards facing' device: surprisingly airway maintenance is often unimpaired, though airway resistance is likely increased and airway protection decreased. Surprisingly, misplacement is not always evident until removal. Good technique will reduce misplacement and improve function. Insertion success and seal pressures are similar to the cLMA. A variety of adjuncts to insertion have been proposed (e.g., tracheal tube or bougie inserted inside or forceps outside the airway tube), most of these increase the longitudinal rigidity of the device but do little to prevent axial rotation. The fLMA is particularly suited for intraoral (maxillofacial and ENT surgery) and nasal surgery. Unlike the cLMA, the fLMA airway tube can be moved as necessary to improve surgical access without displacing the mask. The cuff of the fLMA provides good protection of the larynx from pharyngeal secretions. An example of this is in tonsillectomy where tracheal soiling is reduced when using a fLMA in comparison to a tracheal tube. Head and neck movement have little effect on the position of the mask over the larynx and recovery is smoother than with a tracheal tube with less coughing, laryngospasm, airway obstruction and hypoxia. All these features make the fLMA the airway of choice for many operations on the face or within the mouth, nose or ears. For intraoral and tonsillar surgery it is essential that the fLMA is fully inserted: the proximal cuff should not be within the oral cavity where it might interfere with surgical access.

Despite these potential advantages great care must be taken when surgical access is close to the airway. Displacement of the fLMA may lead to airway leak or obstruction. In particular placing a Boyle–Davis gag for tonsillectomy may lead to loss of the airway in 5–10% of cases. The fLMA is a suitable airway for ophthalmological surgery. In addition to providing good surgical access the fLMA causes less rise in intraocular pressure and is associated with fewer coughing and airway complications during emergence than use of a tracheal tube.

All LMs

Intubating LMA (ILMA) (Fastrach™)

The intubating LMA (ILMA) was designed by Dr Archie Brain and introduced into practice in the late 1990s. It is designed to provide a dedicated airway and allow placement of a moderate size tracheal tube, in both easy and difficult airways. The short rigid anatomically curved stem of the ILMA leads to easy insertion, even by novices but its cost and the potential for mucosal trauma limit its routine use. Use of the ILMA for difficult airway management is described elsewhere (see Chapter 14).

Standard LMs: single use and reusable

Since 2003 many manufacturers have produced competitors to the cLMA both in single use (largely PVC) and reusable form (both PVC and silicone). As the term laryngeal mask airway (LMA) is registered the newer devices are referred to as laryngeal masks (LMs). The manufacturers propose the main driving force for the introduction of single use devices has been concerns over sterility of cleaned reusable

devices. This has been a particular issue in the United Kingdom since 2001 with concerns over elimination of proteinaceous material and the risk of transmission of prion disease (variant Creutzfeldt Jakob disease, vCJD). The scientific rationale for a change in practice to single use LMs on the basis of infection risk is, at best, questionable. The financial opportunities of the cLMA market are another obvious reason for the proliferation of such devices.

For patent reasons all LMs differ from cLMAs and there is also much variation between LMs. All LMs except those made by original manufacturers of the cLMA do not have the grille at the distal end of the airway tube. Some have angulated stems and some enlarged masks. Particularly with the larger sizes there is a possibility of entrapping the tongue and drawing it backwards during insertion and of obstruction by a down-folded epiglottis once inserted. For cost reasons most single use LMs are made with a PVC cuff which increases the rigidity of the device. Silicone devices, both single use and reusable, are now also available. Nitrous oxide does not diffuse into PVC cuffs. Generally there is no robust evidence to advise whether the currently available single use LM devices perform similarly to equivalent LMAs nor to advise which LM performs best. What the limited evidence does show is that all LMs and LMAs are not equivalent. Of 27 currently available devices only two have substantial publications to compare efficacy with the cLMA; for one device the body of evidence strongly suggests poorer performance than the cLMA while for the Ambu Aura LM evidence from about 400 patients suggests equivalence. For the other 25 there appears to be a vacuum of published evidence.

A recent publication from the NHS centre for evidence-based purchasing illustrates the difficulty in determining the relative merits and demerits of these competitors to the cLMA: the document listed more than 25 alternative standard LMs and reported a total of 18 comparative trials between devices. Some of these studies are of poor quality. This contrasts to the >2500 publications on the cLMA alone.

Single use fLMAs

A number of single use flexible LMAs and LMs have been introduced in the past few years. For most devices performance is assumed, as performance evaluations and comparative trials have not been performed.

In the United Kingdom the Department of Health currently advises that all airway equipment used for tonsillectomy should be single use and this is endorsed by the Royal College of Anaesthetists and other professional bodies. NICE (National Institute of Clinical Excellence) did not consider laryngeal mask airways when examining the risk of transmission of vCJD. In this climate the single use fLMA is likely to have a significant role.

Laryngeal tube

The Laryngeal Tube (LT) consists of a slim airway tube with a small balloon cuff attached at the tip (distal cuff) and a larger asymmetric balloon cuff at the middle part of the tube (proximal cuff). The cuffs are inflated through a single pilot tube and balloon, through which the cuff pressure can be monitored. When the device is inserted, it lies along the length of the tongue. Proximal and distal cuffs sit in the oro-pharynx and oesophageal inlet, respectively. Inflation creates a seal and ventilation occurs through orifices between the cuffs.

It is designed for use during spontaneous breathing, controlled ventilation and for airway rescue.

At present the LT is an alternative to the cLMA for controlled ventilation. Its role during spontaneous ventilation has yet to be established and it cannot be recommended for anaesthesia with spontaneous ventilation due to the high frequency of airway obstruction. No advantages of the LT over the cLMA and PLMA during controlled ventilation have been demonstrated.

A single use version of the LT is available (LT-D). It has not been extensively evaluated.

Cost approx £70.

Airway management device (AMD™)

The Airway Management Device consists of a translucent silicone tube with a distal and a mid-shaft cuff, superficially resembling the Laryngeal Tube. The cuffs and the device itself are asymmetric in cross-section and this feature aims to reduce or eliminate rotation of the device once inserted. Each cuff is inflated via a separate pilot balloon. Between the cuffs is an oval ventilation orifice. The distal cuff has a channel within it designed to enable access to and drainage of the upper oesophagus but its function is questioned. When placed correctly, the distal cuff lies at the top of the oesophagus and the proximal cuff lies in the upper laryngo-pharynx or oropharynx. The oesophageal cuff occludes the oesophagus and the pharyngeal cuff pushes the base of the tongue forward

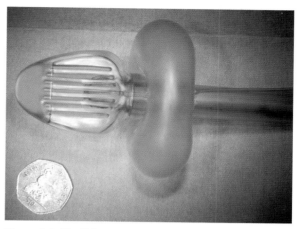

Figure 9.4. The Cobra.

and lifts the epiglottis. The two cuffs therefore straddle the larynx and allow delivery of gas from the tube via the ventilation orifice. The device, which is made in three sizes, is designed for both spontaneous and assisted ventilation.

Several studies have assessed performance of the AMD. Insertion is generally atraumatic and post-operative complications are infrequent. However cohort and comparative studies with the cLMA have shown insertion success of approximately 70%. Airway obstruction (in up to 30% of cases) may occur at any stage of anaesthesia from insertion to emergence requiring early removal of the device in 15–20% of cases.

CobraPLA™

The Cobra Perilaryngeal airway (CobraPLA) is a relatively new single use supraglottic airway (Figure 9.4). The distal end (somewhat resembling a cobra head, so lending the name to the device) consists of a soft plastic head designed to seat in and seal the hypopharynx, with the anterior surface abutting the larynx. The anterior surface of the head consists of a grille of soft bars through which gas exchange takes place. The bars are soft enough to allow instrumentation of the larynx and upper airway if required. A proximal balloon with pilot cuff is designed to elevate the tongue base and seal the oropharynx. The proximal end of the tube is a 15 mm standard connector for attachment to the breathing circuit.

Aspiration has been reported with the CobraPLA. With the exception of a modest increase in airway seal, benefits over the cLMA are not evident.

83

Second generation SADs

These comprise the

- ProSeal LMA
- Laryngeal tube suction II (reusable and disposable versions)
- Gastro LT
- i-gel
- LMA Supreme
- Streamlined liner of the pharynx airway
- Combitube and Easytube

ProSeal Laryngeal mask airway

The ProSeal LMA (PLMA) was introduced to the UK in January 2001. It was designed by Dr Archie Brain based on the classic laryngeal mask airway (cLMA). It was the first major modification of the cLMA and was designed to improve controlled ventilation, improve safety and enable diagnosis of mask misplacement.

Modifications include a softer, larger bowl, a posterior extension of the cuff, a drainage tube running parallel to the airway tube and an integral bite block. The modifications improve the seal with the larynx, enable leaking gas to vent via the drain tube and facilitate passage of an orogastric tube. The drain tube allows early diagnosis of misplacement of the PLMA, which is not possible with the cLMA (Figure 9.5).

Correctly placed, the PLMA lies with the drain tube in continuity with the oesophagus and the airway tube in continuity with the trachea. As the pharyngeal and oesophageal seals are both increased this creates functional separation of the alimentary and respiratory tracts. The drain tube vents gas leaking from the mask into the oesophagus and prevents gastric distension. It also vents regurgitated stomach contents.

Sizes 1½–5 are available with the paediatric sizes (1½–2½) lacking the posterior extension of the cuff. Size selection is as for other LMA devices. The PLMA is supplied with a cuff-deflator, which is recommended to assist complete deflation of the device and flattening of the device tip, prior to insertion. Complete deflation avoids deflection of the epiglottis or entry of the tip into the glottis.

The PLMA may be inserted with or without an introducer that is supplied with it. Without the introducer the technique is the same as that for the cLMA and with the introducer is as for the ILMA. There is no convincing evidence that one method is preferable. Particular care must be taken when removing the

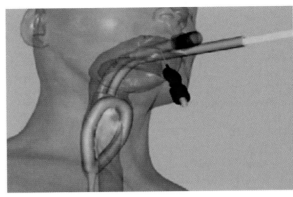

Figure 9.5. The PLMA showing the oesophageal access channel.

Algorithm for PLMA insertion and positioning

Note any resistance or hold up during insertion. This suggests folding over of the mask tip.

Inflate cuff to 60 cmH$_2$O

Assess depth of insertion. >50% bite block should usually be beyond the incisors.

Start controlled ventilation while assessing for unobstructed inspiratory and expiratory flow, observing capnometry and spirometry. Poor compliance or reduced expiratory flow may indicate mechanical obstruction of the vocal cords.

Place gel (or a film of soapy liquid) over the drain tube. a) If this blows (or inflates) immediately with ventilation (or oscillations of the film are seen in time with the pulse) the PLMA may be sited in the glottic opening. Pressure on the chest leading to displacement of the gel confirms this. b) Blowing of the gel with applied pressure of less than 20 cmH$_2$O suggests the PLMA needs advancing further. The airway may be advanced to resolve a leak, otherwise it should be removed and re-inserted.

Unexpectedly high inflation pressures may also indicate folding over of the tip.

If hold-up was noted during insertion further tests to exclude tip folding should be used even if ventilation is successful. Press briefly on the suprasternal notch. This raises the pressure in the oesophagus and if this pressure rise is not transmitted to the drain tube the tip of the mask may be folded over. Inability to freely pass an OGT 30 cm to the tip of the drain tube may be used to confirm this. If the tip is folded over the PLMA should be re-inserted.

introducer to avoid dental damage. After insertion the cuff is inflated. While maximum volumes are published by the manufacturers, inflation to an intra-cuff pressure of 60–70 cmH$_2$O is preferred. An OGT

Table 9.2. Diagnosis of misplacements or confirming correct function of the PLMA

Position	Bite block position	Pressure on chest	Suprasternal notch pressure	Airway seal	Other
Correct position	>50% (often <25%) visible at mouth	–		Median 32 cmH$_2$O	Able to pass OGT with ease
Tip in glottis	–	Gel blows off drain tube	–	–	Obstructed airway
Mask folded over	>50% may be visible	–	–	May be high or low	Resistance on insertion. Airway may be obstructed Unable to pass OGT
Tip in pharynx	>50% visible	–	–	Low (<20 cmH$_2$O)	

can be passed through the drain tube when indicated. The manufacturers recommend this is well lubricated and not refrigerated.

An important alternative method for PLMA insertion involves prior placement over a gum elastic bougie (or gastric tube) into the oesophagus, over which the PLMA drain tube is then railroaded.

When correctly positioned the tip of the PLMA (corresponding to the distal end of the drain tube) lies behind the cricoid cartilage. There are three important misplacements possible with the PLMA. A small amount of gel placed over the drain tube enables diagnosis of misplacements. This in turn allows early correction of position and optimal function.

If the PLMA is placed too proximally ventilated air is vented via the drain tube. If the tip is placed in the glottis, a forced exhalation (pressure on the chest wall) leads to gel displacement from the drain tube and airway obstruction may occur. If the PLMA tip folds over during insertion the functionality of the drain tube is lost. This misplacement is readily diagnosed by inability to pass an OGT to the tip of the PLMA. Gel or soap placed over the proximal drain tube orifice allows diagnosis of misplacements or confirmation of correct function (Table 9.2). It is unclear whether the PLMA is prone to misplacement more commonly than the cLMA but diagnosis is easier.

Successful insertion and ventilation rates of above 95% can be achieved. First time insertion rates are somewhat lower (85%) than for the cLMA (92%) and time taken for insertion a few seconds longer.

However use of a bougie guided technique leads to almost 100% first attempt success rates, without an increase in trauma or sequelae.

Median airway seal pressure with the PLMA is approximately 32 cmH$_2$O (cLMA 16–20 cmH$_2$O) and exceeds 40 cmH$_2$O in about 20% of cases. Results are similar whether the PLMA is used in paralysed or non-paralysed patients. The improved seal allows successful ventilation in many cases where this would not be achieved with the cLMA. The PLMA exerts less mucosal pressure than the cLMA for any given cuff pressure or laryngeal seal.

Orogastric tube passage is successful in close to 100% of correctly placed PLMAs. Ease of passage of an OGT correlates with fibreoptic position of the PLMA over the larynx. Where there is doubt over correct positioning of the PLMA, an OGT should be passed and if this fails the PLMA should be re-sited.

The PLMA is designed to decrease regurgitation risk and decrease the likelihood of aspiration if regurgitation occurs. There is extensive robust evidence from bench work, cadaver and clinical studies to support these claims, but they are unproven and probably unprovable. Cadaver studies show an oesophageal seal of 70–80 cmH$_2$O and efficacy of the drain tube in venting regurgitated fluid. There are several reported cases of regurgitated matter being vented by the drain.

Considering all the available evidence the PLMA lessens the risk of aspiration compared to the cLMA and there is an argument for its routine use. However the PLMA should not be used for cases of significant aspiration risk.

Complications associated with the PLMA include oesophageal breathing, gastric insufflation and airway obstruction. It is unclear whether these occur more frequently with the PLMA than the cLMA. Minor complications are more common when the PLMA is used with spontaneous ventilation.

There are several studies comparing PLMA performance with other SADs. In all of these to date the PLMA performs as well as or better than other SADs.

Based on the available evidence the PLMA is an appropriate SAD for use in several 'extended roles' *in selected patients*. These roles include use in moderately obese patients, for laparoscopic surgery, selected open abdominal surgery, as an adjunct for difficult intubation and a rescue device after failed intubation. Use in such cases mandates careful assessment of risk and benefit, a good understanding of the device and its limitations, experience in lower risk cases and excellent technique.

Other advanced uses reported include use in the super-obese as a bridge to intubation, and for prone and emergency surgery. Areas of interest outside the operating theatre include use in ICU and during resuscitation. Most of these areas have not been adequately explored yet.

The recommended product life is for 40 sterilisations.

Cost is currently £100, which includes introducer tool and deflator device.

The laryngeal tube suction II

In 2002 a new version of the LT was introduced, the LT-suction (LTS), with a drain tube running posterior to the airway tube to allow gastric tube placement and prevent gastric inflation during ventilation. While the design aimed to increase device safety (a similar step to that from cLMA to PLMA) the change in design led to a much more bulky device that was harder to insert and potentially traumatic: thereby losing two of the LT's major advantages. In 2005 the LTS was further modified (LTS-II) with the addition of a slim profile tip and asymmetric oesophageal balloon. Like the LT the LTS-II is re-usable after sterilisation up to fifty times. Size selection and insertion technique for the LTS-II are identical to the LT.

Considerably more work will be needed before a role of the LTS-II during routine anaesthesia can be established.

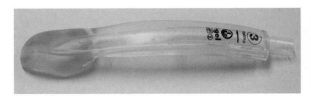

Figure 9.6. The i-gel.

A single use version of the LTS-II exists called the LTS-D.

Gastro LT

The Gastro-LT is a laryngeal tube designed for use in upper gastrointestinal endoscopy. The drain tube has been expanded to a size that will accept a gastrointestinal endoscope and the airway tube reduced to minimal calibre.

i-gel

The i-gel is a relatively new, single use SAD (Figure 9.6). Its shape partially resembles the inflated PLMA, but it is a cuffless device made of a medical grade elastomer gel (styrene ethylene butadene styrene). Features (and potential benefits) include a short wide-bore airway tube with no grilles (low resistance to gas flow and good access to the airway as a conduit), an elliptical shaped stem (stability), 'anatomically' shaped bowl (improved pharyngeal seal), an integral bite block (prevention of obstruction) and a drain tube (safety against regurgitation). Paediatric sizes have been recently introduced but are considerably less well evaluated.

Insertion is performed in the sniffing position and requires that the i-gel is lubricated *on all surfaces* before insertion. Due to its bulk good mouth opening and jaw thrust assist insertion. Standard insertion mimics cLMA insertion with the passage of the i-gel following the roof of the mouth and posterior pharynx until stopped by cricopharyngeus muscles. A rotatory insertion technique is also described in which the device is inserted laterally and when resistance is felt it is rotated and advanced into place.

What research there is confirms that the i-gel is remarkably easy to insert, both by experienced and novice users. This is because of a combination of remarkably low frictional properties and the fact there is no cuff to inflate. The pharyngeal seal is approximately 24–28 cmH$_2$O in most cases but in a few is considerably lower and ventilation is not possible. This low seal is apparent in about 1–5% of uses and in these cases the lack of a cuff is an impediment to effective use: due to the lack of a cuff little can be done in these cases except chose another size device. Several authors report that the 'thermoplastic' nature of the elastomer leads to an increase in seal pressure over time as the device warms. This is not a consistent finding and it is also noted with cuffed devices as the device adapts to the shape of the pharynx and vice versa.

The i-gel, like the SLMA (see below), offers the potential for improved ease of use, improved ventilation and increased safety compared to the cLMA, in a disposable SAD.

The i-gel has become increasingly popular and its performance characteristics and design make it a genuine alternative to the cLMA. Gastric access is as reliable as for the PLMA, though the drain tube is smaller. Cases of airway rescue and use of the i-gel to facilitate fibreoptic-guided intubation are reported: the i-gel has a wider–bored stem than the cLMA and will easily accept a 7.0 mm ETT. The stem is also shorter and care must be taken not to intubate the right main bronchus if it is used as a conduit.

The i-gel is a rather poor alternative to the fLMA for oral and ENT surgery due to the bulky, rigid stem. Whether it is appropriate to expand the uses of the i-gel in a similar manner to the PLMA is as yet unproven but it is notable that it has a lower pharyngeal (ventilation) and oesophageal (protection from regurgitation) seal than the PLMA.

Regarding oesophageal seal the i-gel has been shown to have a much lower oesophageal seal than many other SADs (in cadavers) (i-gel 13–21 cmH_2O compared to cLMA 30–50 cmH_2O, PLMA 50–80 cmH_2O, LT and LTS II up to 70–80 cmH_2O). However the same studies demonstrate that regurgitant fluid is effectively vented by the drain tube, unless it is blocked. Of note the manufacturers state that the low oesophageal seal is due to the truncated tip of the i-gel, in turn designed to reduce compression of the tissues of the oesophageal sphincter and so reduce dysphagia. On the available evidence it appears that an orogastric tube should not be placed in the drain tube during use, as if the drain tube is occluded the oesophageal seal may not protect the airway: if used it should then be removed. Cases of protection from aspiration with the i-gel are reported as is one case of partial aspiration.

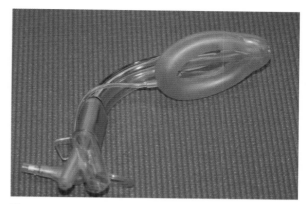

Figure 9.7. The Supreme.

Complications reported with the i-gel are few. Laryngopharyngeal trauma and pain after use appear very infrequent indeed. Transient nerve injuries and lingual congestion have been reported but their frequency appears low.

LMA Supreme

The LMA Supreme (SLMA) is a single use PVC SAD designed to combine the most useful elements of the PLMA (improved airway seal, drain tube, integral bite block) with those of the ILMA (rigid anatomical stem enabling reliable insertion without needing to place the hands in the patient's mouth) (Figure 9.7). Only adult sizes are available at present. The manufacturers recommend it is used for the same indications as the PLMA. However it cannot be considered to be 'a single use PLMA' as there are several important differences. These include increased rigidity of stem and mask, a rigid bite block, a drain tube that runs within the airway itself dividing the tube airway into two narrow (5 mm) channels and the bowl of the mask that includes patented 'fins' (designed to prevent occlusion of the airway by the epiglottis).

Insertion should be performed with the patient in the 'semi-sniffing position' and is otherwise the same as ILMA insertion. Once inserted, correct depth of insertion (and sizing) is indicated by a tab on the upper surface of the device: this should sit 0.5–2.0 cm from the upper lip. The tab is also designed for fixation of the device using adhesive tape.

The SLMA has been far less completely clinically evaluated than other LMAs. What evidence there is suggests it is extremely easily and reliably inserted, even by novices. Once inserted ventilation is reliable and the pharyngeal seal, at approximately 24–28 cmH$_2$O, is higher than the cLMA but lower than the PLMA. The airway sits over the larynx as frequently as the cLMA or PLMA. An orogastric tube can usually be passed via the drain tube. It has been used for both airway rescue and during chest compressions for cardiopulmonary resuscitation. In a direct comparison between the SLMA and i-gel in simulated airway rescue the performance of the two devices was equivalent. The narrow and markedly curved airway channels make it poorly suited to use as conduit for intubation. While efficacy in low risk patients is largely established, its safety is not. The quality of oesophageal seal and the effectiveness of the drain tube are yet to be established.

Further comparative evaluations are awaited before it can be recommended for the same extensive a range of indications as the PLMA.

Streamlined liner of the pharynx airway (SLIPA)

The streamlined liner of the pharynx airway (SLIPA) is a single use SAD of novel design: a soft plastic blow-moulded airway with the shape mimicking a 'pressurised pharynx' (Figure 9.8). In appearance the SLIPA slightly resembles a boot. It has no cuff, is hollow and is designed to sit with the toe of the boot in the hypopharynx. Lateral prominences in the mid-portion of the airway are designed to sit in the pyriform fossae displacing the tongue base anteriorly, so improving airway seal, reducing airway obstruction by the epiglottis and stabilising the device's position.

The SLIPA is included in the second generation SADs on the basis of design only. The inventor claims that the hollow interior of the SLIPA provides a protective reservoir with the capacity to accommodate 50–70 ml of fluid in the case of regurgitation. Bench work (perhaps designed to favour the SLIPA) suggests that this might offer a benefit over the cLMA (capacity approx 5 ml), but there are no clinical data to support this.

There are six sizes and while size selection is based on height the aim is to match the maximum diameter of the SLIPA with the maximum diameter of the larynx (measured as the maximum width of the thyroid cartilage in millimetres).

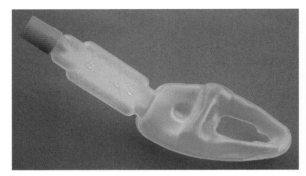

Figure 9.8. The SLIPA.

Early cohort and comparative trials by the inventor showed satisfactory insertion performance (90% first attempt insertion success and a pharyngeal seal comparable or above the cLMA). A few small independent trials have been performed showing adequate insertion success and pharyngeal seal. One trial suggested increased gastric inflation. Trauma and bleeding are potential concerns. There are no data available regarding oesophageal seal and no clinical trials addressing airway protection.

Combitube and Easytube

The Combitube consists of a rigid double lumen tube with dual cuffs. The distal portion of the tube looks like a cuffed tracheal tube with a small cuff attached. The Combitube can be inserted into the trachea and is then indeed used as a tracheal tube with the breathing circuit attached to the 'tracheo-oesophageal tube'. When the distal tube is inserted into the oesophagus the distal cuff is inflated to occlude the oesophagus and a larger proximal cuff lies at the level of the base of the tongue. This high volume cuff is inflated to stabilise the tube position and occlude the oropharynx. Ventilation is then achieved through the 'pharyngeal tube' via ventilation holes sited between the two cuffs. The Combitube has depth of insertion markings to aid positioning.

There were originally two sizes (37F and 41F) for small and larger adults. A smaller size (26F) was recently introduced along with other modifications aimed at reducing the incidence of trauma. The Combitube is not recommended for patients of less than 1.5 m height. Inserted blindly it (almost) invariably enters the oesophagus. Alternatively it can be placed with a laryngoscope in whichever position is desired.

When the distal tube is placed in the oesophagus oxygenation may be improved compared to tracheal placement as a result of delayed expiration through the pharyngeal orifices and the subsequent development of PPEP.

The Combitube is in essence a fore-runner of devices such as the AMD and the family of LTs.

Clinical reports, particularly studying paramedics and emergency medical technicians in North America, have shown the Combitube can be very successful when used as a rescue device after failed tracheal intubation. During blind placement the distal tube is placed in the oesophagus in approximately 98% of cases. Therefore this should be assumed unless shown otherwise. The use of the Combitube during routine anaesthesia is highly controversial. There is no strong argument for its use over other available SADs. The Combitube is for single use and some 10 times more expensive than equivalent devices. There have been reports with high incidences of mucosal trauma during routine use of the Combitube. On balance the Combitube cannot be recommended for airway management during routine anaesthesia. There is a tension between the need to learn to use the device for emergency cases (5 elective uses are recommended by the manufacturer) and the potential trauma associated with routine use (in one study of insertion with the neck immobilised 67% failed blind insertion, 47% blood on device, and 40% sore throat). Oesophageal rupture has been reported. The Combitube remains significantly less popular in the UK than in North America for management of failed emergency tracheal intubation.

The Combitube is designed for single use and costs approximately £30, $50.

The Easytube is a very similar, but more recently introduced device.

In cadaver studies the Combitube and Easytube, (placed in the 'oesophageal position') maintained a higher oesophageal seal than any other SAD (120 cmH$_2$O). The drain tube effectively vented liquid.

Key points

- The cLMA has established that the use of SADs is effective and safe method an airway management in both elective and for some emergency situations.
- SADs are established methods for management of the difficult airway.

- The safety of SAD devices in patients with an increased risk of regurgitation is still uncertain.
- The cLMA can be used for positive pressure ventilation but there is an increasing risk of gastric inflation with inflation pressures above 20 cmH$_2$O. The pLMA or LMA Supreme are preferable.

Potential conflict of interest

I have been paid by the LMA Company and Intavent Orthofix (manufacturers of cLMA, PLMA, SLMA) for lecturing. I have received free equipment for evaluation from many manufacturers of airway equipment. I am not, and have never been, employed by any medical manufacturing company.

Further reading

Asai T, Shingu K. (2005). The laryngeal tube. *British Journal of Anaesthesia*, **95**, 729–736.

Bercker S, Schmidbauer W, Volk T, et al. (2008). A comparison of seal in seven supraglottic airway devices using a cadaver model of elevated esophageal pressure. *Anesthesia and Analgesia*, **106**, 445–448.

Caponas G. (2002). Intubating laryngeal mask airway. A review. *Anaesthesia and Intensive Care*, **30**, 551–569.

Centre for Evidence-Based Purchasing. (2008). *Buyers Guide. Laryngeal Masks*. NHS Purchasing and suppliers agency. July, 2008.

Cook TM. (2003). Spoilt for choice? New supraglottic airways. *Anaesthesia*, **58**, 107–110.

Cook TM, Lee G, Nolan JP. (2005). The ProSeal laryngeal mask airway: A review of the literature. *Canadian Journal of Anaesthesia*, **52**, 739–760.

Eschertzhuber S, Brimacombe J, Hohlrieder M, Keller C. (2009). The laryngeal mask airway Supreme–a single use laryngeal mask airway with an oesophageal vent. A randomised, cross-over study with the laryngeal mask airway ProSeal in paralysed, anaesthetised patients. *Anaesthesia*, **64**, 79–83.

Keller C, Brimacombe J, Bittersohl P, Lirk P, von Goedecke A. (2004). Aspiration and the laryngeal mask airway: Three cases and a review of the literature. *British Journal of Anaesthesia*, **93**, 579–582.

Keller C, Brimacombe J, Kleinsasser A, Loeckinger A. (2000). Does the ProSeal laryngeal mask airway prevent aspiration of regurgitated fluid? *Anesthesia and Analgesia*, **91**, 1017–1020.

Keller C, Brimacombe J, Rädler C, Pühringer F. (1999). Do laryngeal mask airway devices attenuate liquid flow

89

between the esophagus and pharynx? A randomized, controlled cadaver study. *Anesthesia and Analgesia*, **88**, 904–907.

Schmidbauer W, Bercker S, Volk T, Bogusch G, Mager G, Kerner T. (2009). Oesophageal seal of the novel supralaryngeal airway device i-gel in comparison with the laryngeal mask airways Classic and ProSeal using a cadaver model. *British Journal of Anaesthesia*, **102**, 135–139.

Theiler LG, Kleine-Brueggeney M, Kaiser D, et al. (2009). Crossover comparison of the laryngeal mask supreme and the i-gel in simulated difficult airway scenario in anesthetized patients. *Anesthesiology*, **111**, 55–62.

Verghese C, Brimacombe J. (1996). Survey of laryngeal mask airway usage in 11,910 patients: Safety and efficacy for conventional and non-conventional usage. *Anesthesia and Analgesia*, **82**, 129–133.

10

Tracheal tubes, tracheostomy tubes

Viki Mitchell and Anil Patel

The placement of a cuffed tube in the trachea offers the highest level of airway maintenance and protection, and is often the most appropriate route for provision of mechanical ventilation. This chapter concentrates on characteristics of the tube rather than the means of inserting it into the trachea. A wide variety of designs is available (Figure 10.1) with marked differences in tube material, shape of bevel and cuff, or presence of Murphy eye.

History

Intubation of the trachea via the larynx was first described by Macewen of Glasgow in 1878 but only began to gain popularity in the 1920s with the description of blind nasal intubation by Rowbotham and Magill. This technique was quick, accurate and gained early control of the airway. Magill made his own tubes, which he cut from lengths of rubber tubing, bevelling the ends and smoothing the tips with sandpaper before storing them in a biscuit tin to attain the desired curve.

Various materials are used in the construction of tracheal tubes and each has its own properties (Table 10.1). Traditional mineralised red rubber tubes are still in use but began to be replaced with plastic tubes in the 1950s. Plastic tubes are made of polyvinyl chloride or polyurethane, offer a number of advantages and are widely used. Polyurethane can be made thinner than PVC without any loss of strength which makes it particularly suited to cuff manufacture. Silicone tubes are available but less widely used as they are more expensive to manufacture. Polyvinyl chloride and polyurethane tubes may be siliconised as part of the manufacturing process. In the past, some materials used in the manufacture of tracheal tubes have shown evidence of tissue toxicity. Implant testing (IT) or cell culture are mandatory to exclude

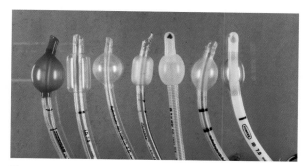

Figure 10.1. Various tracheal tubes from left: Sheridan armoured, Microcuff, Microlaryngeal tube, Gliderite, Fastrach ILMA tube, Mallinckrodt armoured, Portex ivory.

toxicity when a new material is used; without it the device cannot be marketed.

Design

Standard tubes have a preformed curve that approximately conforms to the anatomy of the pharynx and which aids insertion and resists kinking of the tube in situ. The cross-section is round as both oval and ellipses are more prone to kinking. The distal tip is cut at an oblique angle (bevelled) so that the aperture opens to the left if the tube is held in the right hand. The angle of the bevel varies but is usually between 38 degrees and 56 degrees. The left-facing bevel allows visualisation of the tip of the tube as it passes through the cords when introduced with the right hand. 'Hold up' of the tube due to impaction of its tip on the right arytenoid sometimes occurs during railroading of the tube over a fibrescope, bougie or stylet and is a feature of the left facing bevel. This problem can be overcome if the tube is rotated anticlockwise in order to change the orientation of the bevel. Some manufacturers have developed tubes with hooded, blunted or flexible tips

Core Topics in Airway Management, Second Edition, ed. Ian Calder and Adrian Pearce. Published by Cambridge University Press.
© Cambridge University Press 2011.

Table 10.1. Characteristics of materials from which tubes are manufactured

Material	Characteristics
Mineralised rubber	Soft and springy
	Can be sterilised and reused
	May become blocked with inspissated secretions
	Opaque
	Rubber fatigues over time and may kink
	Cuff characteristics: high pressure, low volume
	Cuffs tend to inflate irregularly and may herniate
	Cannot be used in patients with latex allergy
Plastic (PVC or polyurethane)	Non-irritant
	Single use only
	Inexpensive to manufacture to a high standard
	Easy to sterilise during manufacture
	Thermoplastic – softens when warmed
	Can be transparent, opaque or siliconised
	Less tendency to kink than rubber
	Stiffer than rubber or silicone
	Less elasticity than rubber
Silicone	Soft
	Floppy
	Can be autoclaved
	Expensive to manufacture

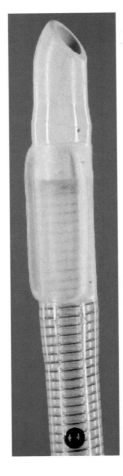

Figure 10.2. The bevel of the special tube for the intubating laryngeal mask.

and these are recommended for use in difficult situations. Of note are the tubes supplied with the intubating laryngeal mask (Figure 10.2) and the Parker Flex tip (Figure 10.3).

Some tubes have a window or Murphy eye cut into the wall near the bevel. This provides an alternative route for gas flow should the bevel become obstructed by impaction against the tracheal wall. It also provides an inadvertent and unwelcome route for fibrescopes, tube exchangers and percutaneous tracheostomies, and means that the cuff cannot be as close to the tip of the tube. The nomenclature is confusing since some authors refer to tubes with a Murphy eye as Murphy tubes and those without as Magill tubes and others refer to all standard curved tubes as Magill tubes whether or not they have a Murphy eye. F.J. Murphy's original tube, developed in the 1940s, was the first tube with a manufactured cuff, it also featured the side vent or eye. The tube may also have an inflatable cuff which, when inflated, seals the space between the tube and the tracheal wall.

Markings

Various markings are seen on the tracheal tube or packaging (Table 10.2). Reference lines, rings or

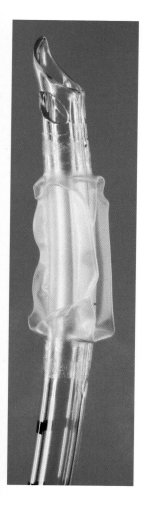

Figure 10.3. The Parker Flex tip. Note the Murphy eye.

Table 10.2. Markings on tracheal tubes

- Tube size in internal diameter in millimetres

- The outside diameter for size 6 and smaller

- The words oral or nasal or oral/nasal

- Name or trademark of the supplier

- Radio-opaque longitudinal line (may be of barium sulphate which increases risk of laser fire by reducing temperature at which ignition of the tube occurs)

- Distance from tip in centimetres marked on the wall

- Do not reuse or single use only if disposable

Additional markings may be added. Reference lines, rings or coloured areas are sometimes used to help position the tube with respect to the vocal cords.
Compliance with CE or International Organization for Standardization (ISO) regulations is marked on the packaging.

Table 10.3. Meaning of symbols found on tube or packaging

	Symbols Key
⊘	Single use, no risk of cross infection
STERILE EO / STERILE GAM	Sterile, ETO or Gamma irradiated
EA	Packed singly
LATEX	Latex free
C	15 mm connector conforming to ISO 5356-1 ensuring full compatibility with circuit connections
BL	Radio-opaque Blue Line for exact location of tube position
I	Manufactured from implantation tested non-toxic Ivory PVC to protect delicate mucosal tissues
NS	Non-Sterile
S	Manufactured from implantation tested Siliconised PVC to protect delicate mucosal tissues
10	Packed quantity

coloured areas are sometimes used to help position the tube with respect to the vocal cords. Materials from which tracheal tubes are manufactured must be tested for biological safety. This is generally established with IT in rabbit paravertebral muscle. Until 1996 tubes were marked with a test number, F-29 or IT on a tube denoting that the material from which it was made had been tested and shown no evidence of toxicity. Single use tubes carry the do not reprocess symbol (Table 10.3). Currently, any product which is marketed in the European Union (EU) must meet the requirement of all relevant EU Directives including biological safety in order to carry the Confirmité Européene (CE) mark and the CE mark is carried on the tube packaging. In the USA the Food and Drug Administration (FDA) does not allow products to be sold unless biological safety has been established.

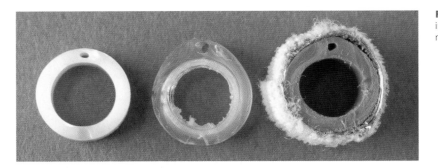

Figure 10.4. All tubes have the same internal diameter: from left microlaryngeal, reinforced, Sheridan laser.

Sizing

Tubes are sized by the internal diameter in millimetres. Due to variations in wall thickness there are significant differences between the external diameters of tubes of the same size (Figure 10.4). Conventional wisdom suggests the use of the widest diameter tube that will pass easily through the cords (or the cricoid ring in a child). Both large and small tubes have a number of advantages and disadvantages (Table 10.4). A large tube reduces resistance to gas flow and work of breathing. In conditions of laminar flow, resistance is inversely proportional to the fourth power of the radius according to the Hagen–Poiseuille equation. Even though flow is often turbulent in vivo, each millimetre decrease in tube diameter increases tube resistance by between 25% and 100%. An increase in the work of breathing parallels the increase in resistance as tube size is reduced, a 1 mm decrease in tube diameter increases the work of breathing by up to 150% depending on the minute volume.

Traditionally, in British anaesthesia, an 8.0 mm tube was placed in adult female patients and a 9.0 mm tube in males. However the use of these large sizes can no longer be recommended. Smaller tubes are easier to insert because the view of the laryngeal inlet is less likely to be obscured during passage of the tube through the cords at direct laryngoscopy. There is less laryngeal trauma on insertion and for the duration of intubation, and there is a lower incidence of sore throat. For provision of anaesthesia, physiologically normal adult patients can be managed perfectly well with size 6.0 and 7.0 mm tubes for both spontaneous respiration and mechanical ventilation.

Length

The tube length from the tip is shown on the outside in centimetres. The correct insertion depth is important

Table 10.4. Comparison of small and large tracheal tubes

	Small tubes	Large tubes
Advantages	Easier to insert	Lower work of breathing in spontaneously breathing patients
	Less laryngeal trauma	
	Lower incidence of sore throat	Tracheal suctioning is easier
Disadvantages	Increased airway resistance	Harder to insert
	Excessive cuff volumes	More laryngeal trauma
	Auto-PEEP	Infolding of cuff may allow tracheal soiling
	Difficult to suction	
	Difficult fibreoptic endoscopy	

to avoid the morbidity of endobronchial placement, inflation of the cuff within the larynx or accidental extubation during the procedure. The position of the tube tip in relation to the carina will be altered by gross movements of the head with head/neck extension causing withdrawal of the tube. Ideally, the tip of an uncuffed tube should be in the mid-trachea so that inadvertent extubation or endobronchial migration are minimised. For a neonate with trachea length 4 cm, the tip should be 2 cm below the vocal cords.

With a cuffed tube, it is important that the insertion depth is sufficient to avoid inflating the cuff within the larynx itself. Many tubes carry depth markers (usually one or two solid black lines) which indicate the correct depth when the markers are placed at the level of the glottis. Depth of insertion is generally referred to by the centimetre marking at the teeth or corner of the mouth.

Cuffs

The cuff and inflation system consists of an inflation lumen in the wall of the tube, an external inflation tube, a pilot balloon and a self-sealing inflation valve. Cuffed tubes are generally used in adult practice to seal the airway to protect it from soiling from above and to prevent gas leaks. Cuff pressure is transmitted to the tracheal wall at the points of contact, and this is termed the lateral wall pressure. To prevent aspiration, lateral wall pressure should exceed the maximum hydrostatic pressure that can be generated by a column of liquid (saliva, vomitus or blood) above the cuff. This hydrostatic pressure depends on the vertical distance from the upper part of the mouth and changes with the position of the patient. This distance is approximately 10–15 cm in the supine patient and 15–20 cm in the erect, necessitating pressures of 20 cmH$_2$O in the supine position and 25 cmH$_2$O in the erect position. The lateral wall pressure cannot be measured directly and is not necessarily predictable from the intracuff pressure. Obstruction to tracheal mucosal blood flow occurs at a lateral wall pressure above 30 cmH$_2$O and total occlusion occurs at 50 cmH$_2$O.

A high cuff pressure reduces the risk of aspiration but at the expense of high lateral wall pressures causing sore throat, mucosal inflammation progressing to ulceration, cartilaginous destruction and tracheal stenosis.

Three factors contribute to the extent of cuff-induced tracheal damage:

- Cuff characteristics
- Cuff pressure regulation
- Cuff inflation technique and medium.

Cuff characteristics

Cuffs may be categorised by their volume and pressure characteristics into two broad groups (Figure 10.5) (Table 10.5).

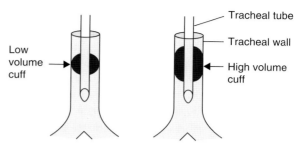

Figure 10.5. The two types of cuff. Difference in seal area with high volume low pressure and low volume high pressure.

Table 10.5. Advantages of high volume, low pressure cuffs

- Low tracheal wall pressure at occluding pressure spares mucosal perfusion
- Cuff inflates evenly on all sides giving a large area of seal
- Tube stabilised in the centre of the trachea and tip is not pushed against tracheal wall
- Wide margin of error in selecting tube size allowing smaller tube and reducing laryngeal damage
- Redundancy of the cuff permits small up and down movements of the tube without tube displacement so abrasive movement of the cuff against the trachea is reduced

Low volume, high pressure

Early red rubber tubes had a small resting diameter, a low residual volume and low compliance. A high intracuff pressure is required to achieve a seal within the trachea. There is a small area of contact within the trachea and the cuff distends and deforms the trachea to a circular shape. In this sort of cuff most of the pressure is needed to overcome cuff wall compliance (i.e., to stretch the cuff), so the pressure exerted against the tracheal wall is lower than intracuff pressure but the relationship between the two is non-linear. The use of a tube diameter close to that of the trachea permits low volume inflation and relative tracheal mucosal protection but increases the potential for laryngeal damage because the diameter of the tube is greater and trauma to laryngeal structures during insertion or friction injury to cords while the tube is in place is more likely. Recognition of the deleterious effects of early cuffs led to the development of high volume, low pressure cuffs in the 1970s.

95

High volume, low pressure cuffs

Modern tracheal tube cuffs have a large resting volume and diameter and a thin compliant wall which allows a seal to be achieved without stretching the cuff wall. When inflated, the thin, floppy cuff adapts itself to the tracheal contour. In this type of tube, cuff size is important. Intracuff pressure reflects lateral wall pressure unless the resting cuff circumference is less than tracheal circumference, in which case it will be stretched beyond its residual volume at seal point and will behave like a high pressure cuff. The optimal cuff is therefore, sufficiently large to effect a seal before being inflated to its residual volume.

Despite these apparent advantages, there is little evidence of benefit in clinical anaesthesia when high volume cuffs are compared to their low volume, high pressure predecessors. This may be due to the fact that although the pressure on the tracheal mucosa may be lower with high volume cuffs, the area of contact is greater. The large, floppy cuff may also obscure the view at direct laryngoscopy increasing the likelihood of trauma on insertion, and once residual volume is exceeded, a 2–3 ml inflation increment is sufficient to cause an exponential rise in cuff pressure resulting in unsafe lateral wall pressures. An additional disadvantage is that, if the cuff circumference is larger than that of the trachea, folds are created when the cuff is inflated and these form channels which allow leakage of fluid through the cuff into the trachea, this may be important in patients in intensive care who are at risk of ventilator-associated pneumonia.

Tracheal tube cuffs and ventilator-associated pneumonia (VAP)

Subglottic secretions accumulate above a tube cuff and may travel along channels within the folds of the cuff wall to the lower respiratory tract causing ventilator-associated pneumonia (VAP) which is a cause of morbidity and mortality in critically ill patients. The following have been used to reduce the incidence of VAP:

1. Tubes with cuffs made from a microthin (10 microns as opposed to 50–80 microns) polyurethane material and a cuff profile which is cylindrical rather than spherical are available. These Microcuff™ tubes provide an effective seal at low cuff pressures but are less prone to infolding and channel formation and may protect against ventilator-associated pneumonia.

2. Preliminary studies using tracheal tubes with a silver ion coating have suggested that they may reduce the incidence of ventilator-associated pneumonia by preventing surface biofilm formation and hampering respiratory tract bacterial colonisation

3. Tubes which incorporate a subglottic secretion drainage channel are available (e,g., Mallinckrodt™ SealGuard™ Evac & PortexBlue Line Ultra® 'Suctionaid'). Drainage of secretions from above the cuff may reduce the incidence of VAP.

4. Continuous automatic regulation of cuff pressure prevents the fluctuations associated with mechanical ventilation and patient posture may have a role.

Cuff pressure regulation

Measurements of cuff pressure are complicated by the fact that the intracuff pressure may not represent the lateral wall pressure especially in a low volume, high pressure device where much of the intracuff pressure is needed to overcome the compliance of the cuff. Despite this, the measurement of cuff pressure is clinically useful in avoiding excessive mucosal pressure since cuff pressure always exceeds lateral wall pressure. In addition, cuff pressure varies with the respiratory cycle (Figure 10.6).

Figure 10.6. Linkage of intracuff with airway pressure (intermittent positive pressure ventilation).

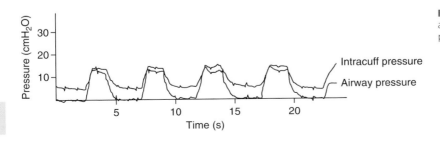

Intracuff pressure

Airway pressure

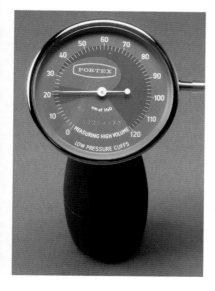

Figure 10.7. Portex intracuff pressure monitor: green segment indicates desirable range.

Table 10.6. Cuff pressures using seal technique for inflation with different inflation media

Cuff pressure to seal (mmHg)	Air	Saline	O$_2$/N$_2$O 'GasMix'
Mean	35.3	22.5	27
Range	9–119	8–41	2–53
SD	31.61	11.27	20.7

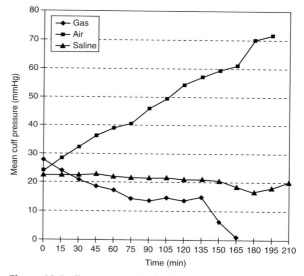

Figure 10.8. Changes in tracheal cuff pressure during anaesthesia with N$_2$O with either air, saline or O$_2$/N$_2$O mix in cuff.

In the spontaneously breathing patient airway pressure and cuff pressure are negative during inspiration. During controlled ventilation, positive pressure is applied to the distal portion of the cuff during inspiration and the air in the cuff is compressed until intracuff pressure equals airway pressure. Several methods have been used for continuous or intermittent measurement of cuff pressure, the most useful being a commercially available cuff pressure monitor (Figure 10.7).

Pressure regulating cuffs

Several cuff systems designed to minimise intracuff pressure changes are commercially available but none has demonstrated significant clinical benefit. The Brandt cuff system pilot balloon allows re-diffusion of nitrous oxide so that a low pressure seal is maintained. The Lanz cuff system consists of a compliant pilot balloon inside a transparent sheath with a pressure regulating valve between them and provides a constant cuff pressure below 3.4 kPa. The valve allows rapid gas flow from the balloon to the cuff but only slow flow from the cuff to the balloon. This prevents leakage of gas when airway pressure rises rapidly in inspiration but prevents cuff pressure rising during nitrous oxide anaesthesia.

The Smith Portex soft seal cuff claims to be less permeable to nitrous oxide limiting the intraoperative rise in cuff pressure, and the Smith Portex Fome-Cuf™ tube features a polyurethane foam filled cuff which exerts a stable lateral wall pressure which is independent of inflation medium and temperature.

Inflation technique and medium

When cuff inflation is carried out using the leak technique, the cuff pressure obtained varies widely (Table 10.6). If inflation is carried out with air, cuff pressure will increase significantly during nitrous oxide anaesthesia as nitrous oxide diffuses into the cuff along a concentration gradient (Figure 10.8). The diffusion of oxygen into the cuff and expansion of air as it warms to body temperature may also contribute to a pressure increase.

Saline provides stable cuff pressures but is more difficult to use than air. Saline is more viscous than air or gas and the cuff must be inflated more slowly than usual to allow time for equilibration of pressure

97

throughout the system. The elasticity of the cuff tends to force saline back into the pilot balloon when filling pressure is discontinued, resulting in a drop in intra-cuff pressure if the process is completed too quickly. Saline is not suitable for reusable tube cuffs as they will explode when autoclaved. Lidocaine has been suggested as an alternative to saline and may offer the additional benefit of a reduction in post-operative sore throat.

If a mixture of inspired gases containing nitrous oxide is used to inflate the cuff, deflation of the cuff may occur. The pressure inside the cuff is above atmospheric pressure and the intracuff partial pressure of nitrous oxide is greater than that of the inspired gas. Nitrous oxide diffuses out of the cuff along a pressure gradient, and the cuff may deflate.

Connectors

Tracheal tubes are attached to the breathing system via tapered male to female 15 mm ISO connectors. The male connector fits the tube via a tapered cone whose diameter is slightly larger than the tube ensuring a secure connection. The tube adaptor (catheter mount) or breathing circuit house the female part of the system with an internal diameter of 15 mm and an outer diameter of 22 mm. An 8.5 mm diameter connector is available for paediatric tubes. Non-ISO connectors such as metal Magill or flexibend connectors are now rarely used.

Special tubes
Polar

Commonly known as RAE tubes (after the designers Ring-Adair-Elwyn, Salt Lake City), polar tubes are preformed so that their ISO connector is distant from the mouth or the nose (Figure 10.9). A bulky angled connector and catheter mount are avoided and the tube can be fixed securely in place with strapping on the chin or forehead with little or no risk of kinking or dislodgement. Both oral and nasal tubes are available in either north- or south-facing pattern with the 'facing' indicating that the tube is preformed to be directed cephalad (north) or caudad (south). North-facing polar nasal tubes (Figure 10.10) are particularly useful in head and neck surgery where access to the oral cavity is required. The main disadvantages are with the fixed length of the intraoral or intranasal section and difficulty with suctioning through a long,

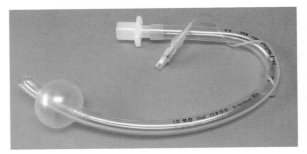

Figure 10.9. South-facing oral RAE tube.

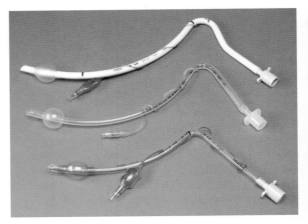

Figure 10.10. Nasal, north-facing polar tubes.

tightly curved tube. They can be converted to conventional tubes by cutting the tube at its bend and re-inserting the ISO connector.

Armoured or reinforced

Standard tubes kink when twisted or compressed. The walls of armoured tubes contain a spiral of metal wire or nylon (Figure 10.11) to prevent kinking or occlusion of the tube when the head or neck are moved. The reinforcement allows the tube to be made of a more elastic material which makes it less traumatic but more difficult to insert as it tends to be floppy with no preformed shape. It is preferable to have the reinforcement welded to the ISO connector to avoid the vulnerable junction of tube and connector, which is liable to kink. The reinforced tubes supplied for use with the intubating laryngeal mask airway (ILMA) are the exception to this rule as the connector must be removed during the passage of the tube through the ILMA.

The external diameter of armoured tubes is greater than ordinary tubes of the same size due to their thicker walls, and the tubes are designed for

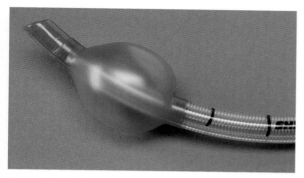

Figure 10.11. Armoured tube: note wire spiral in wall and insertion depth markings.

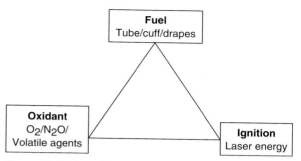

Figure 10.12. Laser fire triangle. All three components of the triangle must be present for an airway fire to occur. If all three components are present during laser surgery it is essential to minimise oxidant source by using the lowest FIO_2 (using air as the diluent) to maintain SpO_2.

oral or nasal intubation, so they are relatively long and inadvertent endobronchial intubation may occur if insufficient attention is paid to positioning. There are circumferential markers to indicate the correct position for the vocal cords. Armoured tubes cannot be cut and must be fixed in place with adhesive tapes.

There are two hazards particular to the use of an armoured tube for oral intubation. As there is no preformed curve there is more potential for longitudinal movement of the tube and complete occlusion may occur if the patient bites on the tube as the reinforcing wire can be permanently deformed. If an armoured tube has been used for an oral intubation it is usual to insert a Guedel airway adjacent to the tube to avoid this complication and to stabilise it.

Laser tubes

Standard and microlaryngoscopy tubes are unsuitable for laser airway procedures due to the high energies contained within the laser beam. Three components (Figure 10.12) are required simultaneously for a laser-induced fire, and a plastic or red rubber tube provides the fuel element. When combined with high concentrations of oxygen, the tube will quickly incinerate within the airway causing fatal damage. Laser tubes have laser resistant properties (so that the laser energy coming into contact with the fuel source is much reduced) but the tubes may ignite with sustained laser energy strikes of sufficient magnitude. In order to be laser proof a tube must be made entirely of metal. All laser tubes have a large external diameter relative to internal diameter and a number of tubes have been used (Table 10.7 and Figure 10.13).

Microlaryngoscopy tubes

These have a small internal and external diameter and are designed specifically for endoscopy procedures of the larynx. A common size is 5.0 mm but both the length and cuff size are appropriate for use in adults (Figure 10.14). They are soft and atraumatic and particularly useful for benign vocal cord lesions where placement is undertaken in a controlled, precise manner with no injury to the glottis. As they warm to body temperature, they soften and may kink at the point at which they emerge from the mouth or nose.

Tubes for monitoring recurrent laryngeal nerve function

Xomed manufactures a tube designed with surface electrodes to monitor vocal cord EMG activity during thyroid or other surgery (Figure 10.15) likely to compromise integrity of the recurrent laryngeal nerve. When correctly placed the blue electrodes lie between the vocal cords and surgical or electrical stimulation of the nerve will be detected by the monitor.

Tubes for paediatric practice

Uncuffed tracheal tubes have been standard for intubation in children under the age of 8 years for the past 50 years. This practice is based on the observation that the paediatric larynx is cone shaped with the narrowest part at the cricoid ring, whereas the adult larynx is cylindrical and the cords are the limiting factor. In theory a tracheal tube which is snug at the cricoid is sealed by the tracheal mucosa, aspiration risk is minimal, and ventilation without a troublesome air leak possible. An audible leak at a pressure

Table 10.7. Laser tubes

Laser tube	Properties
Norton (Oswald-Norton)	Made entirely of steel and therefore laser proof
	Reusable
	Flexible with a spiral wound stainless steel wall, no cuff and a relatively large, rough, external diameter
	Wet packs used to provide a seal for intermittent positive pressure ventilation (IPPV)
Sheridan Laser-Trach	Red rubber
	Single use
	Spiral wrapped with embossed copper foil from the cuff to proximal end of tube*
	Embossing disperses beam
	Outer fabric covering is soaked with water prior to use
Mallinckrodt Laser Flex	Corrugated stainless steel shaft
	Single use
	Two cuffs in case of intra-operative perforation* cuff may be foam filled
Xomed Laser – shield II	Silicone tube wrapped in aluminium foil and overwrapped with Teflon tape
	Smooth atraumatic exterior
	Methylene blue crystals in the cuff allow early detection of perforation*
Bivona	Metallic core
	Single use
	Silicone covering
	Foam filled cuff
	High incidence of sore throat

*Cuff inflation is with saline.

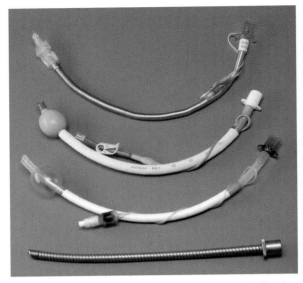

Figure 10.13. Laser tubes: from bottom Norton, Xomed, Sheridan, Mallinckrodt.

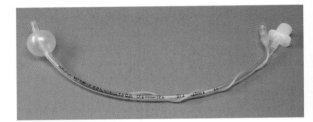

Figure 10.14. Microlaryngeal tube 4.0 mm.

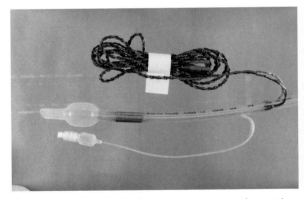

Figure 10.15. Xomed tube for monitoring recurrent laryngeal nerve integrity.

of 20 cmH$_2$o is used to signal that the tube is not too large and that there is minimal risk of distension of the cricoid ring which might lead to mucosal ischaemia, fibrosis and subglottic stenosis.

Table 10.8. Tube sizes for microcuff paediatric tubes

Tube size (ID)	Age/weight
3 mm	Term >3 kg up to <8 months
3.5 mm	8 months to <2 years
4 mm	2 to <4 years
4.5 mm	4 to <6 years
5 mm	6 to <8 years
5.5 mm	8 to <10 years
6 mm	10 to <12 years
6.5 mm	12 to <14 years
7 mm	14 to <16 years

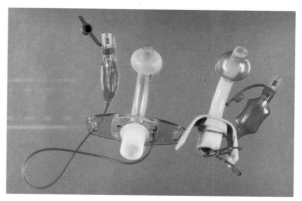

Figure 10.16. Cuffed tracheostomy tubes.

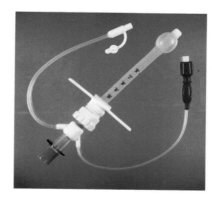

Figure 10.17. Adjustable flange cuffed tracheostomy tube. Note tube for subglottic drainage of secretions.

More recent MRI evidence has suggested that the larynx in children is actually ellipsoidal, and an uncuffed tracheal tube tends to lie against the latero-posterior cricoid wall potentially compromising mucosal blood flow even in the presence of a positive leak test.

The development of tubes specifically designed to suit the paediatric airway with high volume low pressure cuffs made of ultrathin polyurethane and a short cuff length, has challenged conventional practice and cuffed tubes are gaining acceptance. A recent European multicentre study found that the Microcuff cuffed tube was associated with the same low incidence of stridor and a much reduced need for re-intubation than with uncuffed tubes. Accurate positioning of the cuff within the trachea is important, and tubes are designed with depth markers to facilitate this. Cuff pressure monitoring is essential, and a seal pressure of 10 cmH$_2$O may be adequate but it should not exceed 20 cmH$_2$O. Recommended tube size is related to age (Table 10.8).

Tracheostomy tubes

Tracheostomy tubes can be made of metal or plastic, they may be cuffed or uncuffed and of fixed (Figure 10.16) or variable (Figure 10.17) length. Fenestrations or speaking valves can be used to allow the patient to vocalise. They are available with subglottic suction channels to reduce ventilator-associated pneumonia. They are inserted surgically or via a percutaneous dilational technique. Tracheostomy tubes with a 15 mm ISO connector can be connected directly to a breathing circuit. For those without standard connectors, an airway seal can be provided by a laryngeal mask over the tracheostomy, an appropriately sized tube-connector wedged into place or a suitable tube inserted once the patient is asleep.

Sizing

Tracheostomy tube size can be misleading as the number does not always correlate to the internal diameter of the tube. For example: an 8 Portex Blue Line® tube has an internal diameter of 8 mm and an outer diameter of 11 mm. An 8 Portex Blue Line Ultra® has an internal diameter of 8 mm and an outer diameter of 11.9 mm. An 8 Shiley™ Fenestrated tube has an internal diameter of 7.6 cm and an outer diameter of 12.2 mm.

Metal tracheostomy tubes

Generally made of silver which is non-irritant and bactericidal, these tubes are used for patients with long-term tracheostomies. They are uncuffed and

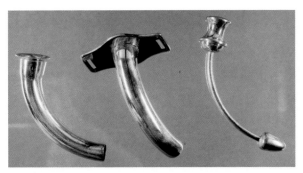

Figure 10.18. Silver tracheostomy tube with obturator and inner tube.

have an obturator for insertion and an inner tube which can be removed for cleaning (Figure 10.18).

Fenestrated tracheostomy tubes

A window or fenestration in the greater curvature of the tube channels air towards the vocal cords enabling speech. When the cuff is deflated, airflow is possible around the tube and through the fenestration as well as through the stoma which reduces the work of breathing and aids weaning from the tracheostomy. Some tubes come with a choice of complete or fenestrated inner tube.

Tracheostomy speaking valves

One way speaking valves can be attached to an uncuffed tracheostomy tube or to a cuffed tube with its cuff deflated.

Laryngectomy (Montandon) tube

This is J-shaped (Figure 10.19) for insertion into the distal trachea following laryngectomy and allows the breathing circuit to be connected at some distance from the stoma. In some versions the cuff is sited at the end of the tube and there is no distal bevel at all to prevent accidental endobronchial intubation.

Key points

- Tube size is internal diameter in millimetres.
- Narrow (small) tubes are easier to insert and cause less morbidity.
- High volume, low pressure cuffs are inherently safer than low volume, high pressure cuffs.
- Intracuff pressure always equals or exceeds lateral wall pressure.

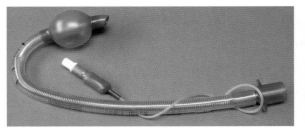

Figure 10.19. Laryngectomy tube.

- If lateral wall pressure exceeds mucosal perfusion pressure ischaemia results.
- Safe lateral wall pressure is 20–30 cmH$_2$O.
- Monitoring intracuff pressure is recommended especially in children.
- Cuff inflation with air results in an increase in pressure during nitrous oxide anaesthesia.
- Cuff inflation with inspired gas mixture results in a decrease in cuff pressure.
- Saline provides stable cuff pressures but is more difficult to use.
- Consider fire triangle when using tracheal tube for laser surgery.
- Tube characteristics may influence the risk of ventilator-associated pneumonia.

Further reading

Bolder PM, Healy TE, Bolder AR, Beatty PC, Kay B. (1986). The extra work of breathing through adult endotracheal tubes. *Anesthesia and Analgesia,* **65**, 853–859.

Chastre J. (2008). Preventing ventilator-associated pneumonia.: Could silver-coated endotracheal tubes be the answer? *Journal of the American Medical Association,* **300**, 842–844.

Crawley BE, Cross DE. (1975). Tracheal cuffs: A review and dynamic pressure study. *Anaesthesia,* **30**, 4–11.

Hannallah MS, Sudyerhoud JP. (1996). Endotracheal tubes and respiratory care. In: Benumof JL (Ed.), *Airway Management Principles and Practice.* St Louis: Mosby.

Jaensson M, Olowsson LL, Nilsson U. (2010). Endotracheal tube size and sore throat following surgery: A randomized study. *Acta Anaesthesiologica Scandinavica,* **54**, 147–153.

Koh KF, Hare JD, Calder I. (1998). Small tubes revisited. *Anaesthesia,* **53**, 46–50.

Kollef MH, Afessa B, Anzueto A, et al. (2008). Silver-coated endotracheal tubes and incidence of ventilator-associated pneumonia: The NASCENT randomized trial. *Journal of the American Medical Association,* **300**, 805–813.

Loesler EA, Hodges M, Gliedman J, Stanley TH, Johansen RK, Yonetani D. (1978). Tracheal pathology following short-term intubation with low- and high-pressure endotracheal tube cuffs. *Anesthesia and Analgesia,* **57**, 577–579.

Mitchell V, Adams T, Calder I. (1999). Choice of cuff inflation media during nitrous oxide anaesthesia. *Anaesthesia,* **54**, 32–36.

Pneumatikos I, Dragoumanis CK, Bouros D. (2009). Ventilator-associated pneumonia or endotracheal tube-associated pneumonia?: An approach to the pathogenesis and preventative strategies emphasizing the importance of endotracheal tube. *Anesthesiology,* **110**, 673–680.

Rai MR, Scott SH, Marfin AG, Popat MT, Pandit JJ. (2009). A comparison of a flexometallic tracheal tube with the intubating laryngeal mask tracheal tube for nasotracheal fibreoptic intubation using the two-scope technique. *Anaesthesia,* **64**, 1303–1306.

Seegobin RD, Van Hasselt GL. (1986). Aspiration beyond endotracheal cuffs. *Canadian Journal of Anaesthesia,* **33**, 273.

Shapiro M, Wilson RK, Casar G, Bloom K, Teague RB. (1986). Work of breathing through different sized endotracheal tubes. *Critical Care Medicine,* **14**, 1028–1031.

Shroff PP, Patil V. (2009). Efficacy of cuff inflation media to prevent postintubation-related emergence phenomenon: Air, saline and alkalinized lignocaine. *European Journal of Anaesthesiology,* **26**, 458–462.

Suzuki A, Tampo A, Abe N, et al. (2008). The Parker Flex-Tip tracheal tube makes endotracheal intubation with the Bullard laryngoscope easier and faster. *European Journal of Anaesthesiology,* **25**, 43–47.

Tonnesen AS, Vereen AS, Arens JF. (1981). Endotracheal tube cuff residual volume and lateral wall pressure in a model trachea. *Anesthesiology, **55**, 680–683.

Weiss M, Dullenkopf A, Böttcher S, et al. (2006). Clinical evaluation of cuff and tube tip position in a newly designed paediatric preformed oral cuffed tracheal tube. *British Journal of Anaesthesia,* **97**, 695–700.

Weiss M, Dullenkopf A, Fischer JE, Keller C, Gerber AC. (2009). Prospective randomized controlled multi-centre trial of cuffed or uncuffed endotracheal tubes in small children. *British Journal of Anaesthesia,* **103**, 867–873.

Websites

http://www.standardsuk.com (British Standards)

BS EN ISO 5366–1:2009 Anaesthetic and respiratory equipment. Tracheostomy tubes. Part 1: Tubes and connectors for use in adults

BS EN 1782:1998 tracheal tubes and connectors

BS EN ISO 14408:2005 tracheal tubes designed for laser surgery.

BS EN 1282–2:1997 Anaesthetic and respiratory equipment. Tracheostomy tubes. Paediatric tubes

http://www.cookmedical.com/ (percutaneous tracheostomy tubes)

http://www.intaventorthofix.com

http://www.kapitex.com (tracheostomy tubes)

http://www.kchealthcare.com/microcuff/ (microcuff tubes)

http://www.myrusch.com (tracheal and tracheostomy tubes)

http://www.nellcor.com (Mallinckrodt tubes)

http://www.parkermedical.com (Parker Flex Tip tubes)

http://www.smiths-medical.com (Portex tubes)

http://www.vbm-medical.com (cuff pressure monitors)

http://www.xomed.com/xomed_physicians.html (recurrent laryngeal monitoring tubes)

Airway damage: iatrogenic and traumatic

Anil Patel

Iatrogenic airway damage

Iatrogenic airway injury is mostly caused by laryngoscopy, visualisation of the laryngeal inlet, the placement of a tracheal tube and long-term intubation. Apart from obvious trauma, lacerations and dental damage the injury may not be immediately apparent and commonly the anaesthetist involved will be unaware of the airway damage caused. There is no period of tracheal intubation before which no injury occurs, and after which injury is inevitable.

Nasal/oral cavity

The placement of a nasal tube past a congested nasal cavity, deviated nasal septum or hypertrophied inferior turbinate can traumatise, avulse or perforate nasopharyngeal mucosa and cause bleeding or infection. The patency of nasal passages, size and type of nasal tube, should be optimised to reduce iatrogenic trauma. Nasal vasoconstrictors and intubation over a guide such as a suction catheter or endoscope may reduce trauma. Prolonged (>24 hours) nasal intubation is associated with sinus infection.

Lacerations to lips, tongue, palate and tonsils have all been described. Throat packs should be placed carefully to minimise abrasions to the soft palate.

Dental trauma

Dental damage still represents the most common cause of a civil action against anaesthetists and occurs during laryngoscopy, particularly during difficult visualisation in patients with restored teeth or poor dentition and gum disease. Careful pre-operative assessment should identify those at risk and appropriate protective teeth guards and techniques used. The upper incisors are most often damaged. In some instances despite all reasonable protection the teeth and gums are so diseased that any instrumentation of the airway will damage or dislodge teeth.

Vocal function

Even short-term tracheal intubation will have a detrimental effect on vocal function as measured by electroglottography, stroboscopic laryngoscopy, acoustic waveform analysis and vocal profile analysis for up to 24–48 hours. Fortunately in the vast majority of patients short-term tracheal intubation does not affect vocal function long-term and within 24–48 hours the voice parameters return to the pre-intubation levels. In an unfortunate unpredictable minority vocal function can be adversely affected long-term which may be incapacitating for professional voice users. Laryngeal resistance and the glottic aperture angle both increase following intubation indicating laryngeal and vocal cord swelling. Routine tracheal intubation affects the larynx anatomically and functionally but fortunately in the majority of patients this is not detectable clinically. In an unpredictable minority these short-term changes can persist. Post-intubation symptoms are decreased by the use of small diameter tracheal tubes (6.0 mm for women and 7.0 mm for men) and facilitating intubation with neuro-muscular blockade.

Iatrogenic laryngeal trauma

Cricoarytenoid joint dysfunction, dislocation, granuloma formation, vocal cord palsy and haematoma can all occur and cause significant morbidity. Any patient with an unexplained persistent sore throat, hoarseness, dysphonia or weak cough should be seen by an ENT specialist for investigation, laryngoscopy and further management.

The closed claims analysis from the United States looking at airway injury during anaesthesia showed

Core Topics in Airway Management, Second Edition, ed. Ian Calder and Adrian Pearce. Published by Cambridge University Press.
© Cambridge University Press 2011.

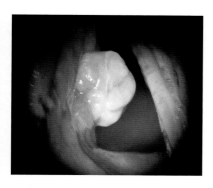

Figure 11.1. Post-intubation granuloma.

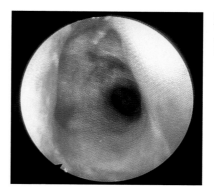

Figure 11.2. Tracheal stenosis caused by intubation.

33% of injuries occurred at the larynx, 19% pharynx, 18% oesophagus, 15% trachea, 10% temporomandibular joint and 5% nasal. Of the laryngeal injuries vocal cord paralysis was the most common (34%) followed by granuloma (17%), arytenoid dislocation (8%) and haematoma (3%). Most (85%) of the laryngeal injuries were associated with short-term tracheal intubation, and most (80%) were associated with routine (not difficult) tracheal intubation.

Iatrogenic laryngeal trauma occurs mostly in patients undergoing routine, non-difficult, short-term tracheal intubation (Figure 11.1).

Iatrogenic unilateral vocal cord paralysis

Unilateral vocal cord paralysis following routine, non-difficult tracheal intubation for peripheral surgery with appropriate tube sizing and cuff pressure monitoring (see Chapter 10) has an incidence of approximately 1 per 1000 procedures. Two thirds of this unilateral vocal cord paralysis occurs on the left and one third on the right vocal cord.

Tracheal intubation-related neuropraxia of the lingual, hypoglossal, and laryngeal nerves have all been described.

For every 1000 patients undergoing routine non-difficult intubation for surgery, approximately 1 patient will develop unilateral vocal cord paralysis as a direct result of the tracheal intubation. In most cases the anaesthetist involved with the intubation will be unaware of these problems because the diagnosis is often some time after discharge.

Iatrogenic airway stenosis

Airway stenosis occurs at any level within the airway following tracheal intubation. The annual incidence of post-intubation laryngotracheal stenosis requiring surgical correction is 1 in 204 000 adults and 4.9 in 100 000 children.

With long-term intubation and mechanical ventilation the incidence of laryngotracheal injuries approaches 90% with long-term sequelae occurring in 11% of these patients (Figure 11.2).

Patients can present with airway compromise many weeks or months after a period of tracheal intubation and may have been misdiagnosed and treated for asthma. Surgical management of these patients involves laser resection, dilation, stent placement, steroid injection, tracheal resection and 'end-to-end' anastomosis and tracheal homografts.

In the paediatric airway the subglottis (cricoid area) is the narrowest part of the airway and intubation can lead to circumferential granulation tissue, scarring and eventual stenosis of the subglottis. The posterior tilt of the cricoid cartilage in neonates may reduce the incidence of interarytenoid injury which is commonly seen in adults.

In adults the glottis is the narrowest part of the airway, and tracheal tubes tend to be most in contact with the posterior glottis. Movements of the tube on the posterior glottis and arytenoids can lead to pressure/ischaemic necrosis of the thin mucosa overlying this area. This can lead to ulceration, perichondritis, granulation tissue formation and scarring. If the scarring affects the inter-arytenoid area bilateral vocal cord immobility can result. Bilateral intubation granulomas can coalesce to fix the vocal cord in adduction. Posterior commissure stenosis can be particularly difficult to treat once it has formed, and as the condition only occurs in the presence of a translaryngeal tracheal tube early tracheostomy reduces its incidence.

105

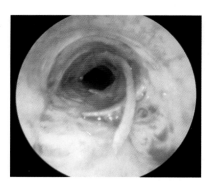

Figure 11.3. Fractured tracheal rings caused by traumatic intubation.

In adults subglottic and tracheal stenosis can be caused by oversized tracheal tubes or overinflated cuffs with high pressures leading to ischaemic necrosis of the tracheal mucosa with ulceration, perichondritis, granulation tissue and scarring (Figure 11.3).

In adults glottic, subglottic and tracheal injury/stenosis can also result from poorly sited tracheostomies close to, or at the cricoid cartilage. Tracheostomy tube cuff pressure monitoring should always be in place to limit the incidence of tracheal stenosis.

Although adult tracheostomies are not without complications themselves and can precipitate airway stenosis, tracheostomy-related airway stenosis often carries a better outlook than laryngeal stenosis.

Pharyngeal or oesophageal perforation

Pharyngeal or oesophageal perforation is a serious complication of aerodigestive tract instrumentation, and is associated with a greater severity of injury and risk of mortality than other iatrogenic airway injuries. Patients present with pain, dysphagia, aspiration and cervical crepitus (surgical emphysema). The principal early sign of perforation is surgical emphysema, but it is not present initially in all cases. If perforation is suspected, the patient must be carefully observed for symptoms and signs. Treatment consists of stopping oral intake, broad spectrum antibiotics and naso-gastric or parenteral nutrition. Sepsis requires urgent intervention with exploration and drainage of purulent collections.

Non-iatrogenic traumatic airway damage

The larynx allows (i) air to flow to the lungs, (ii) phonation and (iii) protects the lower airway during swallowing. Trauma in or around the larynx may compromise one or more of these functions and result in urgent life-threatening airway compromise requiring immediate intervention, or cause longer term problems with the voice (dysphonia), or swallowing dysfunction and the potential for aspiration.

Trauma to the airway can be broadly classified into two types: (i) external laryngeal trauma which includes blunt and penetrating injuries and (ii) internal airway trauma which includes thermal, caustic and iatrogenic injuries.

Laryngeal trauma is rare but acutely life-threatening and if not promptly recognised and treated can cause significant long-term morbidity.

Airway assessment

Whatever the mechanism of injury the initial airway assessment aims to identify those at risk of airway compromise and establish a safe airway with cervical spine protection. Symptoms suggestive of laryngeal trauma can vary widely, but include stridor, pain, dyspnoea, dysphonia, dysphagia and hoarseness. Examination may reveal skin abrasions over the anterior neck, subcutaneous emphysema and crepitus, haemoptysis, bruising, entry and exit wounds, laryngeal tenderness, the loss of palpable landmarks and signs of a pneumothorax.

Immediate intervention and airway control may involve orotracheal intubation or intubation through a large open wound in the airway. An emergency surgical airway under local anaesthetic may be safer for patients where there is concern over the ability to pass a tracheal tube, or where the tracheal tube may exacerbate the laryngeal injury, create a false passage or precipitate total airway obstruction. These patients are difficult to manage and skilled assistance with senior anaesthetic and surgical help should be sought at an early stage. An emergency surgical airway should be via a tracheostomy and avoid a cricothyroidotomy approach as this may cause further injury.

Fibreoptic intubation is difficult following laryngeal trauma because of airway distortion, swelling, oedema, bleeding and the difficulties of passing a fibrescope past areas of airway damage. Fibreoptic intubation is not recommended for the occasional fibrescope user.

If orotracheal intubation is undertaken cricoid pressure should not be performed as this may result in cricotracheal separation and loss of airway patency. A selection of tube sizes, laryngoscope blades, gum elastic bougie, indirect visualising laryngoscopes, skilled help, senior anaesthetist and senior surgeon should be available. In experienced hands indirect visualising laryngoscopes may offer advantages over standard direct laryngoscopy because of reduced (i) neck manipulation and (ii) laryngoscopy generated force and distortion in the laryngopharynx. This may reduce any further laryngeal injury.

If the airway is judged as stable from the history, symptoms and signs then further investigations with flexible nasendoscopy and CT are undertaken. This may reveal unexpected injury and an informed decision over subsequent airway intervention (tracheal intubation or tracheostomy) or conservative management made.

External laryngeal trauma

External laryngeal trauma is uncommon with an estimated incidence of 1 in 1000 trauma victims. In the United States this accounts for between 1 in 5 000 and 1 in 30 000 emergency room visits. External laryngeal trauma should be managed by a multidisciplinary trauma team, and associated cervical and remote injuries should be systematically sought and treated.

Blunt airway trauma

The upper airway is well protected by the mandible superiorly, spinal column posteriorly, sternum inferiorly and the sternomastoid muscles laterally. However anteriorly it is exposed to crushing anterior cervical trauma which compresses the larynx against the spinal cord. Motor vehicle accidents have traditionally been the most common cause of external laryngeal injury when an individual who is not wearing a seat belt is subjected to rapid deceleration with a hyperextended neck thrust against the dashboard or steering wheel. Similarly an exploding airbag may traumatise the larynx. Other injuries arise from sport-related trauma, attempted suicide, strangulation and clothesline injuries where motorcyclists encounter a fixed horizontal object at neck level.

Laryngeal calcification begins from the third decade of life and occurs in men more than women. The greater the calcification of the thyroid cartilage, the less it is able to spring back from compression injuries and the more likely it is to shatter.

The initial airway assessment is as discussed above and for blunt laryngeal trauma the commonest feature is hoarseness (85% of cases), followed by dysphagia (52%), pain (14%), dyspnoea (21%) and haemoptysis (18%).

Associated injuries include open neck injury (18% of cases), maxillofacial fractures (18%), intracranial injuries (17%), cervical spine fracture (13%), chest injury (13%), other facial injury (10%), skull fracture (7%) and open pharyngeal injury (4%).

Various classification systems exist for laryngeal trauma, such as Scaefer-Fuhrmann or Lee-Elishar, and they aim to classify the severity of the damage. In order of increasing significance signs include minor laryngeal haematomas or lacerations, oedema, mucosal disruption, exposed cartilage, non-displaced laryngeal fractures, vocal cord immobility, displaced laryngeal fractures, anterior commissure disruption, two or more laryngeal fractures, unstable laryngeal fractures, and most severely complete laryngotracheal separation.

Management options depend on the severity of the injury and include (a) conservative management with no airway intervention, (b) translaryngeal tracheal intubation, (c) tracheostomy/surgical airway and (d) surgical repair.

Conservative management with no airway intervention involves admission to a high-dependency unit, airway observation, serial flexible nasendoscopy examination, humidified oxygen, antibiotics, corticosteroids, head-up position and proton pump inhibitors. This approach is appropriate for those patients in whom immediate intervention is not required but in whom problems could arise and approximately 40% of patients can be managed in this way. Translaryngeal tracheal intubation and tracheostomy have been discussed. Surgical management involves diagnostic and therapeutic endoscopy, open laryngeal repair, endolaryngeal stenting, management of cricotracheal separation and in rare instances partial or total laryngectomy.

Penetrating injuries of the airway

Penetrating injuries often damage other cervical structures, and the extent of the injury is often dependent on (i) the anatomical 'zone' of injury, and (ii) the weight and velocity of the penetrating object, so that stab wounds often have a better outlook than missile injuries.

Patients with neck trauma who are haemodynamically unstable or who have an obvious injury to the aerodigestive tract will require urgent surgery. However in those who are stable on initial assessment, the 'zone' of injury has traditionally influenced the diagnostic approach. More recently, CT has been advanced as the first-line investigation in stable patients with penetrating neck injuries, with subsequent investigations and endovascular or operative repair being guided by initial CT findings.

Traditionally zone I lies between the clavicles and the cricoid cartilage and accounts for 5% of injuries. The proximity of the great vessels and associated injury often requires translaryngeal tracheal intubation in this group. Zone II lies between the inferior margin of the cricoid cartilage and the angle of the mandible and approximately one-third of patients need emergency airway intervention. Most patients with Zone II injuries require intubation for surgical exploration. Zone III lies between the angle of the mandible and the base of the skull. These patients are traditionally less likely to need airway intervention.

With injuries in zones I and II, oesophageal trauma may initially be asymptomatic but can proceed to cause infections within the neck and mediastinum, and a high index of suspicion should be maintained.

Internal laryngeal trauma

Internal laryngeal trauma can be caused by thermal, caustic and iatrogenic injury. Iatrogenic airway damage, airway assessment and the principles of treatment of airway trauma have been discussed.

Thermal airway injury

Thermal injury to the airway is as a result of inhaling superheated air and these patients can present a major challenge to the anaesthetist requiring a careful history and examination to identify those at risk. A history of a fire in an enclosed space should raise the suspicion of an airway burn or inhalational injury. The face, mouth, nose and pharynx should be inspected for burns and an assessment made for soot in the sputum, nose and mouth as well as an assessment of the airway as described above. All patients should be admitted for observation and prompt immediate intubation undertaken with early signs of airway obstruction.

Inhalational burns occur in 30% of all patients with burns, and 20% of patients with inhalational injury have extensive laryngeal injury. A further 7% of patients with inhalational injury have laryngeal and tracheobronchial injuries. Smoke inhalation accounts for 50% of all fire related deaths.

Oropharyngeal burns cause swelling which is maximal around 12 hours after the burn, which can lead to airway obstruction and is more likely if there are full thickness facial and anterior cervical burns.

Laryngeal burns can lead to a rapid deterioration of the airway due to oedema, and this should be anticipated and acted on early. Fibreoptic or indirect laryngoscopy is performed early to ensure there is no laryngeal oedema. Any sign of airway obstruction should prompt immediate action, and if oedema is seen airway intervention with a tracheal tube or tracheostomy should be undertaken early (do not cut the tracheal tube short).

Dysphonia is present in as many as 70% of patients with inhalational injuries 16 to 25 years after the initial injury.

Caustic airway injury

Ingestion of either alkaline or acidic substances leads to upper aerodigestive tract injury. The majority of injuries are caused by the ingestion of alkaline substances and the larynx is involved in approximately 40% of cases. Injuries of the larynx arise due to chemical irritation of the laryngeal and pharyngolaryngeal mucosa. In those patients that require tracheal intubation nearly all develop glottic airway stenosis requiring a subsequent tracheostomy.

Key points

- Damage to teeth during laryngoscopy is the commonest cause of civil action against anaesthetists.
- Perforation of the aero-digestive tract may lead to deep cervical infection or mediastinitis.
- Surgical emphysema is the cardinal sign of perforation but is not always present initially.
- Sore throat and dysphonia are common after anaesthesia but require investigation after 48 hours.
- Non-iatrogenic airway trauma is rare but often life-threatening. Expert, multi disciplinary opinion is required.

Further reading

Combes X, Andriamifidy L, Dufresne E, et al. (2007). Comparison of two induction regimens using or not using muscle relaxant: Impact on postoperative upper airway discomfort. *British Journal of Anaesthesia*, **99**, 276–281.

Domino KB, Posner KL, Caplan RA, Cheney FW. (1999). Airway injury during anaesthesia a closed claims analysis. *Anesthesiology* **91**, 1703–1711.

Jaensson M, Olowsson LL, Nilsson U. (2010). Endotracheal tube size and sore throat following surgery: A randomized-controlled study. *Acta Anaesthesiologica Scandinavica*, **54**, 147–153.

Jewett BS, Shockley WW, Rutledge R. (1999). External laryngeal trauma analysis of 392 patients. *Archives of Otolaryngology–Head & Neck Surgery,* **125**, 877–880.

Kikura M, Suzuki K, Itagaki T, Takada T, Sato S. (2007). Age and comorbidity as risk factors for vocal cord paralysis associated with tracheal intubation. *British Journal Anaesthesia* **98**, 524–530.

Maktabi MA, Smith RB, Todd MM. (2003). Is routine endotracheal intubation as safe as we think or wish? *Anaesthesiology,* **99**, 247–248.

Morfey D, Patel A. (2008). Airway trauma. *Anaesthesia and Intensive Care Medicine,* **9**, 312–314.

Nottet JB, Duruisseau O, Herve S. (1997). Inhalational burns: Apropos of 198 cases: Incidence of laryngotracheal involvement. *Annales d'oto-laryngologie et de chirurgie cervico faciale,* **114**, 220–225.

Nouraei SA, Ma E, Patel A, Howard DJ, Sandhu GS. (2007). Estimating the population incidence of adult laryngotracheal stenosis. *Clinical Otolaryngology*, **32**, 411–412.

Nouraei SA, Singh A, Patel A, Ferguson C, Howard DJ, Sandhu GS. (2006). Early endoscopic treatment of acute inflammatory airway lesions improves the outcome of postintubation airway stenosis. *Laryngoscope*, **116**, 1417–1421.

Sandhu GS, Nouraei SA. (2009). Laryngeal and esophageal trauma. In: Cummings CW (Ed.), *Cummings Otolaryngology Head & Neck Surgery.* Chapter 70. Philadelphia: Elsevier/Mosby.

Schaefer SD. (1992). The acute management of external laryngeal trauma: A 27-year experience. *Archives of Otolaryngology–Head & Neck Surgery,* **118**, 598–604.

Tanaka A, Isono S, Ishikawa T, Sato J, Nishino T. (2003). Laryngeal resistance before and after minor surgery, endotracheal tube versus laryngeal mask airway. *Anesthesiology,* **99**, 252–258.

Chapter 12

Tracheal intubation: direct laryngoscopy

John Henderson

A properly sited cuffed tracheal tube provides the most reliable airway in management of the unconscious, anaesthetised or critically ill patient. Tracheal intubation is an essential skill but can be difficult and may result in complications, the most serious being hypoxaemic brain damage and death. Soft tissue damage, including fatal mediastinitis, can be caused by traumatic attempts at intubation.

If serious difficulty is anticipated with direct laryngoscopy, facemask ventilation or emergency cricothyroidotomy, the safest management is to secure tracheal intubation under topical anaesthesia of the airway before induction of anaesthesia. However unanticipated difficulty is not infrequent and it is important to have a pre-formulated strategy to cope with this situation. Use of the basic algorithm of the Difficult Airway Society guidelines is recommended. Maintenance of oxygenation must take precedence over all other considerations. Pre-oxygenation should be performed before induction of anaesthesia. When difficulty with intubation is experienced, intubation attempts should be deferred until oxygenation is restored. The risks from trauma must be minimised. Although a significant lifting pressure may be needed in direct laryngoscopy, excessive force should not be used and the maximum number of attempts at any blind technique should be three. The anaesthetist should call for help as soon as difficulty is experienced. When unanticipated difficulty occurs during intubation for elective surgery and visual techniques have failed, the safest plan is to postpone surgery and awaken the patient.

Anatomical basis of direct laryngoscopy for tracheal intubation

Successful direct laryngoscopy depends on achieving a line of sight (LOS) (Figure 12.1) from the maxillary

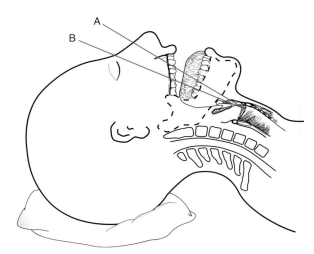

Figure 12.1. LOS with Macintosh (A) and straight (B) laryngoscope. Drawing is based on published scans of patients in the 'sniff' position. The tongue and epiglottis are the principle soft tissue obstructions to the LOS.

teeth to the larynx; management of the tongue and the epiglottis is particularly important (Figure 12.2). The initial patient position normally used is the 'sniff' position, achieved by flexion of the mid neck (C2–C4) and extension of the head (more accurately, the occipito-atlanto-axial complex). Maximum head extension, which rotates the maxillary teeth out of the LOS and facilitates maximum mouth opening, aids laryngoscopy. Neck flexion is achieved by placing the head on a pillow or other bolster. The role of neck flexion is controversial as recent studies have failed to show significant benefit. Excessive neck flexion increases the probability that contact between the laryngoscope handle and sternum will impair insertion. However continued use of the 'sniff' position is recommended as it improves pharyngeal patency. A 'ramped' position, in which both shoulders and head

Core Topics in Airway Management, Second Edition, ed. Ian Calder and Adrian Pearce. Published by Cambridge University Press. © Cambridge University Press 2011.

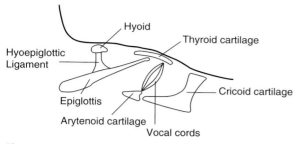

Figure 12.2. Epiglottis and laryngeal cartilages.

are elevated, has been recommended for direct laryngoscopy of obese patients, but there is little evidence that the incidence of grade 3 or 4 (see later) view of the larynx is reduced. However elevation of the shoulders of obese patients may facilitate head extension.

After positioning and creation of optimum pharmacological conditions, the rigid laryngoscope is used to displace soft tissues out of the LOS. Maximum mouth opening facilitates laryngoscope insertion. Both the rotating and sliding components of TMJ function are important and the scissor technique (e.g., right thumb pressing downward and forward from the glossal side of the mandibular teeth while the index or middle finger is stabilised on the maxillary teeth) can be useful. As the laryngoscope is advanced, the tongue is displaced horizontally from the LOS, the mandible and hyoid are moved anteriorly and the epiglottis is elevated (Figure 12.3). A significant lifting force, causing considerable tissue distortion but not damage, may be required in direct laryngoscopy. The vector (magnitude and direction) of this force is adjusted to achieve the optimum view of the larynx. The maximum force is applied close to the epiglottis, and the direction is at right angles to the LOS.

Pharmacology relevant to tracheal intubation

The aim of drug administration for direct laryngoscopy and tracheal intubation is to achieve sufficient tissue relaxation to allow insertion and positioning of the direct laryngoscope and to ensure that the vocal cords are open and non-reactive. These conditions are achieved at a price. Upper airway obstruction increases as consciousness is reduced. Airway patency can usually be achieved by a series of manoeuvres but these are particularly likely to fail in patients presenting with incomplete airway

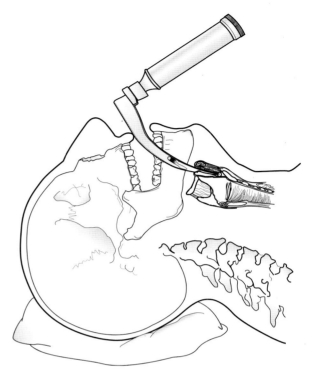

Figure 12.3. Macintosh laryngoscope in optimum position. Maximum mouth opening has been achieved by rotation and advancement of the mandible at the temporo-mandibular joint. The tongue has been displaced to the left of the laryngoscope.

obstruction in whom rapid creation of a surgical airway may then be necessary. Protection against pulmonary aspiration is decreased as consciousness is reduced. The pharmacological approach most frequently used is a combination of intravenous anaesthetic with neuromuscular blockade. Substitution of narcotics for neuromuscular blockade results in poorer conditions, apnoea, difficulty with pulmonary ventilation as a consequence of vocal cord closure and an increased risk of laryngeal damage. Apnoea should *not* be induced (*neuromuscular block or narcotics*) if difficulties are anticipated. Tracheal intubation may also be performed in the patient breathing spontaneously after inhalational induction of anaesthesia. A deep level of inhalational anaesthesia is required, and this may be complicated by hypoventilation, airway obstruction, arterial hypotension, dysrhythmias and pulmonary aspiration. The simultaneous use of topical anaesthesia of the larynx (as used by Magill) facilitates good conditions for tracheal intubation at a lesser depth of inhalational anaesthesia.

111

Table 12.1. Basic essential equipment

- Checked anaesthesia machine (or oxygen source and self-inflating resuscitator)
- Range of anaesthesia masks, SADs, oropharyngeal and nasopharyngeal airways
- Two checked laryngoscope handles
- Range of direct laryngoscope blades (Macintosh and straight)
- Rigid Indirect Laryngoscope ('video-laryngoscope') (one or more types)
- Range of tracheal tubes
- Stylet and introducer
- Syringe for cuff inflation
- Lubricant jelly
- Suction apparatus
- Magill forceps
- Tape to secure tube
- Capnograph

Preparation for direct laryngoscopy

Adequate personnel, drugs and equipment must be available. A minimum list of equipment is shown in Table 12.1. Intravenous access is secured and basic monitoring (ECG, NIBP and pulse oximeter with beep volume turned on and capnograph ready) established. The patient is pre-oxygenated.

Macintosh laryngoscope and technique of laryngoscopy

The Macintosh technique of laryngoscopy depends on indirect elevation of the epiglottis and is the most frequently used direct laryngoscopy technique in most centres. Meta-analysis shows that a view of the larynx may be obtained in 94.2% of patients with this technique.

The patient is positioned with neck flexion, and anaesthesia is induced. Once good conditions have been achieved, full head extension completes the positioning manoeuvres and partially opens the patient's mouth. The Macintosh laryngoscope (size 4 recommended for adult patients) is inserted from right side of mouth to the right of the tongue and advanced carefully, avoiding contact with the palatoglossal arch. As it is advanced, the blade is moved leftwards into the midline to displace the tongue to the left, using

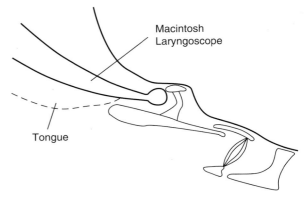

Figure 12.4. Position of epiglottis, tongue and laryngeal cartilages when optimum positioning of the tip of the Macintosh laryngoscope in the vallecula is achieved. The tongue lies entirely to the left of the laryngoscope. Tensioning of the hyoepiglottic ligament results in complete elevation of the epiglottis.

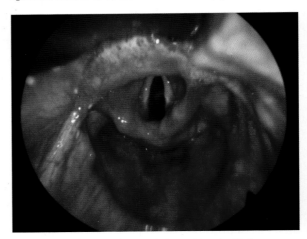

Figure 12.5. Optimum laryngeal view achieved with the Macintosh laryngoscope. In this figure the epiglottis has been allowed to drop a little posteriorly to show the laryngoscope in position in the vallecula.

light lifting pressure to maintain control of the tongue. After ensuring that the lips are not trapped between the laryngoscope blade and the patient's teeth, an increased lifting force is applied to the laryngoscope handle to achieve maximum mouth opening as the laryngoscope is further advanced. As the epiglottis comes into view, the tip of the laryngoscope is advanced into the vallecula and the force applied to the laryngoscope is adjusted to elevate the epiglottis to reveal the laryngeal inlet. The depth of insertion (Figure 12.4) and the lifting force are optimised to achieve the best view of the larynx (Figure 12.5). A considerable lifting force may be necessary (insufficient force is one cause of failure to

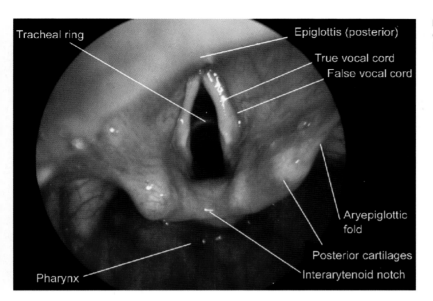

Figure 12.6. Laryngeal anatomy demonstrated with the Macintosh laryngoscope.

expose the larynx). Do *not* lever on the teeth as this action risks dental injury and degrades the view of the larynx (the distal anatomy is pushed anteriorly out of the LOS and the proximal blade is rotated into the LOS). If a good view cannot be achieved without pressure on the teeth, the Macintosh laryngoscope should be abandoned in favour of an alternative technique.

When a good view of the larynx is achieved, the vocal cords, the aryepiglottic folds and posterior cartilages can be identified (Figure 12.6). In other cases, only the posterior cartilages, the interarytenoid notch or the epiglottis may be seen. In the worst scenario, only the palate or posterior pharyngeal wall is seen. Occasionally the oesophagus is seen; it is round and puckered, and has no distinctive structures. Experienced anaesthetists are occasionally misled.

If only a poor view of the larynx is achieved, recheck that the key components (head extension, tongue control and lifting force) of the basic technique are applied correctly. If the view remains poor, the key additional manoeuvre is external laryngeal manipulation (ELM), better described as bimanual laryngoscopy. The thyroid cartilage is manipulated (posterior and lateral movement) with the anaesthetist's right hand (and then the assistant's hand) to optimise the view (Figure 12.7). This ELM is different from cricoid pressure and is a key and integral component of direct laryngoscopy. If a satisfactory view cannot be achieved, consider blind use of an introducer (next section) or, preferably, a different tracheal intubation technique.

When the view of the larynx has been optimised, an assistant retracts the corner of the mouth laterally and the tracheal tube is passed. Do *not* take your eye off the larynx until the tracheal tube has passed into the trachea. Many pass the tracheal tube close to the laryngoscope. However passage of the tube from the right of the LOS (via the corner of the mouth) allows the anaesthetist to better observe progress of the tracheal tube towards and through the laryngeal inlet. The optimum shape of the tracheal tube for this technique is that of an ice-hockey stick. A lubricated stylet can help to produce this shape. It is essential that the tip of the stylet does not protrude beyond the tip of the tracheal tube and that this technique, as all others, is performed gently. Once the tube has entered the trachea, the stylet is removed by an assistant. The tube is passed until the cuff is 2–3cm beyond the vocal cords, often indicated by a line on the tube. The cuff is then inflated to a just-seal pressure, and tracheal position is confirmed. Cuff pressure is then adjusted to 25 cmH$_2$O.

If only the posterior portion of the vocal cords or the interarytenoid notch can be seen, passage of the tracheal tube may be awkward but is not difficult. Passage under vision into the trachea of an introducer, which is then used to guide the tracheal tube into the trachea, is particularly useful in this situation.

Confirmation of tube position is *mandatory* as avoidable deaths from hypoxaemia as a consequence of delay or failure to recognise oesophageal intubation

113

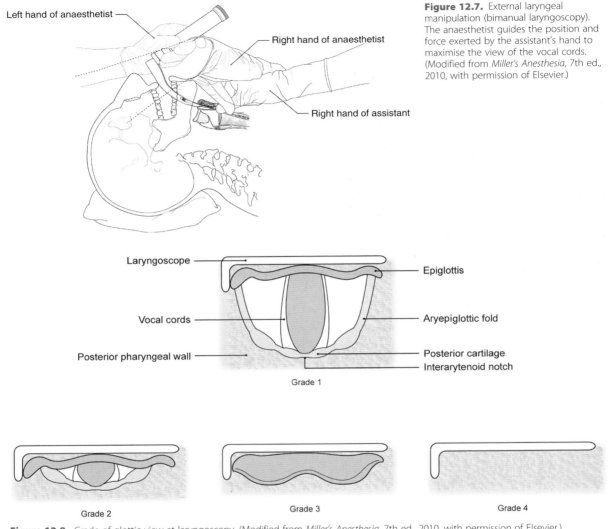

Figure 12.7. External laryngeal manipulation (bimanual laryngoscopy). The anaesthetist guides the position and force exerted by the assistant's hand to maximise the view of the vocal cords. (Modified from *Miller's Anesthesia*, 7th ed., 2010, with permission of Elsevier.)

Figure 12.8. Grade of glottic view at laryngoscopy. (Modified from *Miller's Anesthesia*, 7th ed., 2010, with permission of Elsevier.)

continue to occur. Accidental endobronchial and supraglottic positions also increase the risk of significant morbidity. Confirmation of tube position is considered in Chapter 16. Once satisfactory tracheal tube position is confirmed, it is secured so that it will neither come out nor advance into the right main bronchus. Adhesive or tie tape or both may be used. Record the depth marking on the tube at the patient's teeth or lips.

Finally, it is important to record the best view of the larynx achieved. This information is important in planning safe airway management on a subsequent occasion. The standard description, that of Cormack and Lehane (1984), is illustrated in Figure 12.8:

Grade 1 (most of the larynx visible), Grade 2 (posterior structures of the larynx, including the interarytenoid notch, visible), Grade 3 (only the epiglottis visible) and Grade 4 (no laryngeal structure seen). Grade 3 has been subdivided into 3a in which the epiglottis can be elevated from the posterior pharyngeal wall and 3b when it cannot be lifted. This is an important subdivision as the blind introducer technique does not work well and should not be attempted when the epiglottis cannot be elevated.

Success with the Macintosh technique depends on moving the tongue to the left of the laryngoscope and positioning the laryngoscope tip in the vallecula. When this laryngoscope position cannot be achieved

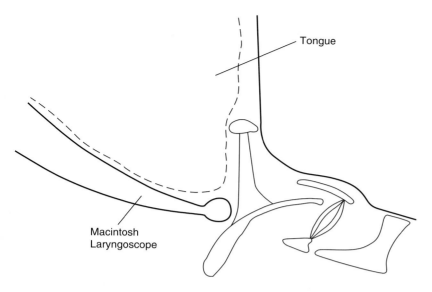

Tongue

Macintosh
Laryngoscope

Figure 12.9. Epiglottis, tongue and laryngeal cartilages when the tip of the Macintosh laryngoscope cannot be positioned in the vallecula. It has not proved possible to displace the base of the tongue to the left of the laryngoscope so that it is trapped between the laryngoscope and the hyoid. The epiglottis is not elevated but is displaced into the LOS. This situation is sometimes erroneously described as 'anterior larynx' or 'floppy epiglottis'.

(Figure 12.9), it is impossible to elevate the epiglottis and to obtain a view of the larynx. The terms 'anterior larynx' and 'floppy epiglottis' are sometimes used erroneously in this situation. Anatomical causes of difficulty with laryngoscopy include limited mouth opening, awkward dentition, macroglossia, hypoplastic or narrow mandible, impaired TMJ function and limited head extension. Pathological causes include lesions of the vallecula or epiglottis, particularly lingual tonsil hypertrophy. A final common pathway of difficulty with the Macintosh laryngoscope may be failure to displace the base of the tongue laterally so that the tip of the laryngoscope fails to enter the vallecula and instead displaces the epiglottis further into the line of sight. Indirect elevation of the epiglottis, the novel feature of the Macintosh technique, is also its fundamental flaw.

There are two important variations on the Macintosh laryngoscope (Figure 12.10). The McCoy laryngoscope uses a lever to flex the tip of the laryngoscope blade. It can improve the view of some Grade 2–3 patients. The left-entry Macintosh laryngoscope is designed for insertion into the left of the mouth. It can be useful in patients with missing upper left maxillary teeth.

Blind tracheal intubation with the Macintosh laryngoscope

Blind use of an introducer ('bougie') with an angulated tip has long been a standard technique of tracheal tube

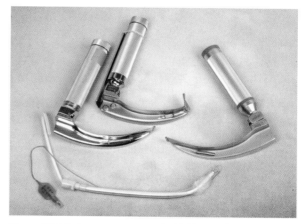

Figure 12.10. Laryngoscopes used with Macintosh technique. Left to right are: Standard Macintosh (size 4), McCoy with tip elevated and left-entry Macintosh. The styleted tracheal tube has been preformed in the shape of an ice-hockey stick. The stylet must be plastic coated and must not protrude beyond the tip of the tracheal tube. This shape can help to guide the tip of the tube to the larynx. Use of a stylet when the larynx is not seen may be more traumatic and less reliable than use of an introducer such as the Eschmann and is not recommended.

passage when the larynx cannot be seen with the Macintosh laryngoscope. The Macintosh laryngoscope is kept in the midline. The larynx should lie behind the epiglottis. The introducer is curved so that it should pass behind the epiglottis and then come anteriorly to pass between the vocal cords. It is passed gently from a position lateral to the midline. The most useful signs of passage into the trachea are a sensation of clicks as the introducer hits the tracheal cartilages

115

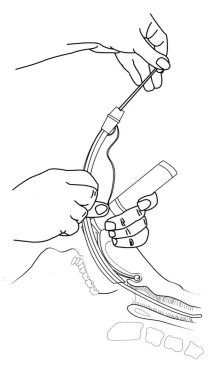

Figure 12.11.
Passage ('railroading') of a tracheal tube over an introducer. The Macintosh laryngoscope has been kept in the optimum position. The assistant holds the proximal end of the introducer while the anaesthetist advances the tube. (Reproduced with permission from *Management des schwierigen Atemwegs*, Dörges und Paschen, Eds., 2004, Springer Verlag.)

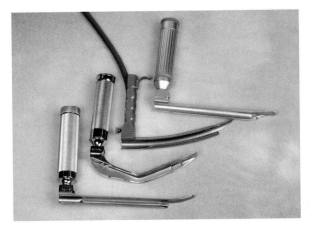

Figure 12.12. Laryngoscopes used with paraglossal straight laryngoscopy technique. Left to right: Miller, Belscope, Piquet-Crinquette-Vilette (PCV) and Henderson. Although the PCV has a gentle curve, it is possible to obtain a LOS through the lumen. The PCV and Henderson have a semi-tubular cross-section to facilitate passage of the tracheal tube.

and increased resistance to passage ('hold-up') when the tip reaches the carina; these signs should always be sought. Their detection is more likely with a gentle technique. The tracheal tube is then passed over the introducer ('railroaded') into the trachea (Figure 12.11). The laryngoscope position is maintained to create the most direct route and highest success rate and the tube is rotated 90 degrees anticlockwise (bevel down) if there is resistance to passage. Use of a narrow tracheal tube facilitates railroading.

A high success rate for the blind introducer technique has been claimed but such reports rarely include the number or duration of attempts. Blind techniques carry a risk of failure and of tissue trauma. The risk of blind techniques is particularly high when the cause is an undiagnosed laryngeal lesion. Multiple blind attempts at tracheal intubation are associated with morbidity and mortality. The number should be limited to three and ideally be zero. Eventual blind tracheal intubation after several attempts should be regarded not as a success but a 'near miss' and some centres do not use blind techniques. There is now evidence of high success rates with the straight laryngoscope, flexible fibreoptic laryngoscope and rigid

indirect laryngoscope when the Macintosh technique fails. If a few attempts with alternative techniques are not successful, elective surgery should be postponed and subsequent awake flexible fibreoptic intubation performed. Use of a supraglottic airway device (SAD) instead of tracheal intubation for elective surgery in such patients places them at risk if the SAD malfunctions.

Straight laryngoscope (paraglossal technique)

Direct laryngoscopy with the straight laryngoscope (Figure 12.12) was the first technique (Elsberg, 1910) to allow tracheal intubation under vision. Factors which contribute to the better view achieved with the straight laryngoscope (in comparison with the Macintosh laryngoscope) are more effective displacement of the tongue from the LOS and more reliable elevation of the epiglottis (Figure 12.13). There is much evidence from prospective studies and case series of the greater efficacy of the straight than the Macintosh laryngoscope. The straight laryngoscope may have particular niche roles in patients with lesions in the region of the vallecula or epiglottis, hypoplastic mandible and in patients with a gap in the right upper dentition (Figure 12.14). The technique is different from the Macintosh technique and effort and commitment are required for its mastery. Differences from the Macintosh technique will be highlighted.

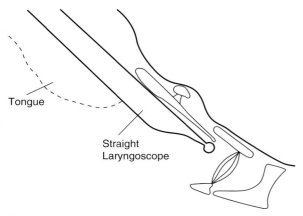

Figure 12.13. Management of tongue, epiglottis and laryngeal cartilages with the straight laryngoscope. In comparison with the Macintosh laryngoscope, tongue control is better and elevation of the epiglottis more reliable.

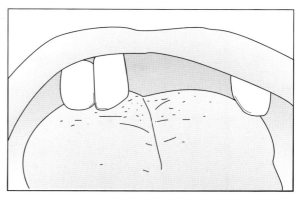

Figure 12.14. Dental pattern associated with difficulty with the Macintosh laryngoscope. Passage of the straight laryngoscope through the upper right gap in dentition is usually straightforward and effective.

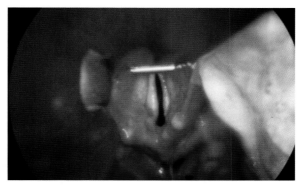

Figure 12.16. View achieved with the straight laryngoscope. The tip is posterior to the epiglottis and close to the anterior commissure. In some patients, the right aryepiglottic fold overlies the right vocal cord to some extent when the laryngoscope is passed from the side of the mouth.

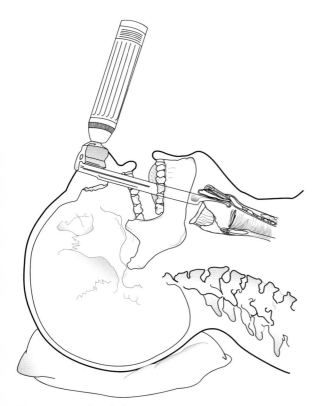

Figure 12.15. Straight laryngoscope in optimum position. The laryngoscope is positioned in the right side of the mouth. Maximum mouth opening has been achieved by rotation and advancement of the mandible at the temporo-mandibular joint. The tongue has been displaced to the left of the laryngoscope. The tip of the laryngoscope is posterior to the epiglottis and close to the anterior commissure of the vocal cords.

Maximum head extension facilitates insertion of the laryngoscope and ensures minimal contact with the maxillary teeth. The laryngoscope is inserted to the right of the midline and passed along the paraglossal gutter to the right side of the tongue. The laryngoscope is kept to the right of midline and may be moved further laterally when laryngoscopy proves difficult. The tip of the laryngoscope is passed posterior to the epiglottis, and sufficient lifting force is applied to achieve maximum elevation of the epiglottis (Figure 12.15). The tip should finish close to the anterior commissure of the larynx (Figure 12.16), so that an inadvertent backward movement of the laryngoscope will not result in loss of elevation of the epiglottis. This position may also facilitate passage of the tracheal tube. If the vocal

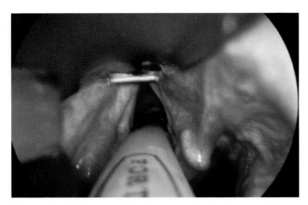

Figure 12.17. Visual confirmation of tracheal intubation with the straight laryngoscope.

cords are not seen, bimanual laryngoscopy is the key manoeuvre. If the vocal cords are still not seen, it is likely that the laryngoscope tip is in the right pyriform fossa and the combination of rightward movement of the larynx and leftward rotation of the laryngoscope tip will bring the latter behind the epiglottis. If the tip lies in the oesophagus (deliberate passage into the oesophagus is not recommended), it will be posterior to the cricoid cartilage and the hand on the larynx senses rolling of the larynx on the tip of the blade.

The tracheal tube is passed when the optimum view of the larynx has been achieved. Tube passage can be awkward with the Miller laryngoscope, but is preferable to blind intubation with the Macintosh laryngoscope. When learning the technique or if an incomplete view of the larynx is achieved, an introducer should be passed into the trachea under vision, with subsequent railroading of the tube. Use of stylet to achieve slight angulation of the tube tip helps negotiate around the flange of the Miller laryngoscope and is useful when a good view of the larynx is achieved. Blind passage of an introducer is not recommended with the paraglossal straight laryngoscopy technique. Verification of the tracheal tube position (Figure 12.17), cuff inflation and securing the tube are identical to the Macintosh technique.

Role of alternative techniques

Many alternative techniques can facilitate tracheal intubation under vision in patients in whom this is not possible with direct laryngoscopy. Expertise in at least one alternative visual technique should be acquired and skills maintained; the necessary equipment should be available. Alternative visual techniques of particular

value include rigid indirect laryngoscopes (Chapter 15) and flexible fibreoptic intubation through conduits such as SADs (Chapter 13). Anaesthetists with these skills should not need to use blind techniques, and tracheal intubation under vision should be achieved in most patients within a couple of attempts.

Nasotracheal intubation

Nasotracheal intubation is necessary when the oral route is not available. Nasotracheal tubes are longer and narrower than the oral tube which would be used in any particular patient. Immediate risks include nasal trauma, haemorrhage and submucosal passage of the tube in the nasopharynx, the latter sometimes leading to pharyngitis. The cuff may be damaged. Nasotracheal intubation may not be possible in some patients with narrow nasal passages. The nasal route should be used in patients with a history (old or new) of basal skull fracture *only* if there is no alternative. A history of trans-sphenoidal pituitary surgery is a contraindication to blind passage of a nasal tube.

The risk of damage to nasal polyps and turbinates can be reduced by passage through the nasal cavity under vision (flexible fibreoptic laryngoscope) but traditional techniques of nasotracheal intubation are still widely used. Whenever possible, the nasal mucosa should be shrunk with a vasoconstrictor before induction of anaesthesia.

Rowbotham and Magill (1921) developed the technique of blind nasal intubation in the patient breathing spontaneously. Deep inhalational anaesthesia was used originally but the technique can be performed in the awake patient under topical anaesthesia. Advancement of the tracheal tube is guided by changes in breath sounds at the proximal end of the tube (amplification by a whistle can be very helpful) and by palpation of the neck. Blind nasal intubation may still be useful when flexible fibreoptic laryngoscopy fails or is not available. Blind nasal intubation in the apnoeic patient has a low success rate and its use is not recommended in the patient undergoing elective surgery.

Nasotracheal intubation is most frequently performed after administration of intravenous anaesthetic and paralysis of the patient. A long narrow cuffed tube (not larger than 7.5 mm for males and 7.0 mm for females) is warmed before use. Passage should be performed gently. The tube is passed along the floor of the nasal cavity. Passage of a soft catheter through the nasopharynx, over which the tracheal tube is then passed, can reduce the risk of submucosal passage of the tube. Gentle rotation of a narrower tube or use of the other nasal cavity should be considered if there is resistance to passage. The tube is advanced between the palate and posterior pharyngeal wall, towards the larynx.

A laryngoscope (direct or indirect) is used to facilitate nasotracheal intubation under vision and it should be positioned once the tube tip has reached the oropharynx. Head extension may be used to bring the tip of the tracheal tube anteriorly. Further advancement of the tracheal tube may be facilitated by head and neck flexion, which aligns the axis of the tip of the tube with that of the trachea. An alternative technique is to use Magill forceps to grasp the tracheal tube (avoiding the cuff) and guide it into the trachea. An assistant then advances the tube.

Key points

- Quantify and record an airway assessment for every patient before induction of anaesthesia.
- Do not use muscle relaxants or narcotics if you suspect any problems with tracheal intubation, mask ventilation or rescue techniques.
- Assemble suitable equipment and personnel before inducing anaesthesia.
- The first attempt at tracheal intubation should be the best.
- Always check and optimise: head extension, mouth opening, tongue control, lifting force and ELM.
- Always optimise the view of the larynx before passing the tracheal tube under vision.
- When the introducer is used blindly, be gentle in order to minimise the risk of trauma and to facilitate verification of tracheal position. No more than three attempts should be made.
- Develop a good range of airway skills. The Macintosh laryngoscope, introducer and laryngeal mask are not enough for every patient.
- The straight laryngoscope offers unique advantages and there is good evidence of its value.
- Nasotracheal intubation may cause trauma. It should be performed gently, ideally under fibreoptic control.

Acknowledgements

Michelle McNicol created the drawings in this chapter.

Further reading

Achen B, Terblanche OC, Finucane BT. (2008). View of the larynx obtained using the Miller blade and paraglossal approach, compared to that with the Macintosh blade. *Anaesthesia and Intensive Care*, **36**, 717–721.

Asai T, Liu EH, Matsumoto S, et al. (2009). Use of the Pentax-AWS in 293 patients with difficult airways. *Anesthesiology*, **110**, 898–904.

Bennett JA, Abrams JT, Van Riper DF, Horrow JC. (1997). Difficult or impossible ventilation after sufentanil-induced anesthesia is caused primarily by vocal cord closure. *Anesthesiology*, **87**, 1070–1074.

Cook TM. (2000). A new practical classification of laryngeal view. *Anaesthesia*, **55**, 274–279.

Felten ML, Schmautz E, Delaporte-Cerceau S, Orliaguet GA, Carli PA. (2003). Endotracheal tube cuff pressure is unpredictable in children. *Anesthesia and Analgesia*, **97**, 1612–1616.

Heidegger T, Gerig HJ, Ulrich B, Kreienbuhl G. (2001). Validation of a simple algorithm for tracheal intubation: Daily practice is the key to success in emergencies–an analysis of 13,248 intubations. *Anesthesia and Analgesia*, **92**, 517–522.

Henderson J. (2009). Airway management in the adult. In: Miller R, Eriksson L, Fleisher L, Wiener-Kronish J, Young W (Eds.), *Miller's Anesthesia*. Philadelphia: Elsevier.

Henderson JJ. (2000). Questions about the Macintosh laryngoscope and technique of laryngoscopy. *European Journal of Anaesthesiology*, **17**, 2–5.

Horton WA, Fahy L, Charters P. (1990). Factor analysis in difficult tracheal intubation: Laryngoscopy-induced airway obstruction. *British Journal of Anaesthesia*, **65**, 801–805.

Lee L, Weightman WM. (2008). Laryngoscopy force in the sniffing position compared to the extension-extension position. *Anaesthesia*, **63**, 375–378.

Mencke T, Echternach M, Kleinschmidt S, et al. (2003). Laryngeal morbidity and quality of tracheal intubation: A randomized controlled trial. *Anesthesiology*, **98**, 1049–1056.

Ovassapian A, Glassenberg R, Randel GI, Klock A, Mesnick PS, Klafta JM. (2002). The unexpected difficult airway and lingual tonsil hyperplasia: A case series and a review of the literature. *Anesthesiology*, **97**, 124–132.

Peterson GN, Domino KB, Caplan RA, Posner KL, Lee LA, Cheney FW. (2005). Management of the difficult airway: A closed claims analysis. *Anesthesiology,* **103**, 33–39.

Semjen F, Bordes M, Cros AM. (2008). Intubation of infants with Pierre Robin syndrome: The use of the paraglossal approach combined with a gum-elastic bougie in six consecutive cases. *Anaesthesia,* **63**, 147–150.

Shiga T, Wajima Z, Inoue T, Sakamoto A. (2005). Predicting difficult intubation in apparently normal patients: A meta-analysis of bedside screening test performance. *Anesthesiology,* **103**, 429–437.

Chapter 13

Tracheal intubation: flexible fibreoptic

Mridula Rai and Mansukh Popat

The first fibreoptic guided tracheal intubation was described by Dr Peter Murphy in 1967 while he was a registrar at the National Hospital, Queen Square, London. He was inspired by an article in the *Lancet*, which described the use of a flexible choledochoscope to view the bile duct and used a similar instrument to intubate the trachea. Since then the flexible fibrescope has revolutionised the management of patients with known anatomical difficulties in tracheal intubation and is a widely practiced technique, which every anaesthetist should attempt to master.

The instrument has many characteristics which make it an 'ideal' intubating device (Table 13.1).

A successful fibreoptic intubation is an interplay of several factors, which are detailed below:

- Understanding the equipment
- Learning basic manipulations and hand eye coordination
- Mastering upper airway endoscopy
- Tube selection and railroading techniques.

Understanding flexible fibreoptic equipment

The modern day flexible fibreoptic scope consists of the following parts (Figure 13.1).

Body: This is held in the palm of either hand, the thumb of the same hand is used to manipulate the control lever and the index finger to activate the working channel. The control lever is pressed down to move the tip of the scope anteriorly and vice versa. The conical connection between the body and the insertion cord facilitates loading of a tracheal tube.

The body has an eye piece which can be focused by a diopter ring to produce a sharp image.

Table 13.1. Characteristics of flexible fibreoptic instruments that make them ideal intubating devices

1. Flexibility conforms easily to normal and difficult airway anatomy
2. Continuous visualisation of airway during endoscopy
3. Less traumatic than rigid laryngoscopes
4. Latest equipment is lightweight and portable
5. Can be used with other intubating techniques (e.g., direct laryngoscopy)
6. Can be used with ventilatory devices (e.g., LMA)
7. Can be used for oral or nasal intubation
8. Can be used on patients of all age groups
9. Can be used in asleep or in awake patients
10. Definitive check of tube position in trachea
11. Ability to use camera and monitor for teaching

On looking down the eye piece a pointer is seen which helps to orient the operator to the anterior direction of the tip. The body also has a port which can be used for suction or to instill drugs or oxygen down the working channel of the scope.

Insertion cord: This is the part of the scope which is advanced into the trachea and acts as a flexible guide to railroad the tube and facilitate intubation. Its outer diameter determines the size of the smallest tracheal tube that can be easily passed over it. This is usually 1 mm greater than the diameter of the insertion cord, e.g., most adult scopes with insertion cord diameter of 4 mm will allow a tracheal tube of 5 mm or larger to easily pass over it. It is 55–60 cm long to allow railroading of the tracheal tube once its tip is positioned in the trachea.

Core Topics in Airway Management, Second Edition, ed. Ian Calder and Adrian Pearce. Published by Cambridge University Press.
© Cambridge University Press 2011.

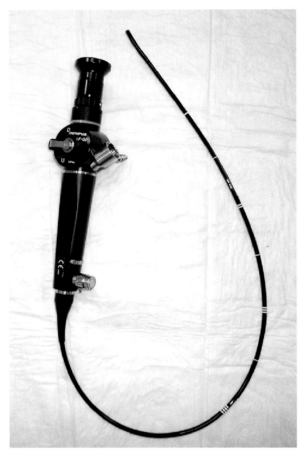

Figure 13.1. A modern intubating fibreoptic laryngoscope (Olympus LF2). The tracheal tube is mounted on the long insertion cord and the length of the cord allows access to the trachea before starting railroading of the tube.

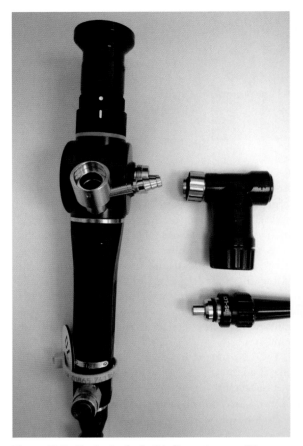

Figure 13.2. The body of a flexible fibreoptic scope (Olympus LF-GP). The battery casing and light guide cable are interchangeable.

The insertion cord contains the image and light transmitting fibreoptic bundles. The image transmitting bundle is coherent and contains around 8000–10 000 fibres.

The insertion cord also contains the working channel which extends proximally from the working channel port in the body of the fibrescope to the tip at its distal end. The working channel facilitates suction, instillation of drugs and oxygen and passage of guide wires. The power of the suction depends on the diameter of this channel. A typical adult scope has a 1.5 mm channel, which is adequate but not very powerful.

Light source: Fibrescopes are powered by an external light source, usually a halogen lamp enclosed in a casing. This is connected to the body by a light guide cable. Modern scopes also have an interchangeable battery casing that replaces the light guide cable

and contains a lithium battery that can last for about 60 minutes (Figure 13.2).

A simple flick of the battery casing acts as an on-off switch. This arrangement affords versatility and portability to the equipment. It should be possible to move, within a very short time, the fibrescope from one operating theatre to another, to the intensive care unit or to the trauma room where it can be used in an emergency.

Camera and monitor: A camera and monitor facilitates training in fibreoptic endoscopy and intubation. The camera control unit (CCU) is the 'box' to which is connected a camera lead. The other end of the camera lead has a camera head that is connected to the eyepiece of the fibrescope. The CCU is powered by the fibreoptic light source and receives signals from the camera lead which are then transmitted to a closed circuit television (CCTV) monitor (Figure 13.3).

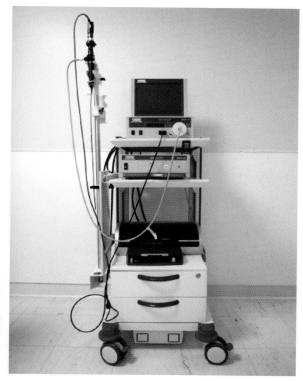

Figure 13.3. The flexible fibreoptic scope connected to a camera control unit which transmits images to a closed circuit television monitor.

Setting up fibreoptic equipment

Example of a simple checklist for fibreoptic equipment:

- Ensure that the fibrescope has been cleaned and disinfected before every use.
- Check the mechanical function by ensuring the tip moves in the appropriate direction when the control lever is moved and that there is no slack between the control lever and tip motion.
- Attach the suction catheter to the working channel port and ensure that the suction works when the suction valve is activated.
- Plug the light guide cable to the light source and switch it on.
- Defog the lens by wiping it with an alcohol swab.
- Keep the tip of the fibrescope at about 1 cm from an object (usually a letter on a machine) and adjust the diopter ring so that a clear sharp image appears in the eyepiece.
- Lubricate the insertion cord (but not the tip), load the tracheal tube on the conical

section of the body and secure it with a small piece of tape.
- The fibrescope is now ready to use.

The following steps are relevant if a CCU is used with the fibrescope:

- Check connections between CCTV and CCU and at the mains and switch on the CCTV.
- Switch on the CCU and connect it to the fibrescope with the camera cable.
- Adjust the orientation mark (e.g., 12 o'clock) and lock the camera head onto the fibrescope.
- Adjust the diopter ring on the camera head for final focusing so that a sharp image is focused on the CCTV monitor.
- Perform white balance.

The above description is for the most basic CCU and CCTV. The anaesthetist must familiarise himself/herself with the camera equipment by following the manufacturer's instructions.

Learning basic manipulations and hand eye coordination skills

Holding the fibrescope

The endoscopist holds the body of the fibrescope in the palm of one hand (left or right) and the insertion cord with the thumb and index finger of the other hand. The thumb of the hand that holds the body manipulates the control lever and its index finger activates the working channel when required. The insertion cord is held straight and taut at all times (Figure 13.4).

If the insertion cord is allowed to bow or become slack then rotation movements of the body will not be effectively transmitted to the tip of the fibrescope.

Manipulating the tip of the fibrescope

There are three ways in which an endoscopist can manipulate the tip of the fibrescope towards the desired target (Figure 13.5). These are advancement (or withdrawal), tip deflection and rotation. Advancing the whole fibrescope moves it towards the target. Sometimes withdrawal is required if the fibrescope has been advanced too far. The control lever on the body moves the tip of the fibrescope in a vertical plane (anteriorly or posteriorly) only. When the control lever is pressed down the tip bends anteriorly

(a)

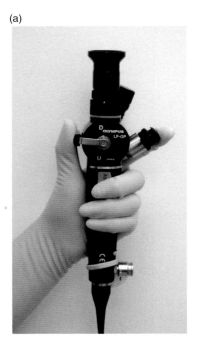

(b)

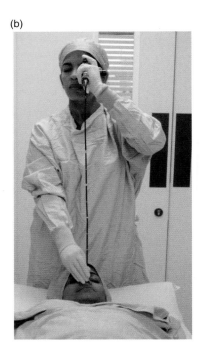

Figure 13.4. (a) The body of the fibreoptic scope is held in the palm of one hand. The thumb manipulates the control lever and the index finger can be used to activate the suction channel. (b) The insertion cord is held straight and taut at all times.

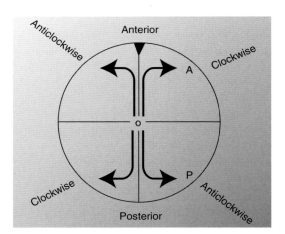

Figure 13.5. Two- dimensional illustration of tip manipulation. The visual field is represented by a circle with four quadrants. The orientation marker is at the 12 o'clock position. Anterior tip deflection and rotation of the body in the clockwise direction are required to move the tip of the fibrescope from O (neutral position) to target A and posterior tip deflection with anticlockwise rotation of the body will move the tip from O to target P.

are achieved by rotation of the body of the fibrescope towards the target while maintaining tip deflection. In practice, a good endoscopy technique involves performing the three basic manipulations simultaneously in order to bring the tip of the fibrescope towards the target. When viewed in the eyepiece or on the monitor, an orientation marker indicates the direction (clockwise or anticlockwise) in which the tip is moving.

Learning manual dexterity and hand eye coordination on models

During fibreoptic endoscopy the 'eye' is at the objective lens in the tip of the fibrescope, unlike direct laryngoscopy, where the movement of the laryngoscope handle and blade are observed with the naked eye. Hence mastering fibreoptic skills requires not only a thorough understanding of the working principles of the instrument but a lot of practice in manipulation skills. Initial practice is best gained on teaching models. Several types of models are available but the main objective is to give the operator a chance to understand how the different manipulations at the

(or away from the endoscopist), and when the control lever is moved up the tip faces posteriorly (or towards the endoscopist). The sideways movements of the tip

(a)

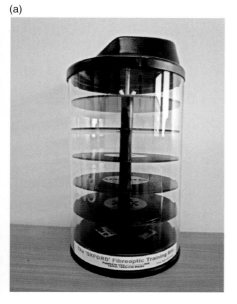

(b)

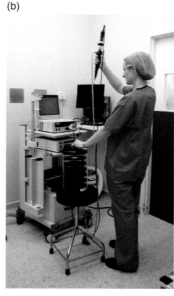

Figure 13.6. (a) The 'Oxford' Fibreoptic Teaching Box. (b) A trainee practising fibreoptic manipulation skills on the Oxford box in the anaesthetic room.

body of the fibrescope are translated to the tip. An indication of achieving perfect manual dexterity and hand eye coordination is a state when one is not consciously thinking of the manipulations while performing them. The mind does the job. It is like learning to drive a car where initially one has to think each time and then the movements become reflex. It is important to thoroughly master these skills on teaching boxes and models before using a fibreoptic scope on patients. The common models used for teaching fibreoptic manipulation skills are the various 'hit the hole' boxes. We have developed one such device, the 'Oxford' Fibreoptic Teaching Box (Figure 13.6).

Position of the endoscopist and the patient

The anaesthetist should be comfortable when performing fibreoptic endoscopy. A platform must be used instead of standing on tip-toe and trying to get enough height to keep the insertion cord straight. If this is not done, then fatigue of the arms will rapidly ensue and inevitably the insertion cord will slacken and bow. A common problem is of the operator moving his/her own body rather than the body of the fibrescope! Although entertaining to onlookers, this should be avoided.

The operator may choose to stand behind the head or in front of or on either side of the patient while facing them. The patient may be supine or lying on the side or sitting upright. Some endoscopists strongly advocate standing at the side of the patient for both awake and asleep intubations.

Mastering upper airway endoscopy

Fibreoptic endoscopy involves guiding the tip of the fibrescope from the nose or the mouth into the trachea under continuous vision. Both nasal and oral endoscopy and intubation can be performed with the operator standing at the head end of the patient (commonly used in anaesthetised supine patients) or facing the patient (commonly used for awake patients in the semi-sitting or upright position). It is important to appreciate the differences in the observed anatomy in the two positions and also as seen through an eyepiece or on the monitor.

Nasotracheal fibreoptic endoscopy

The nose is very vascular and needs to be prepared with a topical vasoconstrictor solution prior to endoscopy, e.g., xylometazoline or ephedrine nasal drops. Awake patients need a combination of local anaesthetic and vasoconstrictor such as cocaine or lignocaine with phenylephrine.

Tips for performing nasopharyngeal endoscopy (See Figure 13.7)

- Check the orientation of the image displayed is correct *before* entering the nostril.
- Insert the tip of the scope just inside each nostril (anterior rhinoscopy) and select the more patent nostril (Figure 13.7).
- Gently advance the tip of the scope and identify the triangular airspace bounded by the inferior turbinate, nasal septum and the floor of the nose.
- Follow the airspace, which generally gets bigger as the scope is advanced towards the nasopharynx until the posterior pharyngeal wall can be seen.
- In anaesthetised patients a jaw thrust is required at this point to open the airspace as the scope enters the oropharynx. The soft palate (and sometimes the uvula) and base of tongue come into view and the epiglottis can be seen at a distance.
- The tip is directed underneath the epiglottis and a full view of the laryngeal inlet is seen.
- The scope is advanced through the glottic opening into the trachea where the tracheal rings are identified and advanced to bring the carina into view.

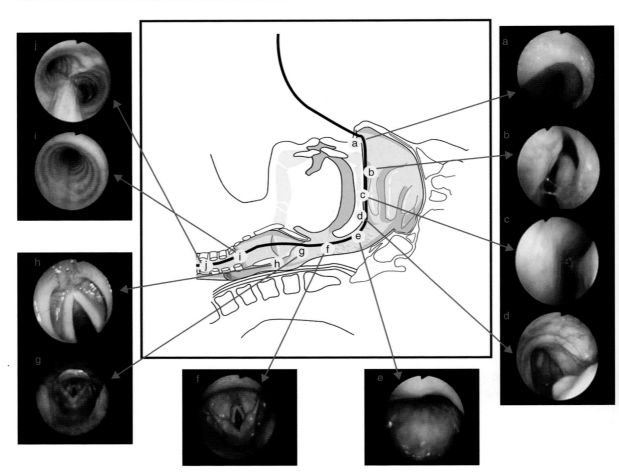

Figure 13.7. (centre) Upper airway anatomy during nasotracheal fibreoptic endoscopy. The endoscopist is standing behind a supine patient. (a) The right nostril is selected. (b) The tip of the fibrescope is advanced in the triangular space bounded by the nasal septum (left) inferior turbinate (bottom) and the lateral wall of the nose (right) of the visual field. (c) The fibrescope tip above the inferior turbinate which is to the right of the visual field. (d) The posterior opening of the nasal cavity is indicated by the disappearance of the inferior turbinate (at the 5 o'clock) position. The posterior pharyngeal wall is seen at the centre of the visual field. (e) The soft palate is seen in the upper part and the base of the tongue in the lower part. (f) Epiglottis in view. (g) Laryngeal inlet with vocal folds, vocal cords, cuneiform and corniculate cartilages. (h) True and false vocal cords. (i) Trachea with tracheal rings. (j) Carina with openings of right and left main bronchi.

Orotracheal fibreoptic endoscopy

The bigger airspace in the oral cavity makes it difficult to keep the fibrescope in the midline. The angle to the glottis is also more acute and can make negotiation of the tip of the scope difficult. These problems are overcome by using an oral 'route guide' such as the Berman, Ovassapian, VBM oropharyngeal airway or an LMA. The Berman Airway is the most commonly used device in the UK and is available in three adult sizes (Figure 13.8).

The fibreoptic scope is passed through the tubular stem of the airway and the epiglottis is visualised. The scope is advanced further through the glottis into the trachea and the tube railroaded. The Berman Airway can then be 'peeled' off (Figure 13.9).

In the awake patient the airway also serves to prevent the patient biting on the scope and causing damage. In practice we find that because of its length the Berman airway almost always causes gagging in the awake patient. We find that this problem can be overcome by cutting the distal 1 to 1.5 cm of the Berman airway.

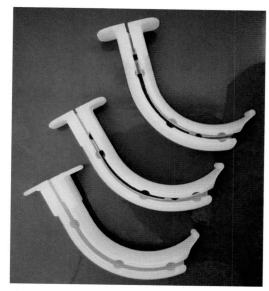

Figure 13.8. Berman Airway.

Tips for performing oropharyngeal endoscopy
- Insert the tip into the mouth and advance the scope keeping the tip in the midline.
- The tongue is seen on the top of the screen and the hard palate at the bottom.
- Jaw thrust and/or lingual traction may be required to keep the airspace open in anaesthetised patients, and the epiglottis is seen at a distance and then, as the scope is advanced, the laryngeal inlet comes into view.
- From this point the procedure is similar to that described in nasopharyngeal endoscopy.

Tracheal tube selection and railroading

The final stage of fibreoptic intubation involves railroading the tracheal tube and removing the fibrescope from the tube. Failure is likely to occur due to impingement of the tube tip on anatomical structures (usually the arytenoid cartilages) in its passage. Certain features may decrease the incidence of impingement and improve the success rate of fibreoptic intubation. These are as follows.

Size of tracheal tube: Relative to the size of the scope. The larger the gap between the insertion cord and the tube the higher will be the rate of impingement. There is a tendency to select a larger size of tracheal tube for the oral route which may explain a higher reported rate of impingement for the oral as compared to the nasal route.

Design of the tube: Certain tracheal tubes such as the ILMA tube and the Gliderite® are easier to pass as the tip is tapered and does not have a bevel edge. Softer flexible tubes such as flexometallics are preferable to rigid standard tubes (Figure 13.10).

We prefer to use preformed north facing blue Portex RAE 6.0 to 6.5 mm internal diameter (ID) for nasal (if using standard Portex tracheal tubes we warm the tube in sterile normal saline just before loading it on the scope to make it more flexible) and 6.5 to 7 mm flexometallic tubes for oral fibreoptic intubation.

Technique of railroading: Railroading is started once the tip of the scope is within 2–3 cm of the carina. The tracheal tube is usually loaded with the tip of the tube facing the right side or 3 o'clock (neutral position). If there is any resistance (impingement) to advancement of the tube, withdraw the tube back by 1–2 cm and rotate 90 degrees anticlockwise and advance again (Figure 13.11). This will bring the tip of the tube to the 12 o'clock position and the bevel to the 6 o'clock position and allow it to enter the trachea. In practice one can load the tube onto the fibrescope with the tip pre-rotated by 90 degrees anticlockwise as this is associated with lower incidence of impingement than the neutral position.

Once the tube is in the trachea, gently pinch the insertion cord with thumb and forefinger and withdraw the scope until the tip of the tube is visible.

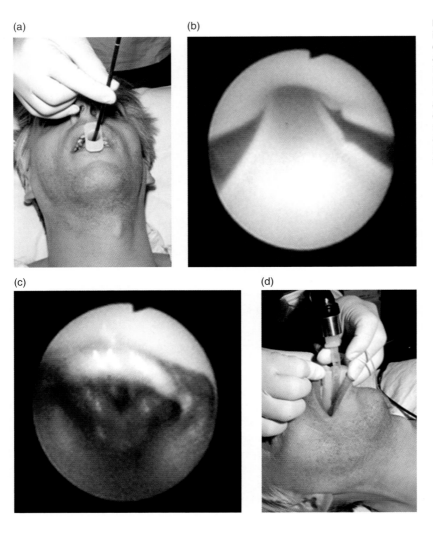

(a)

(b)

(c)

(d)

Figure 13.9. (a) Oral fibreoptic intubation using a Berman airway. The endoscopist is standing behind a supine anaesthetised patient. The fibrescope is inserted through the lumen of the Berman airway. (b) (Internal view) Fibrescope tip in the lumen of the Berman airway. (c) (Internal view) Fibrescope exiting the lumen. The upper flange is seen lifting the epiglottis. (d) The Berman airway is peeled off once the tube has been railroaded over the fibrescope into the trachea.

This will give an estimate of the distance between the tip of the tube and the carina, which should ideally be 3–4 cm. If required adjust the length of the tube in the trachea under vision. Withdraw the scope. Connect the tube to the anaesthetic circuit, and confirm position by capnograph and auscultation.

Clinical application of flexible fibreoptic techniques in difficult airway management

Anticipated difficult airway

Flexible fibreoptic intubation has revolutionised the management of patients with known anatomical airway difficulties. Patients with anatomic abnormalities of the head, neck or upper airway, resulting from surgery, radiation, burn scars, tumours, trauma, infection, arthritis and diseases such as scleroderma and acromegaly can be some of the most difficult to intubate with direct laryngoscopy. In the patient with a known/anticipated difficult airway it is considered the gold standard to secure the airway by awake intubation. Almost all patients, even those in the advanced stages of the conditions listed above, have the ability to breathe when awake. It is only when anaesthesia is induced that airway obstruction becomes a problem and manoeuvres involving the laryngoscope prove to be of restricted use. The logical conclusion is that induction of anaesthesia poses a risk to these patients, and therefore securing the airway while the patients are awake is preferable.

Advantages of awake tracheal intubation
- The natural airway is preserved, spontaneous breathing allows adequate ventilation.
- The airway is relatively protected from aspiration of gastric contents.
- Cardiovascular stability.
- Neurological monitoring may be possible after intubation.
- Good for your coronaries!

Although other airway instruments can be used to secure the airway in awake patients, a flexible scope has significant advantages. These are shown in the Table 13.2.

The safety and efficacy of flexible fibreoptic intubation for awake intubation has been confirmed in many of these scenarios. It must be remembered that operator inexperience is an absolute contraindication for this technique, and the presence of blood and secretions is a relative contraindication. In the patient with obstructed airway, there is concern

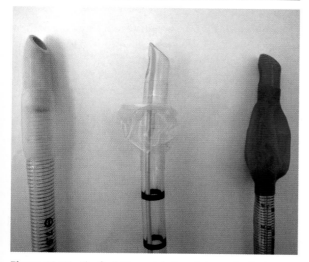

Figure 13.10. The flexibility and design of the tracheal tube influence railroading. The dedicated ILMA tube (left) and flexometallic tube (right) are better suited for railroading than a standard tube (centre).

Table 13.2. Advantages of the flexible fibreoptic scope for awake intubation

1. Flexibility and continuous visualisation allows negotiation of even the most difficult anatomy
2. Can be used for oral and nasal intubation
3. Can be used with other devices such as the LMA/ILMA to aid intubation
4. Ability to apply local anaesthetic through the working channel
5. Immediate definitive tube position check
6. Applicable to all age groups
7. Excellent patient acceptability
8. Very high success rate

(a)

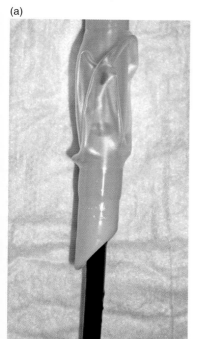

(b)

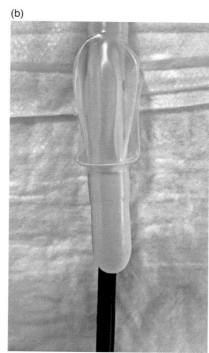

Figure 13.11. (a) Tracheal tube loaded onto the fibrescope in the neutral position. (b) Tracheal tune loaded onto the fibrescope pre-rotated 90 degrees anticlockwise.

that complete obstruction may occur in an already narrow lumen (a 'cork in the bottle' situation). For this reason some anaesthetists tend to avoid fibreoptic intubation in these patients, although an experienced anaesthetist with good endoscopy skills can use the fibreoptic scope to evaluate the airway and decide whether to proceed with intubation (if there is enough space) or ask the surgeon to perform awake surgical airway (if the space is too narrow).

Awake fibreoptic intubation may be desired but not feasible in adults who refuse the procedure, patients with learning disability or altered consciousness and in children. In these patients it is appropriate to try and secure the airway with a flexible fibreoptic scope while the patient is anaesthetised.

Unanticipated difficult airway

It is possible that direct larygoscopy and intubation may be difficult or fail after induction of anaesthesia. The Difficult Airway Society algorithm for unanticipated difficult intubation recommends using fibreoptic assisted LMA/ILMA intubation (Plan B). Experienced anaesthetists may also use the flexible fibreoptic scope as an alternative laryngoscope (Plan A) in the elective situation. A recommendation of Plan C is to awaken the patient, and if it is desired an 'awake' intubation may be performed facilitated with a flexible fibreoptic scope.

Practical fibreoptic techniques

- Awake fibreoptic intubation (oral or nasal)
- Asleep fibreoptic intubation
  - Direct (oral or nasal)
  - Fibreoptic assisted intubation through supraglottic devices (LMA, ILMA, i-gel)
  - Combined techniques
- Retrograde fibreoptic intubation

Awake fibreoptic intubation

Although 'awake' fibreoptic intubation (AFI) is the common terminology used, the patients are usually sedated and the airway is anaesthetised with local anaesthetic. This allows the patients to undergo fibreoptic assisted tracheal intubation with minimal discomfort or pain.

The following considerations are important in ensuring a successful awake fibreoptic intubation:

- Airway evaluation
- Back-up plan
- Explanation and consent
- Premedication
- Monitoring (also sedation)
- Oxygenation
- Conscious sedation
- Topical anaesthesia of the upper airway

Airway evaluation

Two questions need to be answered: Does the patient need an awake intubation? Is the awake fibreoptic intubation going to be easy or difficult?

In our experience of both performing and teaching over 800 awake fibreoptic intubations, we have made the following observations:

Patients with only bony anatomical problems: e.g., TMJ ankylosis, ankylosing spondylitis patients who are predicted to be difficult to intubate with conventional direct laryngoscopy are generally easy to intubate awake using the flexible fibreoptic scope (Figure 13.12)

Patients with some degree of soft tissue airway pathology, with or without bony abnormality but with no clinical signs and symptoms of upper airway obstruction: will generally be easy, but may occasionally be difficult due to presence of 'bulk' of tumour or as a result of previous surgery (Figure 13.13). Blood and secretions may be present and can make topical anaesthesia difficult. A novice operator may find these situations quite challenging.

Patients with soft tissue pathology and presenting with clinical signs of upper airway obstruction (stridor): are the most difficult. There is a real risk of complete airway obstruction (cork in the bottle situation) due to the narrowed airway. Each patient has to be assessed individually, and in some cases an awake fibreoptic intubation may be contraindicated. Sedation is ideally avoided, and the anaesthetist performing the procedure must be an accomplished 'endoscopist'.

Include a back-up plan

Never assume that an AFI will always be successful. It is vital to have a back-up plan. This may involve utilising the expertise of a senior colleague or a surgeon.

Explanation and consent

We find it is useful to explain to the patient what intubation is, why is it indicated and how would it

(a)

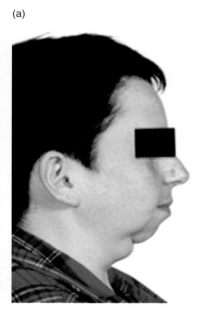

(b)

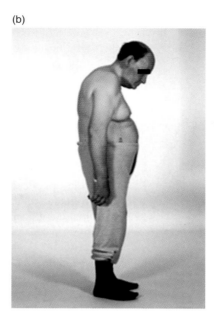

Figure 13.12. Anticipated difficult intubation: Bony deformities. (a) Patient with Stills disease that required an awake oral fibreoptic intubation to secure the airway prior to induction of general anaesthesia. (b) Patient with ankylosing spondylitis and severe spinal flexion deformity.

usually be performed in a patient with a normal airway. Then explain the difficulties that would result if intubation were to be performed after induction of anaesthesia and the safety of an awake fibreoptic technique in their case. Reassure the patient that they do not have to be wide awake during the procedure but will be sedated and comfortable and that a significant proportion of patients have no recall of the event afterwards. The local anaesthetic technique is explained carefully, and the patient is warned that this will reduce the discomfort of the procedure but not provide complete numbness. It is also important to mention that railroading the tube may sometimes be uncomfortable. It is easy to liken the procedure to an upper gastrointestinal endoscopy (with which a lot of patients are familiar) emphasising that the intubating fibrescope is a much thinner tube. The patient is reassured that they will have a general anaesthetic once the tracheal tube is in place. This conversation not only is an explanation of the procedure but more importantly helps to establish a rapport with the patient. Formal consent for the procedure should always follow this discussion. Whether this consent is verbal or written depends on the local hospital policy.

Premedication

Antisialogogues such as hyoscine (0.2 mg IM) or glycopyrrolate (0.2 mg IM) can be given 1 hour prior to the procedure. A dry mouth ensures effective topical anaesthesia of the airway as a result of better contact between the mucosa and the local anaesthetic solution and may also improve the field of vision. Anxiolytic drugs such as temazepam and aspiration prophylaxis (ranitidine or omeprazole) may be indicated in some patients.

Monitoring

Standard anaesthetic monitoring must be applied in the form of continuous ECG, pulse oximetry and non-invasive blood pressure. A capnograph should always be available to check the position of the tube once intubation is complete.

The level of consciousness should be constantly monitored to obtain the desired level of conscious sedation. The goal of conscious sedation is a relaxed and calm patient who is able to respond appropriately to verbal commands or mild physical stimuli. Oversedation will lead to airway obstruction, hypoxia and cardio-respiratory depression. This may result in confusion, restlessness and an uncooperative patient. On the other hand under-sedation and inadequate topical anaesthesia may also cause patient discomfort and restlessness.

Oxygenation

It is important to administer oxygen to the patient during the procedure. During orotracheal fibreoptic

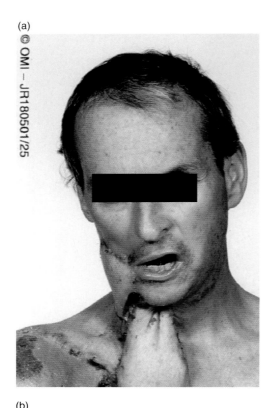

OMI – JR180501/25

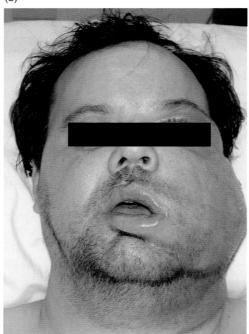

Figure 13.13. Anticipated difficult intubation: Soft tissue deformities. (a) Patient with limited mouth opening due to oral cancer surgery and radiotherapy and multiple free flap procedures. (b) A dental abscess resulting in soft tissue oedema and restricted mouth opening.

intubation, oxygen is best delivered by nasal specs. For nasotracheal fibreoptic intubation, we usually administer oxygen with an ordinary facemask while topical anaesthesia is being applied. After the nasal cavity is anaesthetised, we gently insert a suction catheter in one of the nostrils and connect it to the oxygen delivery tube. Some endoscopists prefer to deliver oxygen via the working channel of the fibrescope during endoscopy.

Conscious sedation

The aim of conscious sedation is to have a relaxed and cooperative patient who will reply to verbal commands and protect their airway. Several drugs such as midazolam, fentanyl, alfentanil, remifentanil and propofol can be used to achieve this goal. We recommend the use of Target Controlled Infusion (TCI) propofol 0.5–1.5 µg/ml or TCI remifentanil 3.0–3.5 ng/ml. TCI allows for easy titration and for a steady state of sedation. Propofol has the advantage of better amnesia and lower incidence of recall for the procedure especially if used in conjunction with a small dose of midazolam 1–2 mg while remifentanil has been shown to provide better conditions for intubation as it suppresses the gag and cough reflex. Over-sedation can result in an uncooperative and hypoxic patient with the potential for loss of the airway, and must be avoided at all costs.

Topical anaesthesia of the upper airway

Topical anaesthesia of the upper airway is central to any awake intubation technique (Figure 13.14). Nerve blocks have been described but are rarely used nowadays. Direct application of the local anaesthetic solution to the mucosa is a more commonly used technique. This can be applied directly through a syringe (lignocaine gel) or as a spray using either devices such as a Moffatiser or a Mackenzie spray.

Alternatively you can spray local anaesthetic through the working channel of the scope (spray as you go along technique, 'SAYGO') (Figure 13.15).

Lidocaine is relatively poorly absorbed (most of it is swallowed) from the nasopharynx. Doses of up to 9 mg/kg have been used (the British Thoracic Society recommends an upper limit of 8.2 mg/kg).

> Tips for performing an awake fibreoptic intubation
> - Secure IV access and commence full monitoring.
> - Administer oxygen via facemask or nasal specs as appropriate.

(a)

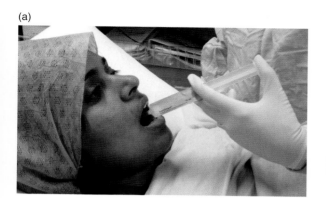

(b)

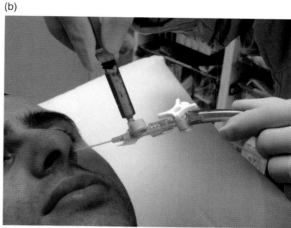

Figure 13.14. (a) Direct application of 2% lignocaine gel to oral cavity via syringe. (b) Direct application of local anaesthetic using a 20G Venflon catheter connected to green oxygen tubing (McKenzie spray technique). Oxygen flowing at 2–4 litres results in a fine jet spray and can be used to apply local anaesthetic to the mouth or nose.

(a)

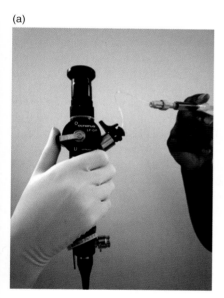

(b)

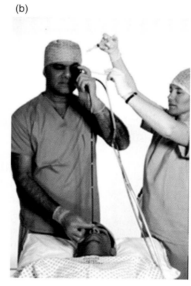

Figure 13.15. The SAYGO technique (spray as you go along). (a) Lignocaine 4% is drawn up in a 2-ml syringe and sprayed through a 16G epidural catheter previously fed through the working channel of the scope. (b) A trained assistant gently dribbles the local anaesthetic after advancing the tip of the epidural catheter beyond the tip of the scope.

- IV glycopyrrolate 0.2 mg +/− IV midazolam 1–2 mg if required.
- Start TCI propofol 0.5 µg/ml or remifentanil 3 ng/ml. Titrate the infusion in increments of 0.1–0.2 to achieve the desired level of sedation.
- Start topicalisation. We suggest 2 ml of cocaine 5% (100 mg) for the nose and lignocaine 4% for the oropharynx using a spray device. The other alternative in common use nowadays is Co-phenylcaine (a proprietary mixture of lignocaine 5% with phenylephrine hydrochloride 0.5%) which has been shown to be as effective as cocaine and has a better safety profile.
- Assess gag reflex by gently suctioning the back of the throat. For the oral route this is the time to insert a Berman airway or a dental guard.
- Ideally the patient should be sitting up and the operator should face the patient. This is more comfortable for the patient and also allows the operator to observe and to communicate with the patient while performing endoscopy
- Start endoscopy via the nasal or oral route.

133

- Once the epiglottis comes into view, slowly advance and spray local anaesthetic under vision through the working channel of the scope (SAYGO). We find that threading an epidural catheter through the working channel allows a more directed spray and much less leakage of the solution. It is important to ensure that the local anaesthetic spray is directed on and around the cords to get good glottic and subglottic anaesthesia.
- The fibreoptic scope is then advanced through the cords into the trachea and positioned just above the carina.
- We always find it useful to warn the patients that this stage may be slightly uncomfortable or may make them cough. The tube is then railroaded over the scope into the trachea making sure that the tip of the scope does not touch the carina during the railroading process.
- If there is any resistance to the passage of the tube, withdraw and rotate 90 degrees anticlockwise as described before.
- Gently withdraw the scope, confirm position of the tube with capnography. Inflate the cuff only when the patient is asleep.

Asleep fibreoptic intubation (fibreoptic intubation in the anaesthetised patient)

Essential requirements are as follows.

- Ensure that the patient is anaesthetised at all times (avoid awareness); this can be achieved by using a TIVA technique
- Oxygenation and ventilation, by using a conduit airway/supraglottic device
- Unobstructed airway, tongue retraction by jaw thrust, Duval's forceps or by using a conduit airway/laryngeal mask airway
- Abolition of upper airway reflexes by local anaesthesia or muscle relaxation

Direct techniques

A fibreoptic intubation can be performed directly via the nose or the mouth as described earlier.

Fibreoptic assisted intubation through supraglottic devices

The fibreoptic scope can also be used to guide a tracheal tube through a supraglottic device such as a laryngeal mask airway (LMA) as described by Silk

et al, or an intubating laryngeal mask airway (ILMA). Intubation through a supraglottic device is suggested in Plan B of the Difficult Airway Society guidelines for unanticipated difficult intubation. It is an excellent rescue technique after failure to intubate with conventional laryngoscopy and in case of an anticipated difficult airway. There are two main advantages to this technique, the supraglottic device can be used to oxygenate and ventilate while performing the technique and the supraglottic device lifts the glottis out of blood and secretions that can make a direct fibreoptic intubation difficult.

Fibreoptic assisted intubation through the LMA

Case reports have described blind intubation through the LMA with a tracheal tube or with the aid of a bougie with reported success rates varying from 30–90%. Blind techniques can cause trauma and bleeding which will render any subsequent attempts at fibreoptic aided intubation useless. Fibreoptic assisted intubation through the LMA is a relatively simple technique the success of which depends largely on choosing the right equipment.

The three main considerations are as follows.

Tube size: It is difficult to pass a tube of more than 6.5 mm ID even through a size 5 LMA. Ideally tubes of 5.5–6.0 mm ID are preferred through a size 3 or 4 LMA.

Tube length: The distance from the distal end of the LMA to the vocal cords is 27–28 cm in males and 26–27 cm in females. Most standard uncut tubes are 27–28 cm and if used to intubate through the LMA may prove to be too short and the inflated cuff may lie at the cords and result in damage. The Mallinckrodt reinforced tubes (Flexilum™) are 33 cm in length and are ideal for this application, but they must be constantly rotated as they are advanced, since it may take several turns at the proximal end to result in a revolution at the distal end (Figure 13.16). Size 5 LMA shafts are too long for even a Flexilum tube and 5 cm should be cut from the end of the shaft before use. Other suitable tubes are the north facing nasal RAE (approx 32 cm in length) or microlaryngoscopy tube (MLT)

Removal of the LMA: Once the patient is intubated it is advisable to deflate the cuff and leave the LMA in situ. Any attempt to remove the LMA is likely to result in extubation as the stem of the LMA is too short to permit this manoeuvre.

Most of the above disadvantages of direct fibreoptic intubation through the LMA can be overcome

(a)

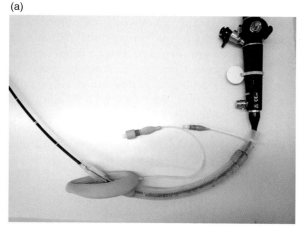

(b)

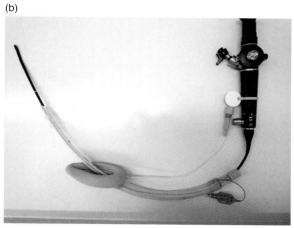

Figure 13.16. (a) Fibreoptic intubation through the LMA. With the tracheal tube fully inserted only about 2–3 cm of the distal end is available for tracheal intubation. This makes it possible for the cuff of the tracheal tube to lie at the cords and cause damage. (b) The problem can be overcome by use of a longer length tube such as the north facing (nasal) RAE tubes. With the tube fully inserted about 8 cm of the distal length is available for tracheal intubation.

by using a two-stage technique using an Aintree Intubation Catheter, or gum-elastic bougie (either guided into the trachea under endoscopic vision, or passed through a tracheal tube and used as an exchange guide).

Tips for performing fibreoptic intubation through the LMA

- Prepare the fibreoptic scope as before and load the tracheal tube onto the scope.
- Insert the LMA.
- Ensure that the LMA is seated well and the patient can be ventilated through it.
- Advance the endoscope through the stem of the LMA and guide it through the bars into the larynx into the trachea until the carina is visible. If the glottis is not visualised when the scope exits the LMA, gently move the LMA from side to side to obtain a view of the glottis.
- Railroad the tracheal tube over the fibrescope into the trachea.
- Confirm the position of the tube with the fibrescope and by capnograph
- Deflate the cuff and leave the LMA in situ. Secure the tube so that it does not slide within the stem of the LMA
- *Note:* It is important to ensure that there is sufficient gel between the fibrescope and the tracheal tube, and during railroading add gel to the tip of the tube to ensure that the tube

slips smoothly over the scope and through the stem of the LMA.

Fibreoptic assisted intubation through the ILMA (Figure 13.17)

The ILMA is a device that has been specifically designed to aid blind intubation and has a reported success rate of up to 96%. However in a small group of patients (10–14%) this can only be achieved after 2–3 attempts or very occasionally not at all, as the tracheal tube persists in entering the oesophagus despite repeated manipulations. Using the fibreoptic scope with the ILMA can help to overcome this problem, and this technique has reported success rates of 100% at the first attempt.

Tips for performing fibreoptic intubation through an ILMA

- Ensure that the ILMA is seated well and the patient can be ventilated adequately through it.
- Insert the ILMA tube until the horizontal mark on the tube is at the edge of the stem of the ILMA (at this point the tip of the tube is just at the epiglottis elevating bar (EEB).
- Pass the endoscope.
- Advance the endoscope through the stem of the ILMA, and guide it so that it sits just inside the distal orifice of the tube.
- Advance the tube under vision, and as the tube lifts the EEB out of the way, the larynx should come into vision.

135

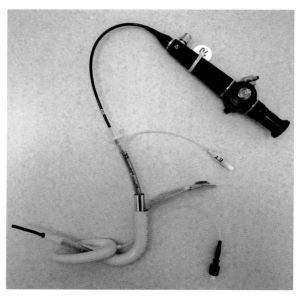

Figure 13.17. Intubating laryngeal mask airway (ILMA) with a dedicated tube. Fibreoptic-guided tracheal intubation through the ILMA has a high success rate and is preferred to the blind technique.

- If the glottis is not visualised gently move the ILMA from side to side to obtain a view of the glottis.
- Advance the scope through the vocal cords into the trachea.
- Railroad the tracheal tube over the fibrescope into the trachea.
- Confirm position of the tube with the fibrescope and by capnograph.
- Proceed to then remove the ILMA as recommended.

Combined techniques

Occasionally copious secretions or massive haemorrhage in the airspace can interfere with fibreoptic endoscopy. In these cases the Macintosh laryngoscope can be 'combined' with the flexible fibreoptic scope. The direct rigid laryngoscope can help to lift the tongue and epiglottis and aid in visualisation of the vocal cords.

Retrograde fibreoptic intubation

In some patients where access to the upper airway is not possible a retrograde fibreoptic intubation technique may be indicated. This technique consists of passing a guide wire through a 20G cannula inserted through the cricothyroid membrane. The guide wire is gently fed through the mouth and onto the distal end of the working channel of the scope until it exits from the working channel port. The fibrescope is now railroaded under vision over the guide wire into the trachea, until the 20G cannula is visible. The cannula and the guide wire are slowly withdrawn through the endoscope, and the fibrescope is advanced to just above the carina. The tube is railroaded over the fibrescope as described

Key points

- Understanding the equipment, knowledge of airway anatomy, good endoscopy skills, correct choice of tubes and railroading techniques are vital to the success of flexible fibreoptic intubation techniques.
- The technique may be difficult when there is serious tissue swelling or disruption, because endoscopy requires that there is an air space and vision can be prevented by blood or other fluids.
- Awake fibreoptic intubation remains as the gold standard for intubation in a patient with an anticipated difficult airway.

Further reading

Asai T, Shingu K. (2004). Difficulty in advancing a tracheal tube over a fibreoptic bronchoscope. Incidence, causes and solutions. *British Journal of Anaesthesia*, **92**, 870–881.

Ashchi M, Wiedemann HP, James KB. (1995). Cardiac complication from use of cocaine and phenylephrine in nasal septoplasty. *Archives of Otolaryngology-Head Neck Surgery*, **121**, 681–684.

British Thoracic Society. (2001). Guidelines on diagnostic flexible bronchoscopy. *Thorax*, **56**, i1–i21.

Cara DM, Norris AM, Neale LJ. (2001). Pain during awake nasal intubation after topical cocaine or phenylephrine/lidocaine spray. *Anaesthesia*, **87**, 549–558.

Cook TM, Asif M, Sim R, Waldron J. (2005). Use of a Proseal laryngeal mask airway and a Ravussin cricothyroidotomy needle in the management of laryngeal and subglottic stenosis causing upper airway obstruction. *British Journal of Anaesthesia*, **95**, 554–557.

Henderson JJ, Popat MT, Latto IP, Pearce AC. (2004). Difficult Airway Society guidelines for management of the unanticipated difficult intubation. *Anaesthesia*, **59**, 675–694.

Jones HE, Pearce AC, Moore P. (1993) Fibreoptic intubation. Influence of tracheal tube design. *Anaesthesia*, **48**, 672–674.

Knolle E, Oehmke MJ, Gustorff B, Hellwagner K, Kress HG. (2003). Target-controlled infusion of propofol for fibreoptic intubation. *European Journal of Anaesthesiology*, **20**, 565–569.

Makaryus JN, Makaryus AN, Johnson M. (2006). Acute myocardial infarction following the use of intranasal anaesthetic cocaine. *Southern Medical Journal*, **99**, 759–761.

Maktabi MA, Hoffman H, Funk G, From RF. (2002). Laryngeal trauma during awake fiberoptic intubation. *Anesthesia and Analgesia*, **95**, 1112–1114.

Marfin AG, Iqbal R, Mihm F, Popat MT, Scott SH, Pandit JJ. (2006). Determination of the site of tracheal tube impingement during nasotracheal fibreoptic intubation. *Anaesthesia*, **61**, 646–650.

Ovassapian A. (1996). *Fibreoptic Endoscopy and the Difficult Airway*. 2nd Ed. Philadelphia: Lippincott-Raven.

Popat M. (Ed.). (2009). *Difficult Airway Management*. Oxford: Oxford University Press.

Popat M. (2001). *Practical Fibreoptic Intubation*. Oxford: Butterworth-Heinemann.

Rai MR, Parry TM, Dombrovskis A, Warner OJ. (2008). Remifentanil target-controlled infusion vs. propofol target-controlled infusion for conscious sedation for awake fibreoptic intubation: Double-blinded randomized controlled trial. *British Journal of Anaesthesia*, **100**, 125–130.

Silk JM, Hill HM, Calder I. (1991). Difficult intubation and the laryngeal mask. *European Journal of Anaesthesiology*, **4**, 47–51.

Wylie S, Calder I. (2008). Flexible fibreoptic intubation. *Anaesthesia and Intensive Care Medicine*, **9**, 358–362.

Websites of interest

Oxford Region Airway Group (ORAG) www.orag.co.uk

Difficult Airway Society (DAS). UK. www.das.uk.com

Tracheal intubation: 'blind' methods

Brian Prater and Adrian Pearce

Direct laryngoscopy is the most common method of tracheal intubation having a high success rate in skilled hands with a low incidence of complications. However all large studies of tracheal intubation have a failure rate due to the inability to gain a direct line of sight to the larynx. In these circumstances tracheal intubation can be accomplished either by 'blind' techniques in which there is no direct or indirect view of the larynx to guide tube placement or 'visual' techniques where an indirect view of the larynx guides tube placement.

There is much to be said for the incorporation of visual techniques, whether direct or indirect, into core practice because of the presumed lower incidence of failure or laryngeal damage associated with intubation attempts. Blind techniques may be seen as 'second-best'. There certainly seems little sense in devising a primary plan of visual-based direct or indirect laryngoscopy with Plan B being a blind technique. But blind techniques developed in the times when there was little technology to build devices alternative to direct laryngoscopes and were remarkably effective in skilled hands. Part of their attraction today is the limited, or absence of, equipment required. This is particularly helpful in developing countries or in developed countries in areas of healthcare, such as pre-hospital or hospital ward, where the range of intubation equipment is limited. Blind techniques may also be valuable when secretions or blood in the airway limit the effectiveness of visual aids. Blind intubation techniques remain within the CCT training syllabus in the UK and can be classified into four groups (Table 14.1).

Blind oral or nasal intubation

The first description of a blind technique was the oral tactile method by Macewen in 1880. This method requires palpation of the larynx with the operator's

Table 14.1. Classification of blind intubation techniques

Technique	Principle
Blind oral or nasal	Advanced by judgement of the location of the larynx aided by digital palpation or by breath sounds
Retrograde	Retrograde introduction of a guide catheter from the trachea or cricothyroid membrane into the mouth, and anterograde intubation over this guide
Light-guided	A light-tipped catheter or stylet is passed blindly into the oropharynx and manoeuvred through the larynx by viewing transillumination
Intubating laryngeal mask	Intubation through a supraglottic airway specifically designed to line-up the stem with glottic aperture

fingers in the pharynx and subsequent guidance of the endotracheal tube into the glottis using the fingers as a guide. Blind oral intubation must be very rarely practiced today except in exceptional circumstances and is no longer taught widely.

Blind nasal intubation, in comparison, remains a popular and successful technique in both anaesthetised and awake patients. A well lubricated tracheal tube of suitable size and length is advanced slowly and gently through the anterior naris into the nasopharynx and supraglottic region. The tube is advanced through the glottis and into the trachea. In the awake, or anaesthetised breathing, patient the passage between the vocal cords can be guided by listening to breath-sounds through the tube or observing reservoir bag movement or capnography. Repeated attempts should be avoided to lessen the chance of

Core Topics in Airway Management, Second Edition, ed. Ian Calder and Adrian Pearce. Published by Cambridge University Press.
© Cambridge University Press 2011.

airway trauma, bleeding and oedema. There are many tips to successful blind nasal intubation (it is a true clinical skill) particularly in subtle movements of the head and neck or part inflation of the tube cuff and a fuller practical description is provided in Chapter 29.

Retrograde intubation

A guide is fed in a retrograde fashion from the trachea in a cephalad direction and intubation completed over the guide in the normal anterograde manner. The term retrograde intubation is a misnomer, and it should perhaps be termed guided blind intubation or translaryngeal intubation. The subject has recently been reviewed (Anaesthesia 2009) describing the various techniques and complications in detail.

The first description and use of the term 'retrograde intubation' was by Butler and Cirillo in 1960. Both anaesthetists for major head and neck resection surgery, they were confronted by the problem of patients requiring surgery in the early post-operative period. Their described technique was to feed a catheter through the healing tracheostomy fistula into the oral cavity and to use this as a guide for advancement of the tracheal tube. Waters, then working in Africa, was the first to describe puncture of the intact cricothyroid membrane and used a Tuohy needle through which he fed 'many yards' of epidural catheter into the oropharynx. The catheter was retrieved from the oropharynx by use of a special hook and used to guide a tube towards and through the glottic aperture. When the tip of the tracheal tube had reached the inner surface of the cricothyroid membrane, the catheter was withdrawn through the mouth (or cut) leaving the tube free to be advanced deeper into the trachea.

Waters was highly successful in awake and anaesthetised patients and established the basic or classic technique which relied on equipment to-hand and the use of the cricothyroid membrane. The cricotracheal ligament may also be used. The epidural catheter is not ideal because it is actually quite difficult to slide a tracheal tube over a narrow guide without the tip of the tube impacting at laryngeal level. There have been a number of innovations and developments since the original description leading to a commercially available retrograde intubation kit.

Cook Medical (www.cookmedical.com) produces three kits for placement of a tracheal tube greater than 2.5, 4.0 and 5.0 mm. They include a catheter which is fed over the wire to stiffen it and provide a wider

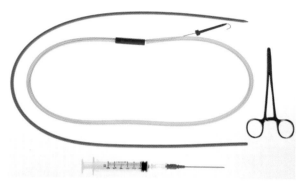

Figure 14.1. The components of the Cook retrograde intubation kit.

support for the tracheal tube. Other described wire-stiffeners are ureteric or radiological stents. The components of the kit are shown in Figure 14.1, Table 14.2 details the steps of the classic retrograde intubation technique and training videos are available on the Internet. The retrograde wire may be found in the oropharynx (against the posterior pharyngeal wall) by gentle direct laryngoscopy and withdrawn with Magill's forceps. It is easier to retrieve the wire if it has a J-tip. An alternative is to keep feeding the retrograde wire until it emerges through the nose. In general, a smaller diameter tracheal tube minimises the chance of hold-up at the larynx.

Fibreoptic assisted retrograde

An amalgamation of blind and visual techniques uses the classic retrograde introduction of a wire through the mouth or nose which is then fed through the working channel of an intubating fibrescope. The fibrescope is advanced along the wire until the view shows the inner surface of the cricothyroid membrane. The wire is withdrawn into the fibrescope taking care not to lose the placement of the tip of the fibrescope just distal to the glottic aperture. Once the wire is fully within the fibrescope, the scope can be passed to the distal trachea and intubation completed as usual over the fibrescope. The wire should be drawn through (into) the fibrescope rather than out through the neck to prevent the contaminated wire seeding oral bacteria into the neck tissues.

If a working fibrescope is available it is probable that a retrograde wire-assisted technique would not be first choice. However if fibreoptic intubation is attempted as the primary plan and fails due to

Table 14.2. Steps in classic retrograde intubation technique

Extend neck

Locate cricothyroid membrane (CTM)

Stabilise larynx with one hand

Insert cannula cephalad through CTM

Feed wire through cannula and advance

Locate wire in oropharynx (fingers, Magill's forceps)

Feed wire-stiffener catheter over wire

Advance tube over catheter until tip abuts CTM internally

Remove wire and advance tube into trachea

inability to locate the glottic aperture, the technique is useful as a back-up plan.

Retrograde pull technique

Another retrograde technique uses the retrograde catheter to pull the tube into the trachea. An epidural catheter or long silk/nylon suture is fed in retrograde fashion and retrieved through the mouth. It is then tied to the Murphy eye of a tracheal tube and used to guide the tracheal tube by pulling it through the glottic aperture. The tube is advanced into the trachea carrying the suture with it. Whilst it is possible for the suture to be cut, it is also useful to leave it attached until after extubation. The suture is still placed to provide a guide for re-intubation if needed.

Complications

Retrograde techniques are relatively contraindicated when neck anatomy is unfavourable, there is infection in the neck, a bleeding diathesis or gross glottic abnormality. Complications include failure, damage to the vocal cords, haemorrhage, infection and surgical emphysema.

Light-guided intubation

The larynx is a superficial structure and the principle of light-guided intubation is that a light-tipped catheter is manoeuvred in the oropharynx until the light can be seen externally in the laryngeal area. A review article explains in detail the development of transillumination since its original description by Yamamura in 1959, but the most recent and well-published

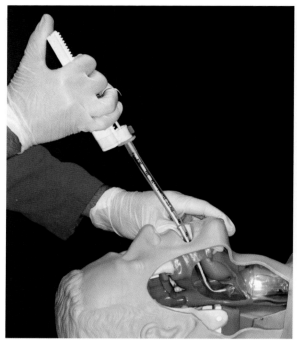

Figure 14.2. Insertion of the assembled Trachlight.

device is the Trachlight. Described in 1995 by Hung the Trachlight incorporates a handle containing batteries, semi-rigid malleable metal stylet and a hollow flexible light wand with bulb at the tip. The device is assembled by placing the lightwand over the stylet and coupling it to the handle. The tracheal tube, with upward orientation of the bevel, is loaded onto the lightwand and secured in the 15 mm mount on the handle. The lightwand is adjusted for tracheal tubes of differing lengths before the distal part of the Trachlight is shaped manually into a hockey stick.

With the patient's head in the neutral position and the Trachlight light switched on the device is introduced into the mouth (Figure 14.2) and manoeuvred in the direction of the cricothyroid membrane. A bright transilluminated light spot is seen (externally) through this membrane when the tip of the instrument is just below the vocal cords (Figure 14.3). When the intubator is certain that the tube tip has passed the vocal cords, the stylet is retracted whilst the tube is advanced. After releasing the tube from the instrument by unlocking the clamp, the Trachlight is pulled out.

The device may be carried in the pocket and used in awake or anaesthetised patients in emergency and elective situations. It became popular in North

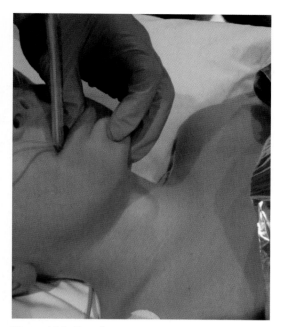

Figure 14.3. Transillumination at cricothyroid membrane.

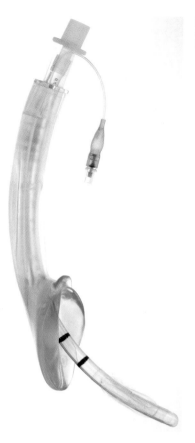

Figure 14.4.
A 7.0 mm tube passed through an i-gel.

America and the Netherlands with a substantial publication base confirming a high success rate. In one study of 206 patients with anticipated difficult intubation there was a 1% failure rate and a mean intubation time of only 26 seconds. Contraindications are the presence of supra- or glottic pathology or inability to view the cricothyroid membrane. It is likely that the era of the Trachlight is past, but a review article from 2001 shows how successful a blind technique can be in skilled hands.

Light-guided intubation has been described through a supraglottic airway, and a recently developed 'blind intubation device' (BID) incorporates a supraglottic airway with oesophageal airway component and catheter with lighted tip. With some modification it may be used also in nasal intubation.

Intubating laryngeal mask

Intubation through a supraglottic airway is a useful effective technique and is included in Plan B for failed direct laryngoscopy in the Difficult Airway Society guidelines. The incorporation of a device providing ventilation, ensuring oxygenation and inhalational anaesthesia, in management of difficult intubation is extremely helpful. The supraglottic airway provides a route for effective alveolar ventilation and is used as the conduit for intubation.

Blind intubation through a classic laryngeal mask has a sub-optimal success rate (50–90%) and other limitations. The size of the tube is limited with a size 3 or 4 LMA accommodating a size 6.0 mm tube and a size 5 mask a size 7.0 mm tube. The tube must be long to allow the length of tube to be sufficient for the cuff to be completely below the vocal cords. Some armoured tubes are satisfactory (although the tube connector may be fixed), and the nasal RAE tube has the required length.

Other later supraglottic airway devices such as the i-gel (Figure 14.4) may be easier to intubate through blindly. The technique is to place the i-gel, check ventilation then advance a well-lubricated appropriately sized cuffed tube through the stem. The i-gel is stabilised with the other hand. Virtually all work with intubation through a standard supraglottic airway indicates that fibrescope-based visual techniques are more successful than blind ones.

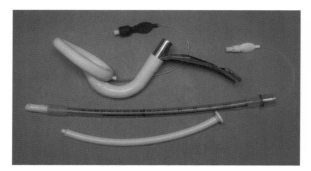

Figure 14.5. Components of the reusable ILMA kit.

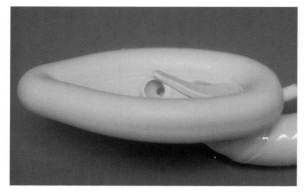

Figure 14.6. The epiglottic elevator bar.

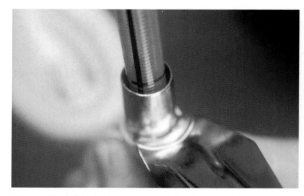

Figure 14.7. The horizontal and vertical lines on the ILMA tracheal tube.

The limitations of blind intubation through the classic laryngeal mask forced Brain to design a specific supraglottic airway for blind intubation. The intubating laryngeal mask airway (ILMA) was described first in 1997 and is supplied as a kit (Figure 14.5). The modifications from the classic laryngeal mask are a highly curved metal stem incorporating a 15 mm connector, a handle to insert and manipulate the device, an epiglottic elevator bar (Figure 14.6), a ramp in the lower part of the stem prior to the bowl to direct the tube and a specially constructed wire-spiralled tube with detachable connector and novel bevel. The bevel was designed to pass easily between the vocal cords, and the design has since proved popular for use with the flexible fibrescope. A stabilising rod was included to facilitate removal of the device over the inserted tube.

It was designed in size 3, 4 and 5 masks with tube sizes 7.0, 7.5 and 8.0 mm, giving a choice of any tube size with all masks. Each tube has a vertical line which should be towards the anaesthetist during insertion to correctly orientate the bevel and a horizontal line (Figure 14.7), which indicates the depth at which the tip of the tube starts to raise the epiglottic elevator bar. The original ILMA was decontaminated by steam sterilisation with the tube used for 10 cycles and the mask 40 cycles. More recently single use ILMA mask and tubes have been available.

The technique of intubation with an ILMA is to select the appropriate mask and tube size for the patient. Generally the size 3 mask is for children 30–50 kg, size 4 mask for adults 50–70 kg and the size 5 adults 70–100 kg. After lubrication the ILMA is inserted by a technique quite unlike the classic laryngeal mask. Holding the handle parallel to, and just over, the sternum the tip of the mask enters the oral cavity and is advanced into place by the handle moving in a semicircular fashion until it lies over the face. The cuff should be inflated to no more than 60 cmH$_2$O. Successful ventilation is confirmed by chest movement and capnography. When this has been confirmed and the patient suitably oxygenated, the breathing system is disconnected and the dedicated lubricated tracheal tube passed through the conducting stem until the horizontal line is at the 15 mm connector. At this point further advancement without undue force leads to elevation of the epiglottic elevator bar and passage into the trachea. When the tube is felt to be in the trachea the cuff is inflated and the breathing system is connected to the tracheal tube connector. Ventilation is once again confirmed by chest excursion and capnography.

If intubation is not successful on the first attempt, the best 'tip' to gain optimal mask positioning relative to the laryngeal inlet is to use a technique devised by Dr Chandy Verghese and called the Chandy manoeuvre. With the ILMA in place the practitioner holds the handle with one hand moving the ILMA back and forth in the sagittal plane whilst assessing the best position for manual bag ventilation with the other hand. The second part involves lifting the handle of the ILMA to move it anteriorly. Another tip is the 'up-down' manoeuvre in which the mask with cuff inflated is removed about 6 cm and re-inserted. This may overcome epiglottis infolding. Intubation is re-attempted with the mask in the optimal position for ventilation. Generally no more than three attempts at blind insertion should be made, recognising that forceful oesophageal insertion may cause damage.

Following successful tracheal intubation (confirmation tests Chapter 16) the mask should generally be removed. The ILMA cuff is deflated and the tube connector removed. The ILMA is removed over the tube in a reverse of the circular motion required for insertion. The stabilising rod is used to aid the process by preventing displacement of the tube from the trachea during mask removal. When possible the tube is grasped by the fingers in the oropharynx and the mask completely removed. The tube connector is replaced and ventilation re-established.

A number of studies have indicated that the ILMA is the most effective method of blind intubation. Ventilation through the mask is possible in virtually all patients, and the rate of successful intubation is 95–99% after three attempts at insertion although first time intubation success rate has been as low as 50–60% in some studies. One strategy to adopt if blind intubation fails is to make it a visual technique. This can be done by placing the fibrescope through the tube or with the CTrach (see Chapter 15).

Key points

- Blind intubation techniques are valuable.
- Blind nasal intubation has a high success rate in skilled hands.
- Retrograde intubation is a rapid and safe technique.
- The intubating laryngeal mask is the most effective blind intubation device.
- Intubation through a supraglottic airway is a core part of UK airway guidelines.

Further reading

Agro F, Hung OR, Cataldo R, Carassiti M, Gherardi S. (2001). Lightwand intubation using the Trachlight: A brief review of current knowledge. *Canadian Journal of Anesthesia*, 48, 592–599.

Caponas G. (2002). Intubating laryngeal mask airway. *Anaesthesia Intensive Care*, 30, 551–569.

Cheng KI, Chang MC, Lai TW, Shen YC, Lu DV. (2009). A modified lightwand-guided nasotracheal intubation technique for oromaxillofacial surgical patients. *Journal of Clinical Anesthesia*, 21, 258–263.

Chung YT, Sun MS, Wu HS. (2003). Blind nasotracheal intubation is facilitated by neutral head position and endotracheal cuff inflation in spontaneously breathing patients. *Canadian Journal of Anesthesia*, 50, 511–513.

Cook Medical Educational Videos. Available at: http://www.cookmedical.com/cc/educationResource.do?id=Educational_Video.

Davis L, Cook-Sather SD, Schreiner MS. (2000). Lighted stylet tracheal intubation: A review. *Anesthesia Analgesia*, 90, 745–746.

Dhara SS. (2009). Retrograde tracheal intubation. *Anaesthesia*, 64, 1094–1104.

Gerstein NS, Braude DA, Hung O, Sanders JC, Murphy MF. (2010). The Fastrach intubating laryngeal mask airway: An overview and update. *Canadian Journal of Anesthesia*, 57, 588–601.

Kapila A, Addy EV, Verghese C, Brain AI. (1997). The intubating laryngeal mask airway: An initial assessment of performance. *British Journal of Anaesthesia*, 79, 710–713.

Lechman MJ, Donahoo JS, Macvaugh H. (1986). Endotracheal intubation using percutaneous retrograde guidewire followed by antegrade fibreoptic bronchoscopy. *Critical Care Medicine*, 14, 589–590.

LMA Fastrach Maneuvres guide. Available at: http://www.lmaco.com/docs/Fastrach_Maneuvers_Guide.pdf.

Reardon RF, Martel M. (2001). The intubating laryngeal mask airway: Suggestions for use in the emergency department. *Academic Emergency Medicine*, 8, 833–838.

Sun Y, Jiang H, Zhu Y, Xu H, Huang Y. (2009). Blind intubation device for nasotracheal intubation in 100 oral and maxillofacial surgery patients with anticipated difficult airways: A prospective evaluation. *European Journal of Anaesthesiology*, 26, 746–751.

Timmermann A, Russo SG, Crozier TA, Eich C, Mundt B. (2007). Novices ventilate and intubate quicker and safer via intubating laryngeal mask than by conventional bag-mask ventilation and laryngoscopy. *Anesthesiology*, 107, 570–576.

Waters DJ. (1961). Guided blind endotracheal intubation. *Anaesthesia*, 18, 158–162.

Weksler N, Klein M, Weksler D, Sidelnick C, Chorni I, Rozentsveig V. (2004). Retrograde tracheal intubation: Beyond fibreoptic endotracheal intubation. *Acta Anaesthesiologica Scandinavica*, 48, 412–416.

Young B. (2003). The intubating laryngeal-mask airway may be an ideal device for airway control in the rural trauma patient. *American Journal of Emergency Medicine*, 21, 80–85.

Chapter 15

Tracheal intubation: rigid indirect laryngoscopy

Ankie E.W. Hamaekers and Pieter A.J. Borg

The commonest method of tracheal intubation is to obtain direct laryngoscopy, which is described in detail in Chapter 12. However, it is not always possible to achieve a direct line of sight to the glottis and intubation may fail or be accomplished only at the expense of major morbidity such as pharyngo-laryngeal trauma, hypoxaemia, cardiovascular instability, aspiration or awareness (see Chapter 11). If direct laryngoscopy is not possible, the feasible alternative ways of tracheal intubation are by:

- Blind intubation (Chapter 14)
- Flexible fibrescope (Chapter 13)
- Rigid indirect laryngoscopy

Rigid indirect laryngoscopy

Indirect laryngoscopy refers to a technique in which a view of the glottis is transmitted through mirrors, prisms, fibreoptic bundles or video technology to the eyepiece of the instrument or a monitor screen. *Flexible* indirect laryngoscopy (flexible fibreoptic intubation) is described in Chapter 13. The term *rigid* indirect laryngoscope (RIL) refers to a device in which the blade, stylet or conduit is sufficiently rigid to allow partial retraction of the oropharyngeal tissues but which also provides an image of the glottis. Rigid indirect laryngoscopy is challenging strongly the supremacy of the flexible fibrescope in dealing with unexpected failed or difficult direct laryngoscopy under general anaesthesia.

The Siker laryngoscope, the first rigid indirect laryngoscope (RIL) to assist intubation, was introduced in 1956. Several other RILs were described in the following years, but none gained wide acceptance in clinical practice. However, numerous rigid indirect laryngoscopes have appeared on the market recently,

Table 15.1. Design and technical features of rigid indirect laryngoscopes

Quality of optics (image resolution)	Portability
Field of view	Cleaning/sterilisation or disposable
Intensity and source of illumination	Costs
Ocular or internal/external display	Range of available sizes
Tube delivery system or not	Anti-fogging system
Angulation of the stylet or blade	Durability
Blade thickness	Preparation time
Flexibility and length of the stylet	Recording system

as if sensing the demise of the flexible fibrescope as the gold standard. The glut is in part due to new technology in miniature cameras, screens and video technology and the preference for single use equipment in airway management. There is currently a wide variety of devices differing in some of the design and technical features summarised in Table 15.1.

No classification of equipment has yet been generally accepted, and we use here a simple scheme:

- Optical stylets
- Bladed indirect laryngoscopes
- Tube-guiding indirect laryngoscopes

The commercially available systems are given in Table 15.2, but devices will be added and removed from this list as technology develops. There is (as yet) no clear

Core Topics in Airway Management, Second Edition, ed. Ian Calder and Adrian Pearce. Published by Cambridge University Press.
© Cambridge University Press 2011.

Table 15.2. Overview of (semi-)rigid indirect laryngoscopes available in Europe

Optical stylets

Bonfils intubation endoscope Karl Storz GmbH & Co. KG, Tuttlingen Germany	Fibreoptic endoscope with a fixed 40-degree distal angle designed for retromolar or paraglossal intubation. Available with an outside diameter of 2, 3.5 and 5 mm. Movable proximal eyepiece, with adjustable diopter correction. Option for O_2 insufflation through the tube holder. 12 000 pixels and a distal viewing angle of 90 degrees.
Levitan FPS scope Clarus Medical, Minneapolis, Minnesota, USA	Short, portable fibreoptic stylet intended to be used in conjunction with a conventional laryngoscope. The TT should be cut to 26 cm to fit on the stylet. The 45 degree curve can be slightly modified to conform to patient's anatomy. A built-in LED provides illumination.
SensaScope Acutronic Medical Systems AG, Hirzel, Switzerland	Hybrid S-shaped fibreoptic stylet (17 000 pixels) with steerable distal tip with a 60 degree bending angle. Remote light source. Camera can be mounted on the eyepiece.
Shikani Optical Stylet Clarus Medical, Minneapolis, Minnesota, USA	High-resolution (30 000 pixels) fibreoptic stylet with a somewhat malleable distal shaft in a 70–80 (can be bent up to 120) degree curvature. Can be used with remote light source, a standard laryngoscope handle or a portable halogen light source. Adjustable tube stop incorporates an oxygen port. Pediatric version available.

Bladed indirect laryngoscopes

Coopdech VLP-100 Daiken Medical Ltd, Osaka, Japan	A CCD camera and LCD monitor-mounted conventional laryngoscope with both paediatric (Miller) and adult (Macintosh) blades. Dedicated blade is reusable and autoclavable. Rechargeable lithium battery.
Glidescope® Video Laryngoscope Verathon Medical, Burnaby, Canada	Video-laryngoscope with a 60 degree angulated disposable blade available in neonatal to adult sizes. The high-resolution camera is connected to a stand-alone monitor.
McGrath® series 5 Aircraft Medical Ltd, Edinburgh, UK	Compact video-laryngoscope with an angulated, 12 mm thick, disposable blade. Length of the blade is adjustable. The 1.7 inch LCD screen is incorporated in the handle.
Truview EVO2™ Truphatek International Ltd, Netanya, Israel	Laryngoscope with a mid-blade angulation and a removable lens system that refracts the distal image by 42 degrees. Proximal eyepiece and camera attachment. Integrated oxygen delivery channel. Pediatric size available.
C-MAC Video Laryngoscope System Karl Storz GmbH & Co. KG, Tuttlinger, Germany	Based on a conventional laryngoscope blade. The CMOS micro video camera provides an enhanced field of view and is connected to a remote 7 inch video screen and incorporates a video recording system. Reusable blade, anti-fogging system.
LaryFlex Acutronic MS, Hirzel, Switzerland	A modified conventional laryngoscope with a channel in the handle for a fibreoptic bundle. Provides an image of 17 000 pixels on a remote screen.

Conduits or laryngoscopes with tube guidance system

Airtraq optical laryngoscope Prodol Meditec SA, Vizcaya, Spain	Disposable laryngoscope with an optical system of lenses, mirrors and prisms. Incorporates a channel to deliver the tube and a heating element to prevent fogging. A wireless camera can be attached. Paediatric sizes available.
Airway Scope AWS-100 Pentax Corporation, Tokyo, Japan	Portable video-laryngoscope with a CCD camera covered by a disposable, anatomically shaped blade with a tube-guiding channel to

Table 15.2. (*cont.*)

	accommodate an TT (6.0–8.5 ID).
Bullard™ Elite Circon – ACMI, Stamford, Connecticut, USA	L-shaped fibreoptic laryngoscope. Incorporates working channel and attached metal stylet to facilitate tube delivery. Battery powered. Video camera attachment on proximal eye piece possible.
LMA CTrach™ Laryngeal mask company, Henley-on-thames, UK	Variation on the intubation LMA with a camera and a click-on video display. Detailed description in Chapter 14.
UpsherScope Ultra™ Mercury Medical, Clearwater, Florida, USA	Portable fibreoptic laryngoscope with J-shaped, curved blade containing a tube-guiding channel for tubes up to 8.0 mm ID. Snap-on camera available. Can be sterilised.

winner, and we present here only an outline of some of the most favoured or heavily marketed devices.

Optical stylets

The (semi-) rigid optical stylets are placed inside the TT and are designed to navigate around the tongue to visualise the laryngeal inlet. The shaft of the stylet may be rigid with a preformed, fixed curve (Bonfils), or malleable with an angle that can be manipulated slightly by hand prior to insertion (Levitan, Shikani), or the shaft may have a flexible tip, that can be adjusted during the intubation procedure by a proximal trigger device (Sensascope). The stylet with mounted TT is inserted in the midline along the surface of the tongue. The uvula and epiglottis should be identified and serve as anatomical landmarks. To create space in the pharynx a firm jaw thrust or tongue pull can be applied or a classic laryngoscope can be used (Figure 15.1). The stylet is steered under the epiglottis and once the laryngeal inlet is clearly visible, the tube can be advanced through the vocal cords into the trachea under endoscopic control. The stylet is withdrawn by a large circular movement towards the patient's chest as the TT is advanced further into the trachea. A common mistake is to advance the stylet too far into the hypopharynx. To avoid this, one should rotate the stylet over the base of the tongue instead of allowing the stylet to sink posteriorly toward the oesophagus. One typical advantage of stylets is the limited mouth opening required, which still allows insertion, laryngoscopy and intubation. They provide, however, a restricted visual field, which can make navigation to the larynx difficult. None of the (semi-) rigid stylets can be used for nasal intubation.

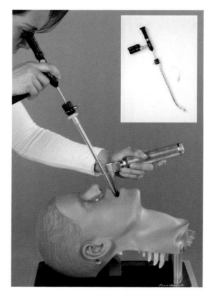

Figure 15.1. The Bonfils optical stylet using the midline approach. A jaw trust or a classic laryngoscope can be used to separate anatomical structures and to create space in the hypopharynx to allow sight beyond the distal lens.

Bladed indirect laryngoscopes

The bladed indirect laryngoscopes can be divided into RILs based on a classic Macintosh blade (Coopdech, C-MAC, Laryflex) or devices with an anatomically shaped, angulated blade (Glidescope, McGrath). They are inserted in the midline and are rotated behind and around the tongue. However the conventional bladed RILs can also be used as a classic direct laryngoscope (Figure 15.2). It permits the operator to directly view the glottis. This makes these devices well suited for teaching direct laryngoscopy and the possibility of a direct view is a potential advantage in case of secretions or blood in the airway.

RILs with a specific angulated blade will provide a view of the larynx on the screen, but the glottis is not

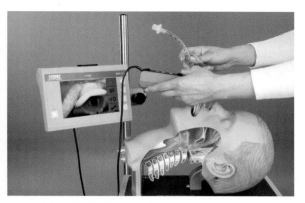

Figure 15.2. The C-MAC video-laryngoscope is based on a Macintosh blade. In most cases a stylet is not necessary.

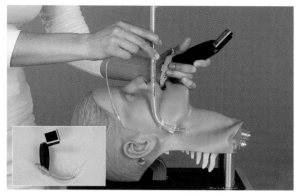

Figure 15.3. When using an angulated laryngoscope, for instance the McGrath video-laryngoscope, a stylet is needed to facilitate TT placement.

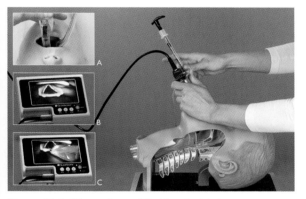

Figure 15.4. When using an TT with stylet it is important to watch the tip entering the mouth directly (a), for only after entering the hypopharynx (b) the tip is visualised on the monitor (c).

visible directly. The TT must be inserted around a corner and this necessitates the use of a stylet (Figure 15.3). When using a stylet it is important to directly observe the placement of the tube into the mouth until the tip becomes visible on the screen (Figure 15.4). Failure to do so can lead to oropharyngeal damage. Optimising laryngeal exposure does not necessarily result in easier intubation and can actually make tube advancement more difficult. Advancement of the tube may be impeded because the TT hits the anterior wall of the larynx due to the curvature of the stylet and the angle between the TT and the laryngeal axis. Withdrawing the stylet and rotating the TT may avoid impingement on the anterior wall of the trachea. Moving the tip of the laryngoscope blade away from the laryngeal inlet provides a broader view and may also aid TT insertion by decreasing the angle between the advancing TT and the larynx.

Indirect laryngoscopes with a tube-guiding system

The RILs with an integrated tube-guiding system to facilitate tube insertion provide easier TT placement, compared to the bladed indirect laryngoscopes, but they also require a larger mouth opening for insertion into the oropharynx and they have a limited potential to manipulate the TT independently. These devices are inserted in the midline and are rotated in the oropharynx until the handle is progressed from a horizontal to a vertical plane. Although the Airway Scope and the Airtraq look quite similar, small differences in blade design, resulting in a different exit angle of the TT, require different insertion techniques (Figure 15.5). The blade of the Airway Scope should pass posterior to the epiglottis, while the tip of the Airtraq is preferentially placed in the vallecula. Once the glottis is visualised the TT can be advanced through the guiding channel. If it is difficult to lift the epiglottis or to direct the TT into the glottis a gum-elastic bougie may be helpful (Figure 15.6). Following successful endotracheal intubation, the TT is pulled laterally and held securely in place as the device is rotated in the reverse direction around the tongue.

One notable indirect laryngoscope with a tube-guiding system functions as a supraglottic airway. This allows easy ventilation around or during attempts at intubation, and the concept must be considered a useful development. The CTrach is effectively an intubating laryngeal mask airway (Chapter 14) with a camera positioned to provide a view of the larynx on a small screen. This view can be used to guide the tube through the glottic aperture. The CTrach has undergone a number of revisions.

147

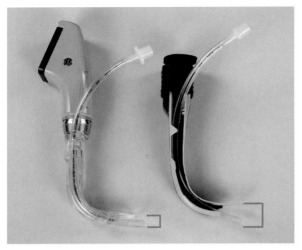

Figure 15.5. The tube-guiding channel of the Airway Scope (left) and Airtraq look quite similar. However the TT leaves the Airtraq in a wider angle than the Airway Scope. This is the reason why the Airway Scope is designed to lift up the epiglottis and the Airtraq is preferentially placed in the vallecula.

Advantages and disadvantages of rigid indirect laryngoscopy

Compared to direct laryngoscopy

As the 'eye' of the optics is located at or close to the distal tip of the RIL one has a magnified and wide-angle view of the vocal cords compared to the tunnel view one obtains with direct laryngoscopy. Where the RIL enables the operator to look around the corner, generally an improved exposure of the glottis can be achieved and RILs have been shown to improve intubation success rates in specific populations with difficult airways. Tube placement during DL is often without visual control as the view of the glottis can be obscured by the TT. RILs allow visually controlled TT placement and visual confirmation of the tube passing between the vocal cords. This helps in avoiding laryngeal injury caused by blind tube advancement. Although an improved view of the glottis enables the practitioner to recognise landmarks, it does not necessarily improve the ease of intubation itself.

RILs eliminate the need to align the axes of the upper airway and in general require less force to achieve a good view of the laryngeal inlet compared to DL. For some of the RILs it has been shown that their use results in less movement of the cervical spine, a reduced incidence of sore throat and improved haemodynamic

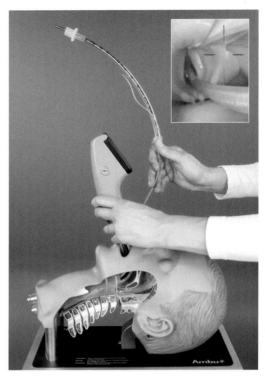

Figure 15.6. In case the view on the vocal cords is limited or advancement of the TT to the glottis is difficult, additional use of the gum elastic bougie may be helpful.

stability. The view in DL is only available for the operator, whilst most RILs have an integrated display or can be attached to an external video monitor permitting several people to view the same object simultaneously. This facilitates teaching and allows an assistant to adjust external laryngeal manipulation which may improve success rate. Furthermore, images can be captured for medico-legal documentation of successful intubation or research purposes.

Secretions and fogging are major obstacles to success for RILs. Adequate suction of the hypopharynx prior to insertion of a RIL is mandatory. Fogging can be reduced by applying an antifogging agent or by warm water immersion of the optics. Oxygen insufflation through the working channel may also clear the optics. Compared to a classic laryngoscope some RILs require extra time for set-up and cleaning.

Compared to flexible fibreoptic intubation

During intubation using a flexible fibrescope the tube is advanced blindly over the scope. Hold-up of the

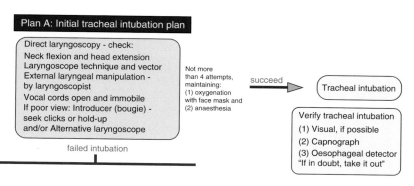

Figure 15.7. DAS difficult intubation Plan A incorporates an alternative laryngoscope.

tube occurs frequently and is often corrected by manipulating the tube without any visual control. RILs permit visually controlled intubation. RILs are more robust and durable, easier to clean, quicker in performance and it has been claimed that they may have a steeper learning curve. The ease of cleaning alone is a major advantage of some RILs in which a single use, disposable insert allows the device to be recycled quickly between patients compared with the protracted sterilisation process for the flexible fibrescope. Although their rigidity makes them easier to navigate to the laryngeal inlet, it does make the RILs less versatile, especially in case of abnormal anatomy.

The flexible fibrescope may be used with equal facility through the nose and mouth and also easily in the awake patient. In addition the flexible fibrescope has a working channel through which local anaesthesia, wires or catheters may be passed. Generally the RILs may only be used orally, although the view may be able to guide nasal intubation. Awake intubation is possible with RILs, but the technique generally involves placing the device in the oropharynx and applying retraction to the base of the tongue. This activates the gag reflex which is the most difficult reflex to obtund with analgo-sedation. Awake intubation remains much easier, more versatile and successful with the flexible fibrescope.

Future and choice of a RIL

The degree to which the RILs have been evaluated varies considerably and as most devices have been modified since their introduction, the literature on device performance must be interpreted carefully. None of the available RILs meets all the criteria of the 'ideal intubation technique' as previously defined by Dr John Henderson. Local availability of other airway management tools and personal skills and preferences must guide the choice for a particular

RIL. The 2008 meta-analysis by Mihai et al is a very useful source of references for the equipment mentioned in this chapter. Despite much enthusiasm for individual techniques the meta-analysis concluded that no device had been shown to be superior to direct laryngoscopy in the normal or abnormal airway. However it is also clear that the specialty is also poor at evaluation of new devices with Frerk suggesting that less than 1% of the uses of a new device may be published in the literature.

It is highly likely that rigid indirect laryngoscopy will become a core skill, not perhaps supplanting traditional direct laryngoscopy, but available to be used early if direct laryngoscopy proves to be even mildly difficult. The guideline produced by the Difficult Airway Society for difficult intubation Plan A (Figure 15.7) includes optimal direct laryngoscopy and the use of an alternative laryngoscope and perhaps it should become much more acceptable to use a rigid indirect laryngoscope than struggle with blind intubation using an introducer. If a patient is found to be a difficult direct laryngoscopy the first management step should be to abandon direct laryngoscopy and choose indirect laryngoscopy. This will usher in a major change in our approach to tracheal intubation and many critical care practitioners have already started incorporating rigid indirect laryngoscopy into their clinical practice.

Key points

- Rigid indirect laryngoscopy can overcome some of the problems inherent to direct laryngoscopy and intubation using a flexible bronchoscope, but it has its own drawbacks. There is no ideal intubation device.
- RILs have a wide field of view 'around the corner' and allow TT advancement under visual control.

- The built-in optics and electronics usually allow viewing of the image by multiple spectators and also allow documentation of successful intubation.
- There are considerable differences in characteristics between individual RILs, resulting in different possibilities and limitations of clinical application.
- The market for RILs is fast-moving. Every year new devices are introduced and existing ones are modified.

Further reading

Arslan ZI, Yildiz T, Baykara ZN, Solak M, Toker K. (2009). Tracheal intubation in patients with rigid collar immobilisation of the cervical spine: A comparison of Airtraq and LMA CTrach devices. *Anaesthesia*, **64**, 1332–1336.

Bathory I, Frascarolo P, Kern C, Schoettker P. (2009). Evaluation of the Glidescope for tracheal intubation in patients with cervical spine immobilisation by a semi-rigid collar. *Anaesthesia*, **64**, 1337–1341.

Cooper RM, Pacey JA, Bishop MJ, McCluskey SA. (2005). Early clinical experience with a new videolaryngoscope (GlideScope) in 728 patients. *Canadian Journal of Anaesthesia*, **52**, 191–198.

Frerk CM, Lee G. (2009). Laryngoscopy: Time to change our view. *Anaesthesia*, **64**, 351–357.

Henderson J. (2007). Laryngoscopy: Past, Present and Future. *Refresher course lectures*. Brussels: European Society of Anaesthesiology.

Howard-Quijano KJ, Huang YM, Materosian R, Kaplan MB, Steadman RH. (2008). Video-assisted instruction improves the success rate for tracheal intubation by novices. *British Journal of Anaesthesia*, **101**, 568–572.

Kaplan MB, Hagberg CA, Ward DS, et al. (2006). Comparison of indirect and video-assisted views of the larynx during routine intubation. *Journal of Clinical Anesthesiology*, **18**, 357–362.

Lopez AM, Valero R, Pons M, Anglada T. (2009). Awake intubation using the LMA-C Trach in patients with difficult airways. *Anaesthesia*, **64**, 387–391.

Malik MA, Subramaniam R, Maharaj CH, Harte BH, Laffey JG. (2009). Randomized controlled trial of the Pentax AWS, Glidescope, and Macintosh laryngoscopes in predicted difficult intubation. *British Journal of Anaesthesia*, **103**, 761–768.

McGuire BE. (2009). Use of the McGrath video laryngoscope in awake patients. *Anaesthesia*, **64**, 912–914.

Mihai R, Blair E, Kay H, Cook TM. (2008). A quantitative review and meta-analysis of performance of non-standard laryngoscopes and rigid fibreoptic intubation aids. *Anaesthesia*, **63**, 745–760.

Norrens RR, Moebus S, Heid F, et al. (2010). Evaluation of the McGrath Series 5 videolaryngoscope after failed direct laryngoscopy. *Anaesthesia*, **65**, 716–720.

Pott LM, Murray WB. (2008). Review of video laryngoscopy and rigid fiberoptic laryngoscopy. *Current Opinion in Anaesthesiology*, **21**, 750–758.

Savoldelli GL, Schiffer E, Abegg C, et al. (2009). Learning curves of the Glidescope, the McGrath and the Airtraq laryngoscopes: A mannikin study. *European Journal of Anaesthesiology*, **26**, 554–558.

Serocki G, Bein B, Scholz J, Dorges V. (2010). Management of the predicted difficult airway: A comparison of conventional blade laryngoscopy with video-assisted blade laryngoscopy and the GlideScope. *European Journal of Anaesthesiology*, **27**, 24–30.

Chapter 16

Misplacement of tracheal tubes

Om Sanehi

Introduction

Misplacement of a tracheal tube is a serious complication. Misplacement is usually into the oesophagus or a main bronchus. Unrecognised oesophageal intubation continues to cause mortality. One might think that it is always possible to tell whether the lungs are being inflated, but experienced anaesthetists know that it can be very difficult. Death or brain damage following accidental oesophageal intubation is devastating, particularly as it is virtually always avoidable.

Rarely, a tube may be placed accidentally in some more exotic location, such as the retropharyngeal or intracranial spaces.

Reasons for confirming tracheal intubation

The prompt recognition of misplacement is important because:

- If not corrected, oesophageal placement will lead to:
  - Hypoxia, brain damage and/or death
  - Insufflation of the stomach when attempting to ventilate the lungs (in children this can lead to bradycardia and in all ages it increases the risk of regurgitation of stomach contents).
- If not corrected, bronchial placement may lead to:
  - Hypoxaemia from shunting of blood
  - Lung or lobar collapse
  - Increased airway pressure and possible baro/volutrauma.

Consequently it is vital to:

- Differentiate between a tube which has passed through the vocal cords from one which is in the oesophagus

- Determine that a tube through the cords is in the trachea and not in a main bronchus.

A variety of tests has been devised to do each of these. The tests reviewed here do not comprise a comprehensive list, but are commonly used, reliable or both. The reliability can be evaluated according to estimates of the frequencies of false positives (related to specificity) and negatives (related to sensitivity, see Chapter 7). These values can give a guide to the efficacy of a test, but misinterpretation of even excellent tests is not difficult when the clinical situation is confusing and deteriorating.

When reading publications on this topic it is important to be clear as to whether the authors are describing their results in terms of the ability of the test to identify correct (tracheal) placement or to identify misplacement (in the oesophagus or bronchus). A 'positive' test might refer to either correct placement or misplacement. In this chapter a positive result always indicates tracheal placement.

Excluding oesophageal intubation
Methods of differentiating between tracheal and oesophageal intubation

Tests to confirm tracheal (as opposed to oesophageal) intubation are listed in Table 16.1. Since manual ventilation through a tube placed in the oesophagus will insufflate the stomach, methods of detecting oesophageal misplacement *prior to* manual ventilation are of great importance and are separated from those requiring manual ventilation.

Core Topics in Airway Management, Second Edition, ed. Ian Calder and Adrian Pearce. Published by Cambridge University Press.
© Cambridge University Press 2011.

Table 16.1. Tests to confirm tracheal (as opposed to oesophageal) intubation

	False positive (Suggests the tube is in the trachea when it is in the oesophagus)	False negative (Suggests the tube is in the oesophagus when it is in the trachea)
Techniques not requiring manual ventilation		
Inspection of the vocal cords		
Immediately after placement of the tube, there is visual confirmation that *the tube is surrounded by the glottic structures*	Infrequent Probably mainly due to migration of the tube after visualisation	None reported
Palpation of the trachea		
As a tube passes through the trachea, an assistant palpating the external trachea may *feel vibrations*	Frequent	Frequent
Oesophageal detector device		
Tracheal placement results in *free aspiration of gas* from the lungs; in oesophageal intubation the walls of the oesophagus collapse around the tube lumen preventing gas flow	Very infrequent	Infrequent The few reported examples relate mainly to *delayed*, rather than absent, aspiration of gas, in patients with airway obstruction (e.g., bronchial intubation, bronchospasm, secretions)
Techniques requiring manual ventilation		
Sounds		
The *absence of a characteristic flatus-like sound* produced during manual ventilation suggests that the tube is correctly placed; presence of such a sound suggests oesophageal placement	Anecdotally frequent	Anecdotally frequent
Compliance		
A '*normal*' *compliance*, (indicated by how hard the reservoir bag must be squeezed for chest expansion) is elicited if the tube is tracheal	Frequent	Frequent
Condensation of water vapour in the tube		
The appearance of condensation in the tube on manual ventilation suggests correct placement	Anecdotally frequent	Infrequent
Visual inspection of the chest		
Good expansion of the chest on manual ventilation suggests correct placement; poor expansion suggests oesophageal intubation	Frequent Abdominal movements may mimic expansion of the chest	Frequent An already hyperinflated chest may exhibit poor expansion

Table 16.1. (*cont.*)

	False positive (Suggests the tube is in the trachea when it is in the oesophagus)	False negative (Suggests the tube is in the oesophagus when it is in the trachea)
Auscultation of the epigastrium		
Manual ventilation through a tube placed in the trachea *does not produce gurgling* heard on auscultating the epigastrium	None reported\nIf the tube is in the oesophagus, there is almost certain to be gurgling	Infrequent
Auscultation of the chest		
Breath sounds auscultated at the axillae suggest correct tracheal placement	Frequent\nOperator-dependent	Frequent\nOperator-dependent
Carbon dioxide detection		
Capnography – *A normal capnogram for at least six breaths* suggests tracheal intubation	Very infrequent\n$CO_2$ in the stomach (e.g., fizzy drinks, prior mouth-to-mouth resuscitation) may cause confusion during the first few breaths but is likely to be washed out by six breaths	Infrequent\nExamples are cardiac arrest, severe bronchospasm and large gas leaks (in all of which CO_2 is not delivered to the capnograph)
Capnometry – detection of CO_2 as indicated either numerically or by a colorimetric change suggests tracheal intubation	Infrequent\nThe lack of a graphical display makes CO_2 in the stomach producing a false positive more of a reality	Infrequent\nSee above
Endoscopy		
Visualisation of the tracheal rings by fibreoptic bronchoscopy can confirm tracheal placement	Unacceptable delay	Unacceptable delay

Techniques not requiring manual ventilation

Visual confirmation

If intubation is accomplished by means of direct or video-laryngoscopy then visual observation that the tube is *surrounded* by glottic structures provides certainty, but in very many cases the view is not sufficiently clear to permit certainty. If a flexible fibreoptic laryngoscope is employed as the method of intubation then the carina provides a reliable landmark. Visual confirmation is the best and simplest method (the only real gold standard for those who like that term), and in situations such as pulmonary agenesis or complete tracheal obstruction, the only practical method.

It is vital to appreciate that if absolute certainty that the tube is surrounded by the glottis is not obtained then the intubator is in a similar position to a pilot who cannot see out of his cockpit, but must rely on his instruments. It can be very difficult to believe instruments if they do not provide the values expected.

Oesophageal detector device

The oesophageal detector device (ODD) depends upon applying a negative pressure to the tube immediately after placement. Commercial devices such as the AMBU^R 'TubeChek' versions A and B are available (Figure 16.1). The B version is a self-inflating bulb and the A an aspirating syringe. 'Home-made' devices can be made by attaching a catheter mount or angle piece to an irrigating syringe bulb, a bulb used for bladder irrigation, or a 60 ml syringe. The junction between the syringe or bulb and the catheter mount must be completely airtight; ensure that aspiration of air is impossible when the orifice is occluded.

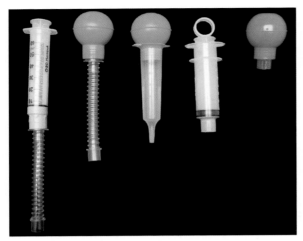

Figure 16.1. Oesophageal detector devices. From left: 1. Wee's original device, a 60-ml syringe attached to a catheter mount; 2. An ODD made from a catheter mount and a surgical irrigating syringe bulb; 3. A surgical irrigating syringe; 4. AMBU^R TubeChek A; 5. AMBU^R TubeChek B. Before using these devices always test that aspiration of air is impossible when the opening is occluded.

The device is attached to the tracheal tube after intubation. With the syringe version, the negative pressure is applied by pulling up on the plunger; the evacuator bulb version merely requires the bulb to be compressed and allowed to re-inflate. Tracheal placement results in rapid, free aspiration of gas from the lungs; the bulb may fill slowly if the tube has been placed in a main bronchus, so the depth of insertion should be checked. Slow filling may also occur if there is severe bronchospasm, there are copious secretions, and in obese patients. If the tube is in the oesophagus, the negative pressure causes the walls of the oesophagus to collapse around the tube lumen preventing gas flow. This means there is resistance to pulling up the plunger in the syringe version, and in the bulb version, the bulb does not re-inflate. Curiously, the ODD has not become a standard of practice, despite having a similar accuracy to capnography. Enthusiasts point to its particular value in cases where there is doubt about the circulation, its ability to give an immediate indication of tube position, and its 100% sensitivity for oesophageal intubation (the device does not fill if the tube is in the oesophagus). Sceptics point out that slow filling may be mistaken for no filling, so that some correctly placed tubes are removed. The device should not be used in children less than 20 kg in weight. The volume of the device (syringe or bulb) should be greater than 30 ml.

Palpation of the trachea

As a tube passes through the trachea, an assistant palpating the external trachea may feel vibrations, likened to a stick being dragged across a corrugated roof and corresponding to the tube touching the tracheal rings. Such vibrations are absent if the tube passes into the oesophagus.

Techniques requiring manual ventilation
Carbon dioxide detection

Capnometers measure carbon dioxide concentration and display it either in a numerical or colorimetric fashion. Capnometers are much more portable than capnographs and are therefore often used in pre-hospital care.

Capnographs produce a graphical trace of carbon dioxide concentration against time (called a capnogram). A capnogram which shows a normal trace for at least six breaths is excellent for excluding oesophageal intubation, although confusing results have been obtained if there has been recent ingestion of fizzy drinks.

With the widespread use of capnographs (which is to be applauded), there has been a tendency to use capnography as the *only* tool to distinguish between tracheal and oesophageal intubation. This is regrettable, as capnography, like all of the other available tests, is less than 100% reliable and is best used in combination with other tests. In reports of disasters following oesophageal intubation it has sometimes been found that a flat end-tidal carbon dioxide trace has been explained away rather than believed. There may be a supposition that the circulation is so poor as to preclude the appearance of expired carbon dioxide (a history or suspicion of anaphylaxis, or known circulatory instability can confuse the issue), and when these doubts are combined with what may appear to be compelling reasons for not removing a tube, such as vomit or blood in the pharynx, it can be tempting to disobey the 'if in doubt take it out' dictum.

Sounds

The characteristic flatus-like sound produced during manual ventilation of a tube placed in the oesophagus is quite different from that produced if the tube is correctly placed, but is not reproduced reliably.

Compliance

Perception of a 'normal' compliance, (indicated by how hard the reservoir bag must be squeezed for chest expansion) is difficult and therefore this is a poor test. Computer-aided techniques have been found to be more reliable.

Condensation of water vapour in the tube

During manual ventilation, 'misting' of the tube often occurs due to condensation on the sides of the tube of water vapour from the lungs. A lack of this misting suggests oesophageal intubation, but its presence does not guarantee that the tube is in the trachea.

Visual inspection of the chest

Once manual ventilation is started, poor expansion of the chest may indicate oesophageal intubation. Although commonly used, this test when used alone is very unreliable.

Auscultation of the epigastrium and chest

Manual ventilation of a tube placed in the oesophagus is reliably accompanied by gurgling heard on auscultating the epigastrium. Breath sounds heard in both axillae suggest correct tracheal placement, but sounds transmitted from inflation of the stomach can easily be mistaken for breath sounds.

Endoscopy

Although fibreoptic bronchoscopy is excellent for differentiating tracheal from oesophageal intubation, in a situation in which oesophageal intubation is suspected, it is likely to lead to unacceptable delay.

Novel methods

Successful identification of tracheal and oesophageal ventilation has been described in small sized studies of the methods below. Larger trials are required to establish their value.

- Computer aided analysis of breath sounds from stethoscopes
- Trans-thoracic impedance measured across defibrillator pads
- An ultrasound device placed on the crico-thyroid membrane can detect the passage of the tube, but cannot detect a stationary tube.

Taking corrective action in suspected oesophageal intubation

It is important to take corrective action promptly for the reasons discussed above. Rapid confirmation of misplacement by direct laryngoscopy should be attempted. Whenever oesophageal intubation is suspected the traditional teaching has been to remove the tube – '*if in doubt take it out!*'. However reluctant one may be to remove a tube (laryngoscopy not easy, actual or high risk of vomiting, intra-oral bleeding, moribund patient) it must be done. The advent of supraglottic airways has made this advice even more sensible.

Passing *an additional* tube, leaving the errant one in situ, has been advocated; the purported advantage being that the original tube may facilitate visualisation of the glottis, and in cases in which the stomach is not empty, the oesophageal tube protects the airway from aspiration of gastric contents.

Excluding bronchial intubation
Methods of differentiating between tracheal and bronchial intubation

Tests to confirm tracheal (as opposed to bronchial) intubation are listed in Table 16.2.

Unfortunately, none of the easily used tests is very reliable, and haemoglobin desaturation is often the reason that bronchial intubation is suspected and detected.

Depth of insertion

In adults correct tracheal placement is usually obtained when about 21–23 cm of tube is distal to the lips.

Compliance

Low compliance of the chest, requiring high airway pressures to inflate the chest (indicated by how hard the reservoir bag must be squeezed), may indicate bronchial placement. However this is only one of many possible causes of decreased chest compliance.

Visual inspection of the chest

Asymmetric expansion of the chest may be the first sign to indicate bronchial intubation.

Table 16.2. Tests to confirm tracheal (as opposed to bronchial) intubation

	False positive (Suggests the tube is in the trachea when it is in a main bronchus)	False negative (Suggests the tube is in a main bronchus when it is in the trachea)
Compliance		
A *'normal' compliance*, is detected if the tube is tracheal, a low compliance if it is bronchial	Frequent	Frequent There are many different causes of decreased chest compliance
Visual inspection of the chest		
Equal expansion of both sides of the chest on manual ventilation suggests correct tracheal placement	Frequent	Frequent
Auscultation of the chest		
Breath sounds heard on auscultating *both axillae* suggest correct tracheal placement and at only one, bronchial placement	Frequent Operator-dependent	Frequent Operator-dependent
Endoscopy		
Fibreoptic bronchoscopic *visualisation* of the trachea confirms tracheal intubation	Operator-dependent	Operator-dependent
Radiography		
The position of the *tube relative to the carina* may be seen on a chest X-ray	Not reported	Not reported

Auscultation of the chest

Unilateral breath sounds suggest bronchial placement. The use of auscultation in this context is very operator-dependent; experienced anaesthetists are far more likely to glean useful information than more junior staff. Computerised analysis of breath sounds, although accurate, is not yet practicable in the clinical setting.

Endoscopy

Fibreoptic bronchoscopy can reliably differentiate between the trachea and a main bronchus, as the trachea has incomplete cartilaginous rings, but it is easy for an inexperienced endoscopist to mistake the divisions of the right main bronchus for the carina.

Radiography

A chest X-ray may be helpful in excluding bronchial intubation.

Taking corrective action in suspected bronchial intubation

If a bronchial intubation is suspected, the tube should be gradually withdrawn and reassessment undertaken.

Excluding misplacement in an exotic space

There are no specific tests to exclude misplacement in positions such as the retropharyngeal space or intracranial space. However there will be a complete inability to ventilate the lungs, which should become apparent very quickly using the standard tests described above. A high degree of suspicion should be maintained in those cases which are susceptible to such misplacements, such as trauma patients. If perforation of the pharyngeal mucosa might have occurred the patient should be given prophylactic antibiotics (cephalosporin and metronidazole) and

Box 16.1 Confirmation of tracheal intubation

1. At laryngoscopy, observe that the tube is surrounded by glottic structures.
2. Apply ODD.
3. Inspect chest expansion.
4. Detect expired CO_2.
5. Auscultate chest and epigastrium.
6. If any doubt, remove the tube and use an SGA.

observed for the possible onset of mediastinitis or deep cervical infection (dysphagia, neck or chest pain, fever).

Developing a routine

There are no perfect tests so it is essential to use a variety of techniques. A recommended sequence is shown in Box 16.1.

Note that this routine has a logical progression, with tests requiring manual ventilation performed after those that do not, although in practice tests 3, 4 and 5 occur concurrently. Some may prefer to omit the ODD if visual confirmation is obtained, but there is much to be said for a fixed routine; regular use of the ODD builds expertise and confidence and ensures the device is actually available when needed.

Confirmation in adverse circumstances

The inclusion of some reliable, *simple* tests in one's routine is essential because there may be situations in which intubation is performed in which more sophisticated tests are not possible. The use of capnography to the exclusion of other tests risks missing oesophageal placement in areas where such a facility is absent – for instance during pre-hospital care, in hospital wards and some accident departments and intensive care units.

Key points

- Unrecognised misplacement of a tracheal tube may have disastrous sequelae, and is avoidable.

- No single test is completely reliable (there is no gold standard), and so a combination of tests should be employed.
- Intuitively, one would imagine that determination of the correct position of a tracheal tube would be a simple matter, but in practice it can be very difficult if there are confounding factors.
- If correct tracheal positioning of a tube cannot be confirmed the safest option is to exchange it for a supraglottic airway.

Further reading

Bozeman WP, Hexter D, Liang HK, Kelen GD. (1996). Esophageal detector device versus detection of end-tidal carbon dioxide level in emergency intubation. *Annals of Emergency Medicine*, **27**, 595–599.

Heath M. (2005). CEMACH report: Oesophageal intubation. *British Journal of Anaesthesia*, **95**, 426.

Kramer-Johansen J, Eilerstjohn J, Olasveengen TM, et al. (2008). Transthoracic impedance changes as a tool to detect malpositioned tracheal tubes. *Resuscitation*, **76**, 11–16.

Ma G, Davis DP, Schmitt J, et al. (2005). The sensitivity and specificity of transcricothyroid ultrasonography to confirm endotracheal tube placement in a cadaver model. *Journal of Emergency Medicine*, **32**, 405–407.

Marciniak B, Fayoux P, Hébrard A, et al. (2009). Airway management in children: Ultrasonography assessment of tracheal intubation in real time? *Anesthesia and Analgesia*, **108**, 461–465.

McCoy EP, Russell WJ, Webb RK. (1997). Accidental bronchial intubation. An analysis of AIMS incident reports from 1988 to 1994 inclusive. *Anaesthesia*, **52**, 24–31.

Nolan JP. (2008). Strategies to prevent unrecognized oesophageal intubation during out-of hospital cardiac arrest. *Resuscitation*, **76**, 1–2.

O'Connor CJ, Mansy H, Balk RA, Tuman KJ, Sandler RH. (2005). Identification of endotracheal tube malpositions using computerized analysis of breath sounds via electronic stethoscopes. *Anesthesia and Analgesia*, **101**, 735–739.

Wolfe T. (2005). *The Esophageal Detector Device*. Summary of the current articles in the literature. Available at: http://www.wolfetory.com/education/eddab.html.

Extubation

Viki Mitchell

Extubation is a critical moment in anaesthesia which few experienced anaesthetists approach with total confidence that their patient will suffer no adverse event, and their own dignity will be unruffled.

In many ways, tracheal extubation should be easier to manage than induction and intubation since the challenge of controlling the airway has already been overcome. However extubation is not simply a reversal of the process of intubation and many factors contribute to conditions which may be unfavourable and a situation in which decision making may be impaired. The risks do not relate exclusively to the airway, cardiovascular instability and changes in venous, intraocular and intracranial pressures may all cause problems.

Extubation remains the 'Cinderella' of management of the difficult airway with few randomised controlled studies. In the UK the Difficult Airway Society Guidelines do not include advice on the management of extubation, although this is included in similar guidelines from Canada and the USA. Articles on the management of extubation are full of opinion and very little in the way of evidence-based medicine. Basic questions such as whether coughing at extubation influences post-operative complications like haematoma formation after neuro, ENT (ear, nose and throat), plastic or eye surgery are unanswered.

However anaesthesia providers are increasingly recognising the importance of the emergence, extubation and recovery period as an important contributor to anaesthetic morbidity, and focusing efforts at improving delivery of a quality service in this area.

Prevalence of problems

Extubation is rarely impossible but on at least one occasion a double-lumen tube has had to be surgically excised. Problems at extubation and recovery account for 14% and 7%, respectively, of all respiratory-related injuries in the American Society of Anesthesiologists (ASA) Closed Claim Project database. These data have revealed a significant reduction in the airway claims arising from injury at induction of anaesthesia following the introduction of guidelines for the management of difficult intubation while airway claims arising from injury at extubation and during the recovery phase have not decreased (Table 17.1).

In the UK it has been shown that respiratory complications occur three times more frequently at extubation than at intubation (Table 17.2). Most of the complications following extubation are minor but can occasionally cause serious injury or death, and Table 17.3 compares the prevalence of complications at induction, extubation and in the recovery room.

Factors producing problems

The post-extubation patient is particularly at risk for morbidity from various factors related to residual anaesthesia or muscle weakness, effects on the airway due to positioning, surgery or intubation and sequelae of arousal. The effects of sympathetic stimulation on the circulation may also be significant.

Inadequate airway patency

- Reduced muscular or soft tissue tone causing pharyngeal collapse.
- Impaired neurological control of complex pharyngeal reflexes.
- Swelling of the soft tissues: oedema or haematoma.
- Vocal cord weakness or paralysis.

Core Topics in Airway Management, Second Edition, ed. Ian Calder and Adrian Pearce. Published by Cambridge University Press. © Cambridge University Press 2011.

Table 17.1. Timing of peri-operative claims (n=156, from Peterson et al, 2005)

Timing	1985–1992 (n = 73)		1993–1999 (n = 83)	
	Claims %	Death %*	Claims %	Death %*
Pre-induction	3	100	1	100
Induction	71	62	63	35
Intraoperative	15	55	14	83
Extubation in OR	8	100	14	83
Recovery	3	50	7	67

*Percent of row resulting in death or brain damage

Table 17.2. Incidence of respiratory complications associated with intubation and extubation (from Asai et al, 1998)

Intubation	4.6%
Extubation	12.6%
Recovery	9.5%

Inadequate reversal of neuromuscular blockade

- Residual neuromuscular blockade impairs the function of respiratory, laryngeal and upper airway muscles and is associated with impaired airway protective reflexes, upper airway obstruction and a decreased hypoxic ventilatory response. Volunteer studies have demonstrated pharyngeal dysfunction with aspiration at train-of-four (TOF) ratios less than 0.9.
- Clinical tests such as head lift and manual or visual assessment of TOF fade have poor sensitivity at detecting residual neuromuscular blockade. Studies have shown that a significant proportion of patients reach recovery with incomplete neuromuscular recovery despite the use of neostigmine reversal and TOF monitoring.
- The introduction of new agents such as sugammadex into clinical practice offers the potential for more rapid and effective reversal of neuromuscular blockade.

Table 17.3. Ranked incidence of respiratory complications from ASA Closed Claims data

Complications during induction	%	Complications at extubation (in operating theatre)	%	Complications after extubation (in recovery room)	%
Coughing	1.5	Coughing	6.6	Airway obstruction	3.8
Difficult ventilation	1.4	Desaturation <90%	2.4	Coughing	3.1
Desaturation <90%	1.1	Breath-holding	2	Desaturation <90%	2.2
Difficult intubation	0.8	Airway obstruction	1.9	Laryngospasm	0.8
Laryngospasm	0.4	Laryngospasm	1.7	Apnoea, hypoventilation	0.8
Oesophageal intubation	0.3	Apnoea, hypoventilation	0.9	Vomiting	0.7
Gagging	0.1	Inadequate reversal	0.5	Breath-holding	0.3
		Vomiting	0.3	Inadequate reversal	0.3
		Masseter spasm	0.1	Bronchospasm	0.2
Patients with one or more complication	4.6%		12.5%		9.5%
95% Confidence intervals	3.3,5.9		10.5,14.6		7.6,11.3

Sequelae of airway stimulation

- Coughing and 'bucking' (a forceful and protracted cough that mimics a Valsalva manoeuvre). These cause abrupt rises in intracavity pressures with increased intrathoracic pressure leading to decreased venous return, decrease in functional residual capacity (FRC) and associated atelectasis. Intracranial, intraocular, venous and arterial pressures all increase.
- Laryngospasm (see below).
- Bronchospasm.
- Negative pressure pulmonary oedema. Typically occurring in young fit adults, an episode of airway obstruction (upper airway obstruction, laryngospasm, occlusion of the tracheal tube or supraglottic airway device by biting) is followed by respiratory distress, haemoptysis and the radiological changes of pulmonary oedema. Treatment includes the application of positive airway pressure, supplementary oxygen and possibly diuretics. Most cases resolve within 24 hours. A bite block prevents occlusion of a tube or SAD by biting, if complete occlusion should occur, deflation of the cuff permits airflow around the device and prevents the generation of extreme negative pressures.

Other problems

- Aspiration. One-third of aspiration events occur after extubation. Protective reflexes may be obtunded and the glottic closure reflex may be impaired for some time after extubation.
- Inadequate ventilatory drive. Opioids and volatile agents blunt response to hypoxia and alter the carbon dioxide (CO_2) response curve.
- Deranged lung function. Increase in dead space as the endotracheal tube is replaced by upper airway volume and residual atelectasis.
- Hypoxaemia. Hypoxaemia results from impaired ventilatory drive, deranged lung function and partial or complete airway obstruction. Arterial oxygen saturation is only 90% in 20–30% of healthy patients extubated without supplementary O_2. The use of nitrous oxide during anaesthesia increases the risk of hypoxaemia due to diffusion hypoxia. The rate of oxygen desaturation with an obstructed airway

will be much more rapid in a struggling, emerging patient than during anaesthesia due to the much increased oxygen consumption.

Conduct of extubation

The evidence to support a universal extubation strategy is lacking, and a survey of extubation practice in the UK showed a wide, unexplained variability. Even the seemingly sensible practice of administering 100% oxygen for several minutes prior to extubation was performed always by only 54% respondents. There is no consensus as to what constitutes a good extubation plan, and as with most aspects of anaesthesia, there are many possible options for managing each clinical situation.

Benumof has proposed the following sound principles.

Extubation should be:

- Controlled
- Gradual
- Step by step
- Reversible.

It is important to remember that extubation is an elective episode. There is a great deal of pressure on the anaesthetist to effect extubation quickly and smoothly at the end of the case but in many respects the situation is less controlled than at induction. Organisational and human factor issues, in particular pressure to complete the case and embark on the next, may compromise decision making.

Equipment, monitoring and skilled assistance should be of the same quality as would be available at induction, and the process should be planned and carried out in a controlled manner with a back-up plan to ensure oxygenation if difficulties are encountered. Every extubation technique should ensure minimal interruption in the delivery of oxygen to the patient's lungs, and should extubation fail, ventilation should be achievable with the minimal difficulty or delay.

Consideration should be given to the following factors that may interact in very different ways for any one individual patient:

- Anaesthesia
- Surgery
- Pathology
- Patient
- Respiratory pattern.

It is useful to ask the questions: is this airway likely to be difficult to manage at extubation? Will it be possible to deliver oxygen to the lungs should extubation fail? Are there any other factors which put the patient at risk? This allows the generation of an extubation strategy using the following basic principles:

- Have a plan.
- Control the airway so oxygen can be given without interruption.
- Avoid the sequelae of airway stimulation.
- Have a back-up plan should extubation fail.

Managing extubation

An appropriate extubation flow-chart is shown in Figure 17.1 which seeks to stratify patients into low-risk and high-risk groups. Generally, adequate spontaneous ventilation should be established. If ultra-short-acting anaesthetic agents have been used (e.g., balanced anaesthetic combining desflurane and remifentanil) return of respiration may occur at the same time as consciousness and in this situation extubation may be performed at the onset of spontaneous respiration. Adequate spontaneous ventilation includes return of adequate ventilatory drive, tidal volume, respiratory rate, breathing pattern and oxygenation with adequate antagonism of residual neuromuscular blockade. Deranged body temperature and pH or surgical factors such as continued oozing may preclude extubation at the end of surgery.

Patient position

There is no consensus on the best position for extubation. The 'left lateral, head-down' position is believed by many to offer a reduced chance of pharyngeal fluids being aspirated, as well as giving the best chance of a naturally clear airway. The position also facilitates re-intubation for the usual left-handed laryngoscopy although intubation in the lateral position is rarely practiced.

However there is now a tendency for the supine, or even head-up position to be used. This may relate to the use of supraglottic airway devices or the increasing prevalence of diseases such as obesity and chronic obstructive pulmonary disease.

The choice of extubation position reflects a balance between the risks of vomiting post-extubation, and subsequent inhalation and soiling of the lungs (favouring the lateral/head-down position), and

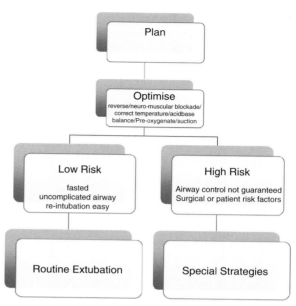

Figure 17.1. Extubation planning flow-chart.

potential respiratory embarrassment and ease of assisting ventilation (favouring the supine/head-up position).

Extubation of the uncomplicated, low-risk airway

The technique of extubation starts prior to removing the tube and should include the following:

- Administering 100% O_2 for a few minutes, aim for an end tidal oxygen concentration >90%.
- Suction of the oro-pharynx under direct vision. The common practice of blind suction is regrettable. Trauma to soft tissue is common. Perforation of pharyngeal mucosa with subsequent mediastinitis has been recorded, bruising and oedema of the uvula secondary to blind suction in the midline causes considerable discomfort post-operatively. If suction cannot be carried out under direct vision, the tip of a rigid sucker should only be inserted into the lateral sulci of the mouth, a soft oro- or nasopharyngeal suction catheter carries less risk of trauma.
- Insert a bite block or oral airway, particularly if the extubation is to be performed 'awake' – to prevent biting of the tube (a particular hazard with reinforced tubes, which may not regain patency after a bite).

161

- Deflate the TT cuff, applying positive pressure to the breathing system reservoir bag.
- Remove the tube and suction any further secretions displaced into the oropharynx.
- Apply mask with high flow O_2 and continuous positive airway pressure (CPAP) as necessary.
- Confirm airway patency and adequacy of ventilation.
- Continue full monitoring during the recovery period.

Deep versus awake extubation

The depth of anaesthesia at the time of extubation is highly important because of the risk of life-threatening laryngospasm. The two 'safe' levels are deeply anaesthetised or awake. Deep extubation refers to extubation in the spontaneous breathing patient who is anaesthetised sufficiently to obtund laryngeal reflexes. It is an advanced technique but offers the advantage of a smoother extubation with less airway stimulation hence reducing coughing, bucking, cardiovascular stimulation, venous, intraocular and intracranial pressure changes.

However this advantage may be offset by an increased incidence of airway obstruction and micro-aspiration. It is important to understand that maintenance and protection of the airway are at risk until consciousness returns. Monitoring must be vigilant and the anaesthetist should be immediately available should airway obstruction develop.

This technique should be reserved for patients in whom it would be easy to control the airway should difficulties be encountered. It should be avoided in patients with a difficult airway, obesity and aspiration risk. To achieve a successful deep extubation the end-tidal sevoflurane concentration needs to be >3%. For this purpose sevoflurane is better than isoflurane, which is better than desflurane.

The technique that usually ensures smooth *deep extubation* is to:

- Establish spontaneous ventilation with the TT in place and an end-tidal sevoflurane of >3% in 90–100% O_2.
- Suction the oro-pharynx under direct vision using a laryngoscope.
- Place an oro-pharyngeal airway or LMA if appropriate.
- Deflate the TT cuff.

Table 17.4. Optimal extubating conditions (from Koga et al, 1998)

	Extubation conditions		
	Optimal	Suboptimal	Poor
Awake	10%	80%	10%
Asleep	15%	80%	5%
LMA	80%	20%	0%

- Ensure there is no reaction to deflation and breathing continues undisturbed.
- Remove the TT in a single smooth action.
- Perform airway manoeuvres as necessary to maintain airway patency and adequate ventilation on 90–100% O_2.
- Any movement of the patient (e.g., theatre table to bed) must be done smoothly and minimising head movement which is likely to promote coughing.
- Close airway monitoring in addition to SpO_2 monitoring must be continued until consciousness has returned.

If *awake extubation* is selected, extubation may initiate coughing and straining but the patient is able to protect and maintain their own airway. The correct stage of anaesthesia is when the patient responds to command. It is easy to remove the tube too early. Awake extubation can also be smooth with careful timing, minimisation of head movement, minimising tube movement and limiting excessive oro-pharyngeal suctioning. Propofol has been shown to obtund airway reflexes to a greater extent than volatile anaesthetic agents. Although it is widely believed that total intravenous anaesthesia with propofol is associated with smoother extubation conditions than volatile anaesthesia, evidence for this belief is scanty.

Exchanging the tracheal tube for an LMA

Peri-extubation insertion of a laryngeal mask airway (LMA) is a useful technique for airway maintenance in the recovery period with less airway obstruction and coughing, and higher saturations than either deep or awake extubation (Table 17.4).

There are two techniques:

- Establish spontaneous ventilation with the TT in place and an end-tidal sevoflurane of >3% in 90–100% O_2, place the LMA and inflate its cuff

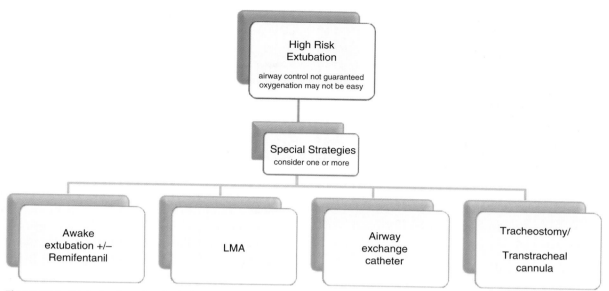

Figure 17.2. Extubation flow-chart for high-risk extubation.

prior to removal of the TT to ensure that the LMA sits behind the epiglottis and laryngeal inlet.

- Alternatively, the tracheal tube can be exchanged for an LMA prior to reversal of neuromuscular blockade.

Extubation of the difficult airway

A difficult extubation is one in which, following extubation, there is difficulty re-establishing oxygenation and ventilation. It may be anticipated when the airway was difficult to manage at induction/intubation or if intraoperative events (such as positioning, surgery or complications of intubation) have adversely affected the airway. Most authorities recommend that the anticipated difficult extubation is undertaken with the patient fully conscious. Undesirable cardiovascular responses can be blunted pharmacologically. Where peri-glottic swelling is a potential issue, a 'cuff-leak' test can be helpful. Ideally there should be an audible air leak as the cuff of the TT is deflated confirming adequate airway calibre. However this does not eliminate the risk of airway oedema developing in the post-operative period.

Difficult extubation strategies

A flow-chart (Figure 17.2) shows the recommended options for extubation strategies in the high-risk patient.

- A remifentanil infusion can be used to reduce undesirable cardiovascular and respiratory responses. The patient remains tube tolerant even after consciousness has returned and can be extubated smoothly once able to obey verbal commands. In a recent study a low-dose remifentanil infusion (mean 0.014 μg/kg/min) maintained during extubation reduced coughing on the tube, non-purposeful movement and tachycardia without compromising recovery from anaesthesia.
- An LMA may provide a useful means of both maintaining the airway in the waking patient and serving as a conduit for fibreoptically guided re-intubation.
- A tracheal tube exchanger can be left in the trachea and provides a conduit for the delivery of oxygen or railroading a tracheal tube should the airway become compromised post-operatively.
- In patients with glottic or supraglottic obstruction, the elective placement of a cannula through the cricothyroid membrane provides a means to guarantee airway control prior to induction of anaesthesia, this can be left in situ for up to 24 hours post-operatively and used for oxygen insufflation or jet ventilation should the airway or respiratory function deteriorate.

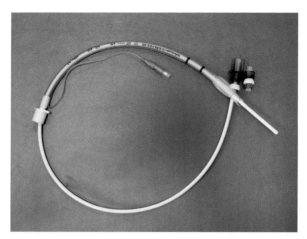

Figure 17.3. Airway exchange catheter.

• If the airway is likely to be compromised for a significant period after surgery, for example after free flap reconstruction of the head and neck, an elective tracheostomy should be considered.

Airway exchange catheters (AEC)

Semi-rigid radio-opaque polyurethane catheters are manufactured by various companies. They are usually 65–85 cm long with a small internal diameter ~ 4 mm (Figure 17.3). They are reasonably rigid to facilitate re-intubation and hollow to facilitate ventilation with removable adaptors allowing passage of the TT over the catheter. A choice of Luer-Lok or 15 mm adaptors permit jet ventilation or attachment to an anaesthetic circuit.

These catheters were originally designed to facilitate safe TT exchange, but experience has demonstrated that they are well tolerated by awake patients even when positioned through the vocal cords in the trachea.

These devices are inserted through the lumen of the TT and into the trachea prior to extubation and as long as the carina is not stimulated by too distal placement of the catheter additional analgesia or sedation is not required to ensure patient tolerance.

These catheters can be left in place for as long as 3 days providing a conduit for TT access to the airway or at least insufflation of oxygen. There are a number of practical points in the use of an AEC (Table 17.5).

Advantages:

• Can be used to oxygenate either by

  insufflation and or
  jet ventilation (but caution needed).

• Can be used as a guide over which a tracheal tube can be railroaded should re-intubation be necessary.

• Can be left in situ for up to 72 hours.

• Generally well tolerated, 5–10% may need lidocaine to prevent coughing.

Hazards:

• May not be tolerated by the patient or coughed out within minutes.

• Failure to railroad a tracheal tube over the AEC (laryngoscopy helpful, anticlockwise rotation of tube prevents hold up at the larynx, a tube with an internal diameter close to AEC is more likely to avoid hold up).

• Complications largely relate to jet ventilation which can cause catastrophic barotrauma and tension pnemothorax. The following precautions increase safety:

  • The distal tip of the catheter should be above the carina (not more than 26cm depth).

  • There should be an annular air space around the catheter within the lower airway so that expiratory flow can occur.

  • Upper airway patency must be maintained to avoid compromising expiratory flow.

  • Jetting pressures must not be excessive.

  • Side holes in the distal catheter may increase safety by decreasing catheter whip, reducing pressures and centring the catheter within the trachea.

• Rupture of the membranous portion of the trachea or the bronchi has been described and is more likely in infants, the elderly and the critically ill. Should never be advanced if resistance encountered and should only be advanced into the trachea.

• Aspiration or impaired cough are theoretical problems but have in practice. One aspiration in a patient who had an AEC in for 18 hours prior to re-intubation but this patient had impaired swallowing (secondary to radiotherapy) pre-operatively.

Table 17.5. Airway exchange catheter troubleshooting

Airway exchange catheters		
Advantages		
Can be used to oxygenate either by Insufflation or Jet ventilation (but caution needed see below)		
Can be used as a guide over which a tracheal tube can be railroaded should re-intubation be necessary		
Can be left in situ for up to 72 hours		

Disadvantages	Solutions
May cause coughing <10%	Lidocaine spray
Failure to railroad a tracheal tube over the AEC	Laryngoscopy: is helpful counterclockwise rotation of tube prevents hold up at the larynx A tube with an internal diameter close to that of the AEC or a blunt level is more likely to avoid hold up
Jet ventilation can cause barotrauma and tension pnemothorax	The distal tip of the catheter should be above the carina (not more than 26 cm depth)
Simple precautions increase safety:	Upper airway patency must be maintained to avoid compromising expiratory flow There should be an annular air space around the catheter within the lower airway so that expiratory flow can occur Jetting pressures must not be excessive Side holes in the distal catheter decrease catheter whip, reduce pressures and centre the catheter within the trachea Rupture of the trachea or the bronchi possible. Do not advance catheter if resistance encountered. Only advance into the trachea
Aspiration or impaired cough are theoretical problems	

Laryngospasm

Laryngospasm is a protective mechanism to prevent foreign material entering the larynx. It is a reflex response mediated by the superior laryngeal branch of the vagus and tends to occur when patients are in light planes of anaesthesia. It can also be provoked by surgical stimulation. It is particularly common after ENT and maxillofacial surgery when blood, secretions and surgical debris may be present. It is more common in children in whom it is particularly unwelcome as hypoxia develops more quickly than in adults.

Mild laryngospasm presents with a degree of stridor, while severe laryngospasm causes complete airway obstruction and is silent. It used to be claimed that the glottis would always relax before the patient dies but it is now clear that this is not true. Laryngospasm can provoke negative pressure pulmonary oedema. Re-intubation and positive pressure ventilation is often required, although some cases can be treated with mask CPAP.

Prevention and treatment

The incidence of laryngospasm is reduced if patients are undisturbed (the 'no-touch technique') while they wake up. Ideally the patient should be in the lateral recovery position and the only touch allowed is the oximeter clip. Various methods have been suggested to reduce the incidence of laryngospasm including

165

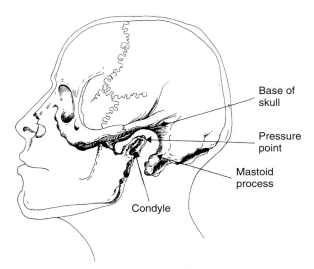

Figure 17.4. The 'laryngospasm notch' bounded anteriorly by the condyle of the mandible, posteriorly by the mastoid process, and superiorly by the base of the skull. (Reproduced with permission from Larson (1998).)

intravenous or laryngo-tracheal lidocaine, doxapram, magnesium and acupuncture.

Simple measures will usually overcome laryngospasm:

- Application of positive end-expiratory pressure (PEEP)/CPAP with 100% O_2. This provides a column of oxygen which will enter the trachea under pressure as soon as the cords part.
- Larson's manoeuvre – jaw thrust with bilateral digital pressure between the posterior border of the mandible and the mastoid process (the 'laryngospasm notch') (Figure 17.4).
- Gentle, pharyngeal suction.
- Propofol (0.25–2 mg/kg) is usually very effective and has much reduced the need for suxamethonium.
- Suxamethonium should always be available; it has a faster onset time in the laryngeal muscles, compared with vecuronium, rocuronium, mivacurium and rapacuronium. An effective dose (1–2 mg/kg) should be used. A major advantage of Succinylcholine is that it is effective when given intramuscularly.

If laryngospasm is not quickly resolved then it is important to rule out other causes of post-extubation stridor such as:

- Soft tissue obstruction
- Throat packs
- Airway oedema (supra- or subglottic)
- Vocal cord dysfunction or paradoxical vocal cord motion
- External compression (haematoma or obstructed venous drainage)
- Aspiration
- Narcotic-induced muscle rigidity
- Laryngo- or tracheomalacia.

Follow-up of a difficult airway

Following difficulties with tracheal intubation or re-intubation, particularly if there have been multiple attempts, it is essential to be vigilant for mediastinitis resulting from airway perforation. Only half of the airway perforations are noted at the time but early diagnosis is crucial as this condition carries a significant risk of mortality.

The symptoms and signs include the triad of:

- Pain- retrosternal or cervical or sore throat
- Pyrexia
- Crepitus

Treatment includes broad spectrum antibiotics, urgent surgical referral, nil-by-mouth and imaging.

Airway Alert form

If there have been any difficulties with bag mask ventilation or tracheal intubation, it is important to explain this orally and in writing to the patient and to provide robust documentation on the anaesthetic notes and in the main hospital clinical record. The simplest method of compiling written information is to complete an Airway Alert form available from the Difficult Airway Society website http://www.das.uk.com/guidelines/downloads.html (Figure 17.5).

An airway alert form should include a summary of airway management, ease or difficulty of bag mask ventilation, grade of laryngoscopy and whether awake fibreoptic intubation is considered necessary for future anaesthetics. It should also include prompts to provide copies for notes, the patient, the General Practitioner, anaesthetic department and to add an alert notice to the front of the notes.

Key points

- An extubation plan should always be formulated.
- Airway complications are more frequent during extubation and recovery than during intubation.

London Hospitals NHS

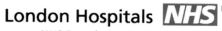

NHS Foundation Trust

Department of Anaesthesia
Road
Town
Postcode
Tel: xxxxxxxxxxx
Fax: xxxxxxxxxxx
E-mail: xxxxxx

AIRWAY ALERT

Name	
Date of birth	
Hospital number	
Home address	
Telephone	
Fax	
Email	

To the patient:

Please keep this letter safe and show it to your doctor if you are admitted to hospital.

Please show this letter to the anaesthetic doctor if you need an operation.

This letter explains the difficulties that were found during your recent anaesthetic and the information may be useful to doctors treating you in the future.

To the GP:

Please copy this letter with any future referral.

Summary of Airway Management

Date of operation:

Type of operation:

		Reasons/comments
Difficult mask ventilation?	YES/NO	
Difficult Direct laryngoscopy?	YES/NO	
Difficult tracheal intubation?	YES/NO	
Laryngoscopy grade	1/2/3/4	

Equipment used:

Other information:

Is awake intubation necessary in the future?

Follow up care (tick when completed)

Copies of letter   Spoken to patient

   One copy to patient   Anaesthetic chart complete

   One copy to GP   Information on front of case notes

   One copy in case notes   Medic Alert or Difficult Airway

   One copy in anaesthetic department   Society referral (Specify)

Name of anaesthetist: Grade: Date:

If you require further information please contact the Anaesthetic Department.

This Form is downloaded from http://www.das.uk.com/guidelines/downloads.html

Figure 17.5. Airway Alert Form.

- Extubation in a deep plane of anaesthesia is an advanced technique.
- If there is doubt about airway control, think about special strategies to minimise risk.
- Low-dose remifentanil improves conditions during awake extubation.
- An airway exchange catheter is a useful aid.
- Follow-up and documentation is essential if airway difficulties have been encountered.

Further reading

Aouad MT, Al-Alami AA, Nasr VG, Souki FG, Zbeidy RA, Siddik-Sayyid SM. (2009). The effect of low-dose remifentanil on responses to the endotracheal tube during emergence from general anesthesia. *Anesthesia and Analgesia*, **108**, 1157–1160.

Asai T, Koga K, Vaughan RS. (1998). Respiratory complications associated with tracheal intubation and extubation. *British Journal of Anaesthesia*, **80**, 767–775.

Benumof JL. (1999). Airway exchange catheters: Simple concept, potentially great danger. Editorial views. *Anesthesiology*, **91**, 342–344.

Benumof J, Hagberg CA. (2007). *Benumof's Airway Management: Principles and Practice*. 2nd ed. Philadelphia: Mosby.

Brull SJ, Naguib M, Miller RD. (2008). Residual neuromuscular block: Rediscovering the obvious, *Anesthesia and Analgesia*, **107**, 11–14.

Debaene B, Plaud B, Dilly MP, Donati F. (2003). Residual paralysis in the PACU after a single intubating dose of nondepolarizing muscle relaxant with an intermediate duration of action. *Anesthesiology*, **98**, 1042–1048.

Epstein SK. (2001). Predicting extubation failure. Is it (on) the cards? *Chest*, **120**, 1061–1063.

Koga K, Asai T, Vaughan RS, Latto IP. (1998). Respiratory complications associated with tracheal extubation. Timing of tracheal extubation and use of the laryngeal mask during emergence from anaesthesia. *Anaesthesia*, **53**, 540–544.

Larson CP. (1998). Laryngospasm – the best treatment. *Anesthesiology*, **89**, 1293.

Lien CA, Koff H, Malhotra V, Gadalla F. (1997). Emergence and extubation: A systematic approach. *Anesthesia and Analgesia*, **85**, 1177.

McConkey PP. (2000). Postobstructive pulmonary oedema – a case series and review. *Anaesthesia and Intensive Care*, **28**, 72–76.

Miller KA, Harkin CP, Bailey PL. (1995). Postoperative tracheal extubation. *Anesthesia and Analgesia*, **80**, 149–172.

Mort TC. (2007). Continuous airway access for the difficult extubation: The efficacy of the airway exchange catheter. *Anesthesia and Analgesia*, **105**, 1357–1362.

Murphy GS, Szokol JW, Marymont JH, Greenberg SB, Avram MJ, Vender JS. (2008). Residual neuromuscular blockade and critical respiratory events in the postanesthesia care unit. *Anesthesia and Analgesia*, **107**, 130–137.

Nair I, Bailey PM. (1995). Use of the laryngeal mask for airway maintenance following tracheal extubation. *Anaesthesia*, **50**, 174–175.

Oberer C, von Ungern-Sternberg BS, Frei FJ, Erb TO. (2005). Respiratory reflex responses of the larynx differ between sevoflurane and propofol in pediatric patients. *Anesthesiology*, **103**, 1142–1148.

Peterson GN, Domino KB, Caplan RA, Posner KL, Lee LA, Cheney FW. (2005). Management of the difficult airway: A closed claims analysis. *Anesthesiology*, **103**, 33–39.

Probert DJ, Hardman JG. (2003). Failed extubation of a double-lumen tube requiring a cricoid split. *Anaesthesia and Intensive Care*, **31**, 584–587.

Rassam S, SandbyThomas M, Vaughan R, Hall JE. (2005). Airway management before, during and after extubation: A survey of practice in the United Kingdom and Ireland. *Anaesthesia*, **60**, 995–1001.

Srivastava A, Hunter JM. (2009). Reversal of neuromuscular block. *British Journal of Anaesthesia*, **103**, 115–129.

Tsui BC, Wagner A, Cave D, et al. (2004). The incidence of laryngospasm with a 'no touch' extubation technique after tonsillectomy and adenoidectomy. *Anesthesia and Analgesia*, **98**, 327–329.

Vaughan RS. (2003). Extubation – yesterday and today. *Anaesthesia*, **58**, 949–950.

Chapter 18

The aspiration problem

Richard Vanner

Pulmonary aspiration

The pulmonary aspiration of gastric contents can cause a pneumonitis with bronchospasm and pulmonary oedema if acidic liquid is inhaled, or less often airway obstruction or massive atelectasis if particulate matter is inhaled. Conversely, if no symptoms, signs or hypoxaemia occurs within 2 hours of aspiration, respiratory sequelae are unlikely. Aspiration occurs in 1 in 4000 anaesthetics for elective surgery and 1 in 900 for emergency surgery. This is despite using a rapid sequence induction with cricoid pressure for patients requiring emergency surgery. Of those patients that aspirate, 64% have no respiratory sequelae, 20% require ventilation on ITU for more than 6 hours and 5% die. If a tracheal tube is used then aspiration is just as likely after extubation as during induction.

Rapid sequence induction

This is the most commonly used anaesthetic technique used to try and reduce the chance of regurgitation of gastric contents into the pharynx and subsequent pulmonary aspiration in those at risk. It is the combination of pre-oxygenation, intravenous induction of anaesthesia, a fast onset muscle relaxant, cricoid pressure and tracheal intubation with a cuffed tube. Although cricoid pressure was first described in 1961, rapid sequence induction was not in widespread use until 1970.

A survey of 209 anaesthetists in the UK in 2001 showed that aspiration can occur despite a rapid sequence induction with cricoid pressure. The anaesthetists reported 99 cases of regurgitation at induction; 15 aspirated and 3 died. Recently 1085 caesarean sections were studied in Australia and New Zealand.

All had rapid sequence inductions with cricoid pressure, there were four cases of regurgitation on induction one of whom had pulmonary aspiration confirmed and survived.

Three reviews on rapid sequence induction and cricoid pressure have all pointed out that there is no evidence that the technique is effective as there are no published randomised controlled trials comparing the incidence of regurgitation on induction with and without cricoid pressure in patients at high risk of regurgitation. It may have been thought to be unethical to perform such a trial.

Which patients need a rapid sequence induction?

It is generally agreed that patients presenting for elective surgery that have fasted of food for 6 hours and clear drinks for 2 hours (and do not fall into the high risk groups below) are at low risk of aspiration and that a rapid sequence induction with cricoid pressure is not needed to prevent the pulmonary aspiration of gastric contents.

Those patients with a higher risk of aspiration during anaesthesia are: those who are not fasted and present for emergency surgery; patients with delayed gastric emptying (bowel obstruction, critical illness, acidosis, pain, opiates and diabetes mellitus); those patients with an incompetent lower oesophageal sphincter (symptomatic oesophageal reflux disease or women more than 20 weeks pregnant); those with oesophageal strictures. It is these higher risk patients that need a rapid sequence induction to reduce the risk of regurgitation and aspiration pneumonitis.

In 2007 a survey of 421 anaesthetists in the UK investigated current practice on indications for rapid

---

Core Topics in Airway Management, Second Edition, ed. Ian Calder and Adrian Pearce. Published by Cambridge University Press.
© Cambridge University Press 2011.

sequence induction. All would use it for a patient with bowel obstruction, 98% for caesarean section, 95% for appendicectomy, 83% for an elective knee arthroscopy in a patient with a symptomatic hiatus hernia and only 25% for an elective knee arthroscopy in a patient with an asymptomatic hiatus hernia. Discussing the latter scenario the authors pointed out that, when oesophagoscopy was performed on a sample population that was asymptomatic for heartburn, 10% were found to have erosive oesophagitis. These patients would be considered low risk without these findings and are usually anaesthetised safely without a tracheal tube. Also, the 5% that do not use a rapid sequence induction in appendicectomy may be justified following the results of a recent study describing the uneventful use of the ProSeal LMA in 102 patients undergoing an acute appendicectomy.

Anaesthetic technique

The patient's airway is assessed beforehand and awake fibreoptic intubation should be performed in someone with a full stomach who is thought to have a difficult airway. However McDonnell et al found that only half of difficult airways in obstetrics are predicted. A nasogastric tube should be inserted and aspirated before induction in the patients most at risk of aspiration, those with a pyloric gastric obstruction, bowel obstruction or acute abdomen. In other patients likely to have a full stomach an orogastric tube can be passed to empty the stomach during surgery before extubation as aspiration often occurs in the early post-operative period. In pregnant patients at term additional precautions are taken to reduce the acidity of gastric contents as otherwise they have a mean pH of 1.4.

Two recent surveys of rapid sequence induction in the UK have shown us current practice. For high risk cases all anaesthetists use pre-oxygenation, cricoid pressure and a cuffed tracheal tube. Pre-oxygenation is most often with a rebreathing circuit with a median oxygen flow of 8 litres/min for 3 minutes. Actually oxygen flow should be at least 8 litres/min with a rebreathing circuit. In healthy patients pre-oxygenation during 20 degree head-up tilt increases the apnoeic time before hypoxaemia from 4 to 6 minutes and is also effective in the morbidly obese, increasing it from 2 to 3 minutes. In pregnant women at term an increased apnoeic time has not been demonstrated

in the head-up position. However the functional residual capacity of the lungs is increased. Taha et al have claimed that an $F_{ET}O_2$ of about 90% can be obtained if the patient takes eight deep breaths in 60 seconds with an oxygen flow of 10 litres/min using either a circle or Mapleson A or D systems.

Thiopentone was the most popular induction agent in 1999, and in the more recent survey in 2007 the most commonly chosen drug was thiopentone in 86% of caesarean sections, propofol in 60% of appendicectomies and etomidate in 46% of bowel obstructions. Opiate drugs are given at induction by the majority of anaesthetists (fentanyl or alfentanil) for all scenarios apart from caesarean section. Succinylcholine was still the most commonly used muscle relaxant in 2007 with rocuronium chosen by only 12% for appendicectomies, 5% for bowel obstructions and 2% for caesarean sections.

Most anaesthetists now wait for signs of loss of consciousness before giving the muscle relaxant. When using rocuronium, induction with alfentanil and propofol will give the best conditions for intubation. Conditions are better than with alfentanil and thiopentone, propofol alone or thiopentone alone. However conditions for intubation are better when using thiopentone and succinylcholine than with alfentanil, propofol and rocuronium. Etomidate is now unpopular in critically ill patients as it inhibits cortisol production for up to 48 hours. Midazolam is frequently used with muscle relaxants by emergency physicians in doses which may be inadequate and it does not have a fast onset of action.

Increasing the dose of succinylcholine from 1 to 1.5 mg.kg^{-1} improves conditions for intubation. Rocuronium 1 mg.kg^{-1} can provide almost as good conditions for intubation in 60 seconds as succinylcholine 1 mg.kg^{-1}. A Cochrane meta-analysis of 37 studies in 2008 stated that 'succinylcholine created superior intubation conditions to rocuronium when comparing both excellent and clinically acceptable intubating conditions'. Also, 'Rocuronium should therefore only be used as an alternative to succinylcholine when it is known that succinylcholine should not be used'. However rocuronium should probably be used instead of succinylcholine in critically ill patients. Fatal hyperkalaemia can occur following succinylcholine in any patient that has been immobilised for more than 4 days, particularly in those with denervation, severe infection or burns. Fatal hyperkalaemia can also occur in acutely ill patients with severe metabolic acidosis (BE – 17) and exsanguinating haemorrhage.

The fast recovery from succinylcholine is sometimes useful in the 'can't intubate can't ventilate' scenario. Although some would argue that laryngospasm may contribute to this scenario and that would not happen with a longer acting drug. Hayes et al found that, in healthy patients spontaneous ventilation usually returned within 5 minutes following preoxygenation, a sleep dose of thiopentone, succinylcholine 1 mg.kg^{-1} and fentanyl 1 μg.kg^{-1}. The oxygen saturation of haemoglobin reduced to 90% in 11% of those patients. With the introduction of sugammadex reversal of rocuronium can be faster than recovery from suxamethonium. In a recent study by Lee et al 16 mg.kg^{-1} sugammadex was given 3 minutes after 1.2 mg.kg^{-1} of rocuronium. Neuromuscular blockade was reversed within another 3 minutes. Sugammadex could be given even earlier than 3 minutes after rocuronium and hopefully will be available in a sterile pre-prepared syringe from the manufacturer.

Cricoid pressure

So is cricoid pressure effective or not? In the 6 years of Confidential Enquiries into Maternal Death in England and Wales from 1964 to 1969 (before the use of cricoid pressure) there were 52 deaths from aspiration. *'In these deaths caused by inhalation of stomach contents, anaesthesia was usually induced with an intravenous barbiturate, the vocal cords paralysed with succinylcholine and the lungs inflated with oxygen'.*

In contrast during the last four triennial reports (in the UK) from 1994 to 2005, there have only been two deaths from aspiration pneumonitis. One patient did not have cricoid pressure applied having been transferred to theatre from the intensive care unit and the other aspirated followed a failed intubation. This is an incidence of approximately 1 in 100 000 emergency caesarean sections under general anaesthesia. All maternity units in the UK now routinely use a rapid sequence induction with cricoid pressure. Of course there are other measures, such as antacid therapy, which have also helped to reduce death from aspiration.

Evidence that it is sometimes not effective is mainly from reports of regurgitation despite the application of cricoid pressure, such as that from Whittington. Evidence that cricoid pressure is effective comes from four cadaver studies in the literature

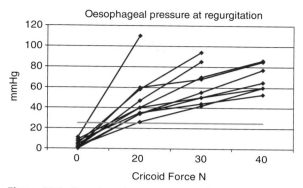

Figure 18.1. Oesophageal pressure measured in 10 cadavers at the moment regurgitation occurred when distending the oesophagus with saline. This was repeated at each increment of cricoid force applied by a cricoid yoke with a force transducer (Vanner 1992). The yellow line at 25 mmHg rep resents the maximum likely gastric pressure (Hartsilver & Vanner, 1999).

(see Figure 18.1) and also case reports of regurgitation seen on release of cricoid pressure but after tracheal intubation, like those from Neelakanta and Sellick.

Some anaesthetists in the UK have suggested that because French anaesthetists do not apply cricoid pressure we should abandon the technique. However in a survey of maternity units in France in 1998, 202 of them replied and of those 88% routinely applied cricoid pressure. Actually, there is also evidence of its effectiveness in a recent randomised controlled trial from France. The incidence of regurgitation was compared in 65 patients who had cricoid pressure applied with 65 patients without cricoid pressure. All patients were at high risk of regurgitation and also had swallowed a methylene blue capsule. No patients regurgitated on induction in the cricoid pressure group compared to three who regurgitated without cricoid pressure ($P < 0.05$).

In an anatomical study Smith et al showed, with both CT and MRI studies, that the larynx can be displaced in a lateral position with cricoid pressure and also that the oesophagus can be imaged slightly lateral to the cricoid cartilage and they explain that this is why cricoid pressure is not always effective. This is misleading as the oesophagus is not behind the cricoid cartilage as it starts caudal to it. To image both structures in the same coronal slice the very inferior edge of the cricoid cartilage has to be found. The position of the oesophagus (which is quite a mobile structure) compared to the cricoid cartilage is therefore irrelevant to the mechanism of cricoid pressure (Rice et al). Actually, it is the hypopharynx

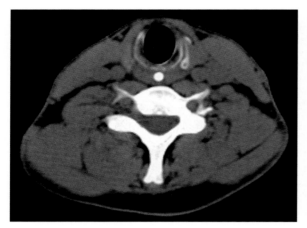

Figure 18.2. CT scan of the author's neck at the level of the cricoid cartilage with a nasogastric tube filled with radio opaque contrast which identifies the lumen of the pharynx (Vanner, 1993).

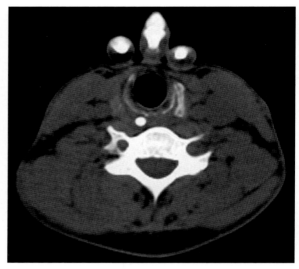

Figure 18.3. As in Figure 18.2 but with cricoid pressure applied (Vanner, 1993). The cricoid has been displaced laterally. Only part of the pharyngeal lumen is compressed onto the vertebrae the rest is compressed onto the pre-vertebral muscles on that side. The pre-vertebral muscles are also compressed on that side when compared to the other side and in Figure 2. The nasogastric tube is squeezed laterally.

within the cricopharyngeus muscle which is behind the cricoid cartilage and is therefore compressed during cricoid pressure. When a manometry catheter was positioned at the level of the cricopharyngeus muscle, cricoid pressure caused a rise in pressure in all 25 subjects studied. As the cricopharyngeus muscle is attached to each side of the larynx the hypopharynx is always behind the larynx and moves with the cricoid when it is displaced laterally with cricoid pressure. Figures 18.2 and 18.3 show that it is not only compressed against the vertebral body but also against the pre-vertebral muscles on either side.

One interesting observation that has emerged from these anatomical studies is the fact that cricoid pressure often (if not always) causes a degree of lateral displacement of the larynx (see Figure 18.3). Lateral displacement can be up to up to 8 mm (Smith KJ – personal communication).

Airway problems with cricoid pressure

Recently 1085 caesarean sections were studied in Australia and New Zealand. All had rapid sequence inductions with cricoid pressure. There were 36 cases of difficult intubation, 4 of those failed to be intubated (2 were a grade 3 laryngeal view and 2 were grade 4). All four had a laryngeal mask airway (LMA) inserted; two had a ProSeal LMA, one a Classic LMA and one an intubating LMA (ILMA). In all four the lungs were successfully ventilated. Intubation was again attempted through the ILMA which again failed.

Hawthorne reported 23 failed intubations in 5,802 caesarean sections under general anaesthesia over a 17 year period, an incidence of 1 in 250. The majority were at night with junior anaesthetists. Fifteen were a grade 3 laryngeal view and six had laryngeal oedema. Seven were difficult to ventilate with a facemask (30%) and two were impossible (9%). Of the two cases with the can't intubate can't ventilate scenario, one had a failed cricothyrotomy and later started breathing (having had succinylcholine) and the other was intubated in the lateral position when cricoid pressure was released. Four other patients had an LMA inserted. In three the lungs were successfully ventilated, but the fourth could not then be ventilated but soon started breathing. One patient became profoundly hypoxaemic with a lowest reading on the pulse oximeter of only 17%. The mother and baby both survived with no ill effects. It seems that the newborn is more damaged by chronic rather than acute hypoxia.

Two consecutive reports from the South West Thames Region reported 56 failed intubations in 13,738 obstetric general anaesthetics, also an incidence of approximately one in 250. All patients survived, most were grade 3 views at laryngoscopy

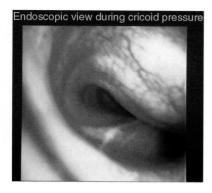
Endoscopic view during cricoid pressure

Figure 18.4. The airway is compressed in 50% of females at 44 N of cricoid force (Palmer, 2000).

and again the majority were at night with junior anaesthetists.

Cricoid pressure can cause problems with the airway. Difficulty with tracheal intubation can be caused by distorting the larynx, particularly if the pressure is applied with excessive force or incorrectly to the thyroid cartilage. When cricoid pressure is correctly applied it often improves the view at laryngoscopy, but it can also make it worse in 14–45% of patients. Insertion of a laryngeal mask is made more difficult with cricoid pressure and ventilation with a facemask is more likely to be obstructed the more cricoid force is applied (see Figure 18.4).

However there has been a randomised double blinded trial comparing the incidence of failed intubation with and without 30 N of cricoid pressure applied in 700 elective surgical patients by Turgeon et al. Failed intubation was defined as failure after 30 seconds with a Macintosh laryngoscope. There was no statistical difference in the two groups, with 15 failures in the cricoid pressure group and 13 in the group without cricoid pressure ($P = 0.7$). The authors state 'The application of cricoid pressure should not be avoided for fear of increasing the difficulty of intubation by direct laryngoscopy when its use is indicated'.

It is important that cricoid pressure is released or adjusted to become Optimal External Laryngeal Pressure (OELP) if intubation is difficult as this may improve the view at laryngoscopy. Most failed intubations are with a grade 3 laryngeal view. Releasing cricoid pressure will certainly correct any lateral displacement for more accurate passage of the bougie under the epiglottis in the midline. If intubation does fail it will allow easier ventilation with a mask and insertion of a laryngeal mask airway. A recent review

(Neilipovitz and Crosby) has described cricoid pressure as a benign practice, since it is completely reversible and can be released if airway problems occur.

Correct technique for cricoid pressure

Although Sellick's original description of cricoid pressure was with the head and neck in the extended position (tonsillectomy position) intubation is easier when a pillow is placed beneath the occiput to adopt the ideal intubating position (the Magill position). The occluding pressure measured within cricopharyngeus during increments of cricoid pressure under anaesthesia is similarly effective between the two positions. The three-finger technique to apply cricoid pressure described by Sellick is actually almost impossible to apply when the patient's head is resting on a pillow. A technique with the forefinger and thumb is much easier (see Figure 18.5).

If a nasogastric tube is already in place before induction of anaesthesia gastric contents should be removed by suction. The tube should be left in place since its presence improves the efficacy of cricoid pressure and not removed as suggested by Sellick. Leave the gastric tube open to atmospheric pressure by connecting it to a bag, then liquid and gas remaining in the stomach can vent and reduce intragastric pressure.

Gastric pressures are less than 25 mmHg during emergency caesarean section with a full stomach. A study of ten cadavers showed that 20 N of cricoid force prevented the regurgitation of oesophageal fluid at a pressure of 25 mmHg in all cases (see Figure 18.1). Therefore 20 N of cricoid pressure is enough force to prevent passive regurgitation into the pharynx. A reasonable recommendation is to apply 10 N (1 kg) to the cricoid cartilage when the patient is awake and to increase the force to 20 N (2 kg) once the patient has lost consciousness. The problem with recommending 20 N is that it has been found that when practicing the correct force on weighing scales, half of the assistants apply less and half more than the recommended level, and that is why 30 N has been recommended previously.

Some also consider that bimanual cricoid pressure is required to support the neck to improve the view of the glottis at laryngoscopy. Three studies have assessed this hypothesis, with apparently contradictory results. It appears that when cricoid pressure is applied using a force of 30 N it usually improves the

173

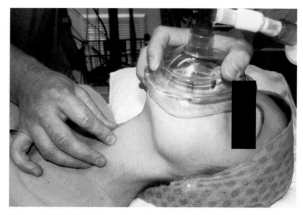

Figure 18.5. Cricoid pressure is more easily applied with the forefinger and thumb when the head is resting on a pillow in the Magill position.

view at laryngoscopy, whereas if too strong a force is used, cricoid pressure is more likely to flex the head and to make laryngoscopy more difficult, requiring neck support to counteract it. It is therefore better not to use bimanual cricoid pressure and to apply less force. The assistant's other hand is useful in passing and helping with the bougie, tracheal tube and inflating the cuff during intubation. If bimanual cricoid pressure is thought to be needed (perhaps when there is a suspected fractured spine – see Chapter 26), more assistants are necessary.

Alternatives to cricoid pressure

The incidence of regurgitation is not known following intravenous induction of anaesthesia with muscle relaxants, without cricoid pressure applied in patients at high risk. Oehlkern and Mort have reported that when the patient is supine it could occur in 2–5%, and this would be more likely if there was ventilation with a facemask or repeated attempts at intubation. The left lateral head-down position has been described for induction by Bourne and if regurgitation occurs it flows out of the mouth and is not aspirated. However McCaul has shown that intubation is more difficult in this position.

The 20 degree head-up position has been described and used during induction of anaesthesia for caesarean section in the late 1950s and early 1960s. In this position the pressure of refluxed gastric contents in the upper oesophagus would be reduced by an amount (in cm H_2O) equal to the height of the cricoid cartilage above the stomach. The apnoeic time before

hypoxaemia is longer following pre-oxygenation in this position. Also, the view at laryngoscopy may be improved in the head-up position. However there have been reports of regurgitation with this technique and no randomised controlled trials have been performed to assess its effectiveness. This does not appear to be an effective alternative to cricoid pressure, so I would suggest that cricoid pressure is still applied even if the 20 degree head-up position is used. As the oesophageal contents would have a lower pressure, the force applied to the cricoid cartilage could be reduced to 20 N (see Figure 18.1). This reduction in force may reduce the incidence of airway problems as these are often proportional to the force applied. The head-up position may give us more confidence to release cricoid pressure if airway problems are encountered.

Failed intubation

During a rapid sequence induction, intubation has failed after two unsuccessful attempts at laryngoscopy both using the gum elastic bougie. The second attempt should be without cricoid pressure and may be with another laryngoscope that the anaesthetist is familiar with, such as the McCoy. Once the anaesthetist has acknowledged that intubation has failed the priority is to ventilate the lungs with oxygen. This is usually done with a facemask with an oral Guedel type airway. If this is successful cricoid pressure could be re-applied to reduce distension of the stomach with gas. If not successful an LMA should be inserted without cricoid pressure. If ventilation is still impossible a cricothyrotomy should be performed.

If ventilation does succeed then a decision needs to be made whether to wake the patient up or not. This is a possibility if the effects of the muscle relaxant recede or are reversed and when the patient is breathing they can be turned into the lateral position. When the patient is awake the options available are to postpone the operation, a spinal anaesthetic or a fibreoptic intubation. In some caesarean sections surgery needs to continue after a failed intubation, and although a spontaneous breathing technique is traditionally recommended, Awan et al have reported the use of a ProSeal LMA with further muscle relaxation.

In critically ill patients waking the patient is often not an option. If the LMA allows ventilation the patient may then be intubated through this device using the Aintree Catheter (Cook Medical) with a

4 mm fibreoptic scope. Although the Classic LMA or the Intubating LMA could be used, the Proseal LMA has the advantage of having a higher seal pressure and can also be used to insert a gastric tube. In the critically ill patient, once the airway is established with a ProSeal LMA an alternative to intubation with the Aintree is to proceed to a percutaneous dilatational tracheostomy so that subsequent unplanned re-intubation would then not be necessary.

Key points

- Rapid sequence induction of anaesthesia with cricoid pressure is usually the technique of choice for those at risk of aspiration despite no randomised controlled trials to give evidence of its effectiveness.

- Aspiration still occasionally occurs despite a rapid sequence induction of anaesthesia with cricoid pressure, particularly if there is difficulty with intubation.

- If a difficult intubation is anticipated awake fibreoptic intubation or spinal anaesthesia should be considered instead.

- Rocuronium may be safer than succinylcholine in the critically ill patient.

- Cricoid pressure should be released, or adjusted to OELP, if there are difficulties with the airway: particularly at intubation with a grade 3 laryngeal view, difficult mask ventilation and during insertion of an LMA.

Further reading

Asai T, Barclay K, Power I, Vaughan RS. (1995). Cricoid pressure impedes the placement of the laryngeal mask airway. *British Journal of Anaesthesia*, **74**, 521–525.

Awan R, Nolan JP, Cook TM. (2004). Use of a ProSeal laryngeal mask airway for airway maintenance during emergency Caesarean section after failed tracheal intubation. *British Journal of Anaesthesia*, **92**, 144–145.

Barnardo PD, Jenkins JG. (2000). Failed tracheal intubation in obstetrics: A 6-year review in a UK region. *Anaesthesia*, **55**, 685–694.

Bourne JG. (1962). Anaesthesia and the vomiting hazard. *Anaesthesia*, **17**, 379–382.

Brimacombe JR, Berry AM. (1997). Cricoid pressure. *Canadian Journal of Anesthesia*, **44**, 414–425.

Brimacombe JR, Berry AM, White A. (1993). An algorithm for the use of the laryngeal mask airway during failed intubation in the patient with a full stomach. *Anesthesia and Analgesia*, **77**, 398–399.

Cook TM. (1996). Cricoid pressure: Are two hands better than one? *Anaesthesia*, **51**, 365–368.

Cook TM, McCrirrick A. (1994). A survey of airway management during induction of general anaesthesia in obstetrics: Are the recommendations of the Confidential Enquiries into Maternal Deaths being implemented? *International Journal of Obstetric Anaesthesia*, **3**, 143–145.

Crawford JS. (1984). *Principles and Practice of Obstetric Anaesthesia*. 5th ed. Oxford: Blackwell Scientific Publications.

Department of Health. (1969). *Report on Confidential Enquiries Into Maternal Deaths in England and Wales 1964–1966*. London: HMSO.

Dixon BJ, Dixon JB, Carden JR, et al. (2005). Preoxygenation is more effective in the 25° head-up position than in the supine position in severely obese patients. *Anesthesiology*, **102**, 1110–1115.

Ellis DY, Harris T, Zideman D. (2007). Cricoid pressure in emergency department rapid sequence tracheal intubations: A risk-benefit analysis. *Annals of Emergency Medicine*, **50**, 653–655.

Fabregat-Lopez J, Garcia-Rojo B, Cook TM. (2008). A case series of the use of the ProSeal laryngeal mask airway in emergency lower abdominal surgery. *Anaesthesia*, **63**, 967–971.

Hartsilver EM, Vanner RG. (1999). Gastric pressure during general anaesthesia for emergency Caesarean section. *British Journal of Anaesthesia*, **82**, 752–754.

Hartsilver EM, Vanner RG. (2000). Airway obstruction with cricoid pressure. *Anaesthesia*, **55**, 208–211.

Haslam N, Parker L, Duggan JE. (2005). Effect of cricoid pressure on the view at laryngoscopy. *Anaesthesia*, **60**, 41–47.

Hawthorne L, Wilson R, Lyons G, Dresner M. (1996). Failed intubation revisited: 17-yr experience in a teaching maternity unit. *British Journal of Anaesthesia*, **76**, 680–684.

Hayes AH, Breslin DS, Mirakhur RK, Reid JE, O'Hare RA. (2001). Frequency of haemoglobin desaturation with the use of succinylcholine during rapid sequence induction of anaesthesia. *Acta Anaesthesiologica Scandinavica*, **45**, 746–749.

Higgs A, Clark E, Premraj K. (2005). Low-skill fibreoptic intubation: Use of the Aintree catheter with the classic LMA. *Anaesthesia*, **60**, 915–920.

Hignett R, Fernando R, McGlennan A. (2008). Does a 30 degree head-up position in term parturients increase functional residual capacity? Implications for general anaesthesia. *International Journal of Obstetric Anaesthesia*, **17**, S5.

Hodges RJH, Tunstall ME. (1961). The choice of anaesthesia and its influence on perinatal mortality in caesarean section. *British Journal of Anaesthesia*, **33**, 572–588.

Koerber JP, Roberts GEW, Whitaker R, Thorpe CM. (2009). Variation in rapid sequence induction techniques: Current practice in Wales. *Anaesthesia*, **64**, 54–59.

Lane S, Saunders D, Schofield A, Padmanabhan R, Hildreth A, Laws D. (2005). A prospective, randomised controlled trial comparing the efficacy of pre-oxygenation in the 20 degrees head-up vs supine position. *Anaesthesia*, **60**, 1064–1067.

Lee BJ, Kang JM, Kim DO. (2007). Laryngeal exposure during laryngoscopy is better in the 25 degrees back-up position than in the supine position. *British Journal of Anaesthesia*, **99**, 581–586.

Lee C, Jahr JS, Candiotti K, Warriner V, Zornow MH. (2007). Reversal of profound rocuronium NMB with sugammadex is faster than recovery from succinylcholine. *Anesthesiology*, **107**, A988.

Lerman J. (2009). On cricoid pressure 'may the force be with you'. *Anesthesia and Analgesia*, **109**, 1363–1366.

Levy DM. (2000). Rapid sequence induction: Suxamethonium or rocuronium? *Anaesthesia*, **55**, 86.

Martyn JA, Richtsfeld M. (2006). Succinylcholine-induced hyperkalaemia in acquired pathological states. *Anesthesiology*, **104**, 158–169.

McCaul CL, Harney D, Ryan M, Moran C, Kavanagh BP, Boylan JF. (2005). Airway management in the lateral position: A randomised controlled trial. *Anesthesia and Analgesia*, **101**, 1221–1225.

McDonnell NJ, Paech MJ, Clavisi OM, Scott KL, and the ANZA Trials Group. (2008). Difficult and failed intubation in obstetric anaesthesia: An observational study of airway complications associated with general anaesthesia for caesarean section. *International Journal of Obstetric Anesthesia*, **17**, 292–297.

Morgan M. (1986). The confidential enquiry into maternal deaths (editorial). *Anaesthesia*, **41**, 689–691.

Morris J, Cook TM. (2001). Rapid sequence induction: A national survey of practice. *Anaesthesia*, **56**, 1090–1097.

Morris C, McAllister C. (2005). Etomidate for emergency anaesthesia; mad bad and dangerous to know? *Anaesthesia*, **60**, 737–740.

Mort TC. (2004). Emergency tracheal intubation: Complications associated with repeated laryngoscopic attempts. *Anesthesia and Analgesia*, **99**, 607–613.

Naguib M, Samarkandi AH, Emad El-Din M, Abdulla K, Khaled M, Alharby SW. (2006). The dose of succinylcholine required for excellent intubating conditions. *Anesthesia and Analgesia*, **102**, 151–155.

Neelakanta G. (2003). Cricoid pressure is effective in preventing esophageal regurgitation. *Anesthesiology*, **99**, 242.

Neilipovitz DT, Crosby ET. (2007). No evidence for decreased incidence of aspiration after rapid sequence induction. *Canadian Journal of Anesthesia*, **54**, 748–764.

Oehlkern L, Tilmant C, Gindre G, Calon B, Bazin JE. (2003). Is cricoid pressure efficient? The first evidence. *Anesthesiology*, **99**, A1235.

Ovassapian A, Salem MR. (2009). Sellick's maneuver: To do or not to do. *Anesthesia and Analgesia*, **109**, 1546–1552.

Ovassapian A, Krejcie TC, Yelich SJ, Dykes MH. (1989). Awake fibreoptic intubation in the patient at high risk of aspiration. *British Journal of Anaesthesia*, **62**, 13–16.

Palmer JH, Ball DR. (2000). The effect of cricoid pressure on the cricoid cartilage and vocal cords: An endoscopic study in anaesthetised patients. *Anaesthesia*, **55**, 260–267.

Perry JJ, Lee JS, Sillberg VA, Wells GA. (2008). Rocuronium versus succinylcholine for rapid sequence intubation. *Cochrane Database of Systematic Reviews*, **2**, CD002788.

Rahman K, Jenkins JG. (2005). Failed tracheal intubation in obstetrics: No more frequent but still managed badly. *Anaesthesia*, **60**, 168–171.

Rice MJ, Mancuso AA, Gibbs C, et al. (2009). Cricoid pressure results in compression of the postcricoid hypopharynx: The esophageal position is irrelevant. *Anesthesia and Analgesia*, **109**, 1546–1552.

Sagarin MJ, Barton ED, Sakles JC, Vissers RJ, Chiang V, Walls RM. (2003). Underdosing of midazolam in emergency endotracheal intubation. *Academic Emergency Medicine*, **10**, 329–338.

Schwartz DE, Kelly B, Caldwell JE, Carlisle AS, Cohen NH. (1992). Succinylcholine-induced hyperkalaemic arrest in a patient with severe metabolic acidosis and exsanguinating haemorrhage. *Anesthesia and Analgesia*, **75**, 291–293.

Sellick BA. (1961). Cricoid pressure to control regurgitation of stomach contents during induction of anaesthesia. *Lancet*, **2**, 404–406.

Smith KJ, Dobranowski J, Yip G, Daupin A, Choi P. (2003). Cricoid pressure displaces the esophagus: An observational study using magnetic resonance imaging. *Anesthesiology*, **99**, 60–64.

Smith KJ, Ladak S, Choi P, Dobranowski J. (2002). The cricoid cartilage and the esophagus are not aligned in close to half of adult patients. *Canadian Journal of Anesthesia*, **49**, 503–507.

Snow RG, Nunn JF. (1959). Induction of anaesthesia in the foot down position for patients with a full stomach. *British Journal of Anaesthesia*, **31**, 493–497.

Sparr HJ, Giesinger S, Ulmer H, Hollenstein-Zacke M, Luger TJ. (1996). Influence of induction technique on intubating conditions after rocuronium in adults: Comparison with rapid-sequence induction using thiopentone and suxamethonium. *British Journal of Anaesthesia*, **77**, 339–342.

Stept WJ, Safar P. (1970). Rapid induction/intubation for prevention of gastric-content aspiration. *Anesthesia and Analgesia*, **49**, 633–636.

Taha SK, El-Khatib MF, Siddik-Sayid SM, et al. (2009). Preoxygenation by 8 deep breaths in 60 seconds using the Mapleson A (Magill), the circle system, or the Mapleson D system. *Journal of Clinical Anesthesia*, **21**, 574–578.

Tourtier J-P, Compain M, Petitjeans F, et al. (2004). Acid aspiration prophylaxis in obstetrics in France: A comparative study of 1988 vs. 1998 French practice. *European Journal of Anaesthesiology*, **21**, 89–94.

Turgeon AF, Nicole PC, Trepanier CA, Marcoux S, Lessard MR. (2005). Cricoid pressure does not increase the rate of failed intubation by direct laryngoscopy in adults. *Anesthesiology*, **102**, 315–319.

Vanner R. (2009). Cricoid pressure (editorial). *International Journal of Obstetric Anesthesia*, **18**, 103–105.

Vanner RG, Asai T. (1999). Safe use of cricoid pressure (editorial). *Anaesthesia*, **54**, 1–3.

Vanner RG, Goodman NW. (1989). Gastro-oesophageal reflux in pregnancy at term and after delivery. *Anaesthesia*, **44**, 808–811.

Vanner RG, Pryle BJ. (1992). Regurgitation and oesophageal rupture with cricoid pressure: A cadaver study. *Anaesthesia*, **47**, 732–735.

Vanner RG, Pryle BJ. (1993). Nasogastric tubes and cricoid pressure. *Anaesthesia*, **48**, 1112–1113.

Vanner RG, O'Dwyer JP, Pryle BJ, Reynolds F. (1992). Upper oesophageal sphincter pressure and the effect of cricoid pressure. *Anaesthesia*, **47**, 95–100.

Vanner RG, Clarke P, Moore WJ, Raftery S. (1997). The effect of cricoid pressure and neck support on the view at laryngoscopy. *Anaesthesia*, **52**, 896–900.

Warner MA, Warner ME, Weber JG. (1993). Clinical significance of pulmonary aspiration during the perioperative period. *Anesthesiology*, **78**, 56–62.

Whittington RM, Robinson JS, Thompson JM. (1979). Fatal aspiration (Mendelson's) syndrome despite antacids and cricoid pressure. *Lancet*, **ii**, 228–230.

Yentis SM. (1997). The effects of single-handed and bimanual cricoid pressure on the view at laryngoscopy. *Anaesthesia*, **52**, 332–335.

Chris Frerk and Priya Gauthama

Introduction

An experienced anaesthetist rarely has significant difficulty in maintaining a patent airway and ventilating a patient's lungs. If significant difficulty is encountered, it may be that the anaesthetist is just able to maintain oxygenation utilising all their skills or it is possible that the patient is consuming oxygen faster than the anaesthetist can deliver it. Various terminologies describe this latter scenario including 'can't intubate, can't ventilate' (CICV) and 'can't intubate, can't oxygenate' (CICO), but for the purpose of this chapter it is defined as 'the lost airway'. Prompt recognition, diagnosis and management are essential in order to have the best chance of a successful outcome. This extreme situation, where ventilation by facemask, laryngeal mask and tracheal intubation has failed, is rare in elective general surgery with an estimated incidence of 1:10 000 to 1:50 000. The incidence is thought to be higher in obstetric anaesthesia with three reports of lost airways in the 2000–2002 Confidential Enquiry into Maternal and Child Health.

The Royal College of Anaesthetists and the Difficult Airway Society conducted a year long audit ending in August 2009 looking at cases of death, hypoxic brain injury and other morbidity associated with lost airways in intensive care units, emergency departments and operating theatres throughout the United Kingdom (expected 2011).

Pathophysiology

An adult patient requires 200–250 ml/min of oxygen to sustain life. After induction of anaesthesia if this amount of oxygen cannot be delivered to a patient's lungs they will use up their reserves over 1–2 minutes (longer if well pre-oxygenated, sooner in the obese or those with increased oxygen requirements) and then they will begin to desaturate. Without intervention to increase oxygen delivery to the lungs the patient will die. How long an individual patient will survive depends on many factors, but increasing experience in the management of non-heart beating organ donation provides evidence that cardiac arrest will probably occur within 5–10 minutes of complete airway obstruction.

Causes of lost airways
Anaesthetic drugs and depth of anaesthesia

Most general anaesthetic agents decrease upper airway tone leading to compromise of the natural airway and minor degrees of difficulty with facemask ventilation around the time of induction of anaesthesia. The loss of tone associated with the use of neuromuscular blocking drugs is considerably greater than that seen with intravenous or volatile anaesthetic agents, potentially leading to greater compromise of the airway.

By complete contrast, difficulty with ventilation around the time of induction of anaesthesia is frequently associated with obstruction at the level of the larynx caused by laryngeal spasm. In this situation ventilation is likely to be *improved* by deepening anaesthesia. Larson has claimed that bilateral digital pressure in the posterior temporomandibular joints (the 'laryngospasm notch') can relieve laryngospasm, but the most effective treatment in this situation is to administer a muscle relaxant drug. Muscle relaxant drugs are also the appropriate treatment for difficult mask ventilation associated with opioid-induced muscle rigidity. Arguments have been made for and against the use

Core Topics in Airway Management, Second Edition, ed. Ian Calder and Adrian Pearce. Published by Cambridge University Press.
© Cambridge University Press 2011.

of neuromuscular blocking drugs in difficult ventilation due to other causes (see Chapters 6 and 25).

Patient characteristics

Kheterpal studied 50 000 anaesthetics and found an overall incidence of 0.15% impossible mask ventilation. Previous radiotherapy to the neck, obstructive sleep apnoea, poor Mallampati grade, presence of beard and male sex were all independent predictors of failure to mask ventilate. Of these patients, 25% were also difficult to intubate. It is important to specifically look for these risk factors in the pre-operative evaluation especially in the anticipated difficult intubation, as the rescue technique of mask ventilation may not be available. In this situation, securing the airway awake is the most sensible course of action.

Anaesthetic trauma

American Society of Anesthesiologists closed claims reviews have shown that a significant proportion of failed ventilation cases occur in patients where some difficulty has been predicted but for whom the anaesthetic plan has not taken account of the potential risks. In two thirds of reviewed cases, repeated non-surgical attempts at tracheal intubation were deemed responsible for the loss of the airway.

External compression of natural airway (e.g., cricoid pressure)

The cricoid cartilage is the only complete cartilaginous ring encircling the trachea. It has been assumed that during a rapid sequence induction, correctly applied pressure (30 N to the cricoid cartilage) will occlude the oesophagus while leaving the trachea patent. The cricoid cartilage is however much more deformable than was previously believed and forces of 30 N can significantly narrow the airway and greater forces may occlude it, particularly in young female patients. In a failed ventilation situation where cricoid pressure is being applied, the pressure should be reduced or removed to determine if this is the cause of the obstruction.

Airway devices

Laryngeal mask airways, tracheal tubes and other airway devices can be misplaced leading to failure to ventilate the lungs. Rarely can they become occluded

in the manufacturing process or during cleaning and resterilising, resulting in a lost airway even though they may be placed correctly. If a tracheal tube or laryngeal mask (or other airway conduit) has been placed and ventilation is then found to be difficult or impossible, the device should be considered suspect, removed and ventilation re-established with a facemask.

Breathing system malfunction, misassembly or occlusion

Although rare as a cause of failed ventilation, serious hypoxic injury and death have occurred as a result of equipment faults. There are reports of stuck valves, faulty scavenging systems and incorrectly assembled breathing systems leading to an inability to ventilate the lungs. Breathing system components, filters, angle pieces and catheter mounts can become occluded leading to serious morbidity or mortality (Luer-Lok caps, plastic from packaging, syringe plungers, rogue pieces of anaesthetic equipment and unidentified gelatinous materials have all been implicated in various reports of lost airways). Breathing system problems can be rapidly confirmed or excluded by connecting a self-inflating bag directly to the anaesthetic facemask, tracheal tube or laryngeal mask airway (excluding all filters, catheter mounts and angle pieces). Equipment faults leading to inability to ventilate the lungs are almost entirely avoidable by performing a thorough pre-operative equipment check. Association of Anaesthetists of Great Britain and Ireland guidelines (*Checking Anaesthetic Equipment*, 3: 2004) recommend that the whole breathing system including a new single use filter, catheter mount and airway device is checked for patency immediately before use on *each* new patient.

Medical problems

Certain medical problems can present under anaesthesia with high airway pressures, decreased or absent CO_2 return and increasing hypoxaemia. If difficulty with ventilation occurs with a tracheal tube that has been seen to pass through the vocal cords and it is not resolved by reverting to a facemask or laryngeal mask then the most likely cause for loss of the airway is a distal airway problem such as bronchospasm or tension pneumothorax. Specific treatment will be determined by the suspected pathology.

Recognition and diagnosis

Loss of the airway is quite apparent once oxygen saturations begin to fall but identifying it before this happens gives more time for a definitive diagnosis to be made and for the correct course of action to be implemented. Early recognition of the problem depends on identifying the pattern of decreased or absent chest movement, an abnormal or absent capnograph trace and unusual airway pressures. Airway pressures will be high when the airway is obstructed, but may be normal or low if the cause of airway loss is a misplaced tracheal tube. These signs are not specific for the cause of the problem but this may be apparent from the timing and or nature of the difficulty.

How to avoid a lost airway

It is obviously preferable to maintain ventilation throughout a general anaesthetic rather than have to rescue a lost airway. The importance of conducting a thorough machine and breathing system check cannot be over-emphasised. Observing a capnograph trace during pre-oxygenation gives final confirmation of facemask seal, patency of the breathing system and correct functioning of carbon dioxide monitoring prior to induction of anaesthesia.

It is important that the anaesthetist considers his or her back-up plans for every anaesthetic and has the equipment, skills and support to enact them if the primary plan is unsuccessful.

An emergency situation only exists when all three routine methods of oxygenation (facemask, laryngeal mask and tracheal intubation) have failed. This is well-recognised and described in failed intubation guidelines produced by the Difficult Airway Society (Figure 19.1). The priority is oxygenation with optimal facemask ventilation using jaw thrust, oral/nasal airways, reduction of cricoid pressure if applied and four handed ventilation (where the primary anaesthetist uses both hands to maintain the airway while an assistant squeezes the bag). If these measures are not successful in maintaining ventilation, attempts should be made to place a laryngeal mask, or other supraglottic airway device (SAD) – (see Chapter 9). If ventilation cannot be reliably established after two attempts at laryngeal mask placement you are facing a lost airway. If a SAD is not available, an alternative may be to place a tracheal tube in the pharynx, inflate the cuff and occlude the nostrils and mouth with the fingers of one hand. This tactic is known as TTIP – tube tip in the pharynx.

One area where there is less agreement is in the timing of administration of muscle relaxants in relation to induction of anaesthesia and facemask ventilation (see Chapter 6). Though checking ease of mask ventilation before administering muscle relaxants has become part of many anaesthetists' routine, it has been questioned by Calder and Yentis. However we believe that checking for ease of facemask ventilation after induction of anaesthesia, before administering muscle relaxants is useful. Knowing that facemask ventilation is easy reduces stress and allows further unhurried decision making if laryngeal mask or tracheal tube placement is predicted to be, or turns out to be difficult. If facemask ventilation is difficult or impossible immediately following induction of anaesthesia, the decision whether or not to administer muscle relaxants should be based on a combination of patient factors, the skill and expertise of the anaesthetic team and the environment/equipment available (Table 19.1).

The decision whether to proceed or awaken if faced with difficult mask ventilation should be made prior to induction of anaesthesia. If the decision has been made to continue with anaesthesia then administering a muscle relaxant is probably appropriate to maximise the chances of successful tracheal intubation or laryngeal mask placement. If the decision has been taken to awaken a patient should facemask ventilation fail then the only indication for administering muscle relaxants would be if there is worsening hypoxia and wake up is not imminent. This would allow a best chance of airway rescue with tracheal intubation before committing to cricothyroidotomy. In defence of Calder and Yentis' position, if the decision has been made not to attempt to wake the patient up no matter what, then indeed there is no benefit to checking facemask ventilation before paralysis. Put simply, by not confirming facemask ventilation the anaesthetist is removing awakening the patient as one of the management options.

There are no guarantees that either proceeding with anaesthesia or attempting to wake the patient will secure oxygenation. The anaesthetist must always

Failed intubation, increasing hypoxaemia and difficult ventilation in the paralysed anaesthetised patient: Rescue techniques for the "can't intubate, can't ventilate" situation

failed intubation and difficult ventilation (other than laryngospasm)

> **Face mask**
> **Oxygenate and Ventilate patient**
> Maximum head extension
> Maximum jaw thrust
> Assistance with mask seal
> Oral ± 6mm nasal airway
> Reduce cricoid force - if necessary

failed oxygenation with face mask (e.g. SpO2 < 90% with FiO2 1.0)

call for help

> LMA™ Oxygenate and ventilate patient
> Maximum 2 attempts at insertion
> Reduce any cricoid force during insertion

→ succeed →

> Oxygenation satisfactory and stable: Maintain oxygenation and awaken patient

"can't intubate, can't ventilate" situation with increasing hypoxaemia

Plan D: Rescue techniques for "can't intubate, can't ventilate" situation

or

> **Cannula cricothyroidotomy**
> Equipment: Kink-resistant cannula, e.g. Patil (Cook) or Ravussin (VBM)
> High-pressure ventilation system, e.g. Manujet III (VBM)
> Technique:
> 1. Insert cannula through cricothyroid membrane
> 2. Maintain position of cannula - assistant's hand
> 3. Confirm tracheal position by air aspiration - 20ml syringe
> 4. Attach ventilation system to cannula
> 5. Commence cautious ventilation
> 6. Confirm ventilation of lungs, and exhalation through upper airway
> 7. If ventilation fails, or surgical emphysema or any other complication develops - convert immediately to surgical cricothyroidotomy

→ fail →

> **Surgical cricothyroidotomy**
> Equipment: Scalpel - short and rounded (no. 20 or Minitrach scalpel)
> Small (e.g. 6 or 7 mm) cuffed tracheal or tracheostomy tube
> 4-step Technique:
> 1. Identify cricothyroid membrane
> 2. Stab incision through skin and membrane Enlarge incision with blunt dissection (e.g. scalpel handle, forceps or dilator)
> 3. Caudal traction on cricoid cartilage with tracheal hook
> 4. Insert tube and inflate cuff
> Ventilate with low-pressure source
> Verify tube position and pulmonary ventilation

> Notes:
> 1. These techniques can have serious complications - use only in life-threatening situations
> 2. Convert to definitive airway as soon as possible
> 3. Postoperative management - see other difficult airway guidelines and flow-charts
> 4. 4mm cannula with low-pressure ventilation may be successful in patient breathing spontaneously

Difficult Airway Society guidelines Flow-chart 2004 (use with DAS guidelines paper)

Figure 19.1. DAS Guidelines flow-chart. Rescue techniques for the 'can't intubate, can't ventilate' situation.

be prepared to face and deal with a lost airway whichever route is chosen. Worsening hypoxaemia in the lost airway patient is an indication for immediate cricothyroidotomy.

Emergency cricothyroidotomy

The cricothyroid membrane is the preferred site for emergency access to the trachea for oxygenation. It has several desirable features (Table 19.2)

Table 19.1. Factors to consider when planning whether to wake a patient up (no relaxant before facemask ventilation) or to continue general anaesthesia (give relaxant)

Increased likelihood to wake patient	Increased likelihood to continue GA
Obstructive sleep apnoea	Low body mass index
Predicted difficult intubation	No predictors of difficult intubation
Anticipated problems are anatomical	Anticipated problems are irritable airways
Elective or urgent surgery	Emergency surgery (e.g., massive haemorrhage)
Inexperienced anaesthetist/team	Anaesthetist and team experienced in advanced airway management techniques
Isolated unit	Support readily available
No advanced airway equipment available	Readily available fibrescope/ videoscope etc Unlikely to wake before critical hypoxia.

Table 19.2. Desirable features of the cricothyroid membrane

Superficial, easily palpable

Rarely calcifies

Relatively avascular

1 cm *below* the vocal cords

Usually large enough to take a 6.0 mm tube

Cricoid ring holds the airway open

Posterior lamina reduces the risk of posterior tracheal wall injury

Table 19.3. Steps in emergency needle cricothyrotomy

Extend the chin and neck to improve access

Place syringe on needle/cannula

Identify CTM and stabilise larynx with one hand

Insert needle through the CTM, aspirating to confirm intratracheal location

Once in the trachea keep needle still

Slide cannula off inserted needle

Remove needle only when cannula fully inserted

Aspirate air freely through cannula to confirm correct placement

Secure the cannula with hand initially or ties around neck later

Apply short burst of high pressure oxygen

Watch chest rise appropriately *and* fall

Maintain upper airway patency with LM or oral airway for exhalation

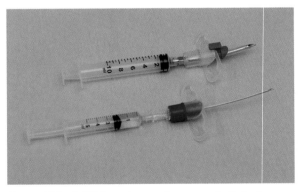

Figure 19.2. A 13G Ravussin cannula over needle (below) compared with the wide bore Quicktrach (above).

and, in general, cricothyroidotomy is quicker than tracheostomy.

What equipment is available?

There are three types of cricothyroidotomy:

1. Percutaneous small cannula devices (2–3 mm internal diameter)
2. Percutaneous large bore devices (4 mm internal diameter or larger)
3. Surgical cricothyroidotomy kits for insertion of standard 6.0 mm tracheal or tracheostomy tubes.

Small cannula devices

A 13G cannula over needle device such as the Ravussin (Figure 19.2) or similar, with an approximate internal diameter of 2 mm is placed through the cricothyroid membrane and directed caudally into the trachea. The steps for insertion are given in Table 19.3 and illustrated in Figure 19.3a–e. These cannulae require high-pressure ventilation (1–4 bar) from a Sanders injector or Manujet jet ventilation system (Figure 19.4). Exhalation occurs through the upper airway, which must be patent. Complications include misplacement of the

(a)

(b)

(c)

(d)

(e)

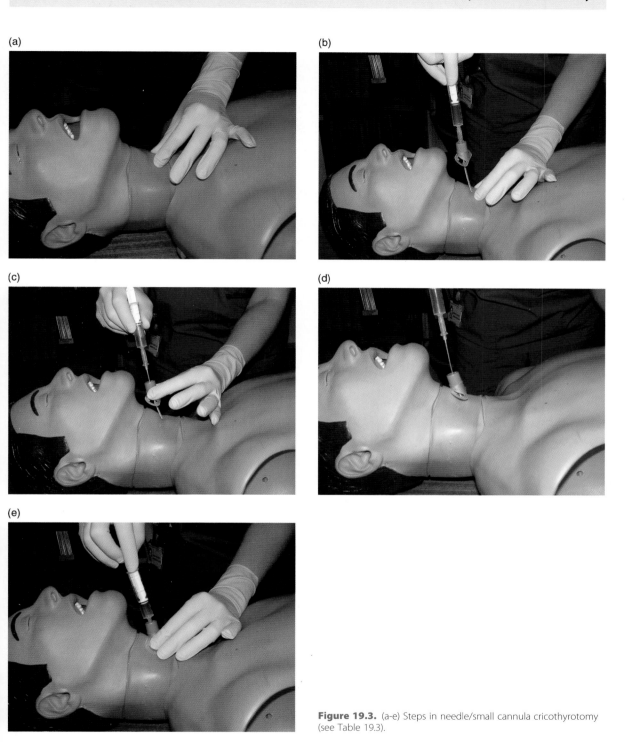

Figure 19.3. (a-e) Steps in needle/small cannula cricothyrotomy (see Table 19.3).

cannula outside the trachea leading to failure of the technique, posterior tracheal wall damage, damage to surrounding vascular structures, surgical emphysema and barotrauma. Capnography is not available to confirm continued correct placement and suctioning is not possible through these small cannulae.

183

Large bore cannula devices

The 2004 DAS guidelines did not include percutaneous large bore devices, however, since 2004 there have been case reports of successful rescue of lost airways with such devices and they would therefore now meet the standard for consideration for inclusion in the guidelines.

The **VBM Quicktrach** is a rigid pre-assembled cannula-over-needle device with an internal diameter of 4 mm. It is available as a cuffed or uncuffed version (Figures 19.5a and 5b). The needle tip is specially designed to cut first and then dilate to 4 mm, avoiding the need for a skin incision. A stopper distal to the needle hub reduces the risk of posterior tracheal wall injury by limiting depth of insertion of the needle. The cuffed version is longer and has a safety clip, which avoids the metal needle being readvanced out of the cannula once it has been retracted. The Quicktrach is inserted with a simple 'push and go' technique (Figures 19.6a–f). The **Portex Cricothyroidotomy kit** is a cannula over needle device with a spring loaded Veress needle, blunt stylet and dilator sitting inside a 6 mm internal diameter cuffed airway. There is a small red flag indicator in the needle hub to indicate intratracheal placement. The **Cook Melker** (Figure 19.7) is a wire guided cricothyroidotomy kit inserted using a Seldinger technique. It is available in a 5.0 mm cuffed and a variety of uncuffed sizes and lengths.

An internal diameter of 4 mm permits adequate inspiratory gas flows to be achieved with pressures generated within a standard anaesthetic breathing system. Passive exhalation occurs through these cannulae, suctioning is possible through them and capnography can be used to confirm placement within the trachea. Cuffed airways are preferred to avoid proximal gas leakage, particularly in patients with poorly compliant lungs and they also offer

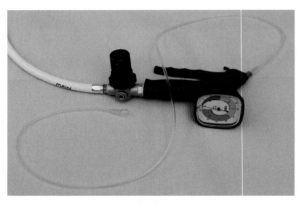

Figure 19.4. Manujet jet ventilation system.

(a)

(b)

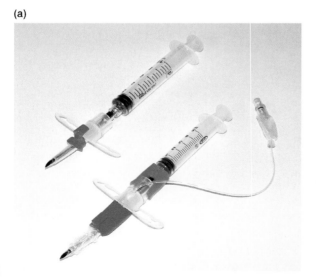
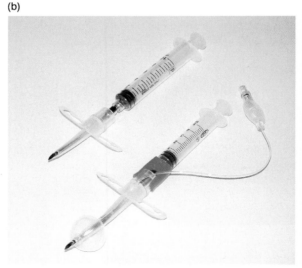

Figures 19.5. (a) The Quicktrach uncuffed (above) and cuffed (below); note red depth guard. (b) The Quicktrach with depth guard removed and cuff inflated (below).

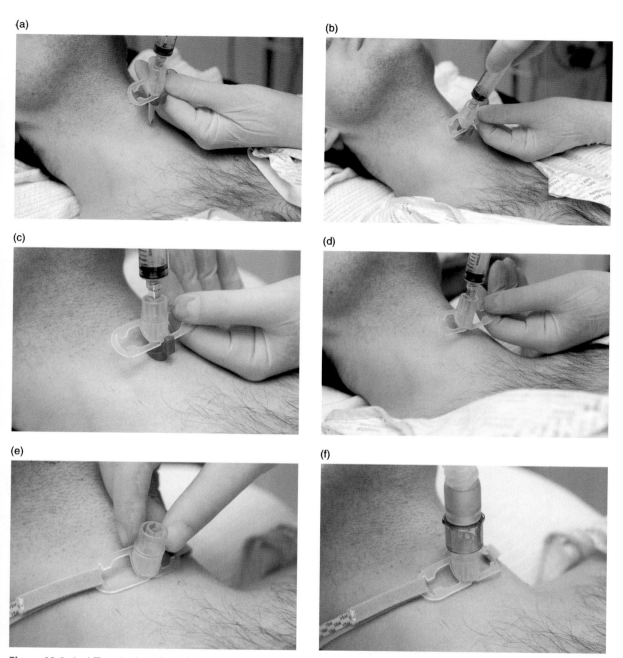

Figure 19.6. (a-c) The cricothyroid membrane is identified and the Quicktrach is inserted until the depth guard reaches the skin. (d) Depth guard removed, needle *not* advanced further but cannula slid into trachea. (e) Needle removed and cannula fixed securely in place by tape. (f) Standard breathing system is attached by 15 mm connector.

some protection from pulmonary aspiration. Complications of these large bore devices include misplacement of the cannula outside the trachea leading to failure of the technique, posterior tracheal wall damage and damage to surrounding vascular structures.

185

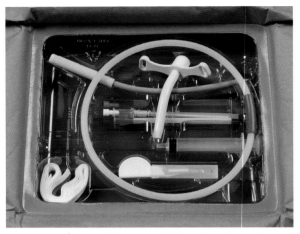

Figure 19.7. Cook Melker wire guided cricothyroidotomy kit.

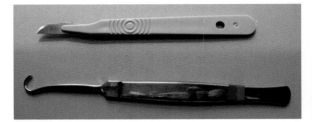

Figure 19.8. Basic surgical cricothyroidotomy kit comprising scalpel and cricoid hook. A standard 6.0 mm tracheal or tracheostomy tube is used.

Surgical cricothyroidotomy

The most basic surgical kit contains a scalpel and a cricoid hook (Figure 19.8). A horizontal incision is made through the cricothyroid membrane, and the scalpel handle is used to dilate the incision. The cricoid hook is then used to hold the anterior wall of the trachea forwards allowing a tracheal/tracheostomy tube to be inserted.

Choosing which technique

One type of cricothyroidotomy kit should be chosen for a hospital and be made available in all areas. There are case reports of successes and failures with small cannula devices, with large cannula devices and with surgical airways. With respect to insertion time and complications there is no clear advantage to any of the three techniques. Manikin and bench testing studies give conflicting results as to the optimal choice of device for emergency airway management, and it has not been shown that laboratory studies are directly transferrable to emergency cricothyroidotomy in clinical practice.

It is a matter of personal choice between cannula over needle devices, wire guided devices and surgical methods. Many anaesthetists are unfamiliar with surgical cricothyroidotomy techniques and may be reluctant to resort to them in an emergency. Wire guided cricothyroidotomy is preferred by some because of familiarity with Seldinger techniques and a perceived decreased risk of complications while others prefer the simplicity of a push and go technique. Although it has been suggested that cuffed devices can be more difficult to insert, several studies show no significant difference in insertion time between cuffed and uncuffed devices.

What is clear is that whichever device is chosen, training is essential to gain familiarity with the device and also to maintain the necessary skills, as the benefits of initial training last only 4–8 months.

What not to use

The Portex Mini-Trach II is designed for tracheo-bronchial suctioning and is neither licenced nor recommended for emergency ventilation.

It is inappropriate to consider using self-assembly kits put together from items found in the anaesthetic room to provide jet ventilation via small cannulae.

Surgical cricothyroidotomy should not be performed in prepubescent children because of the risk of damaging the cricoid cartilage. The tracheal cartilages are soft and pliable in prepubescent children, and the cricoid provides the only circumferential support keeping the upper airway open. In this age group needle cricothyroidotomy with jet ventilation is the recommended strategy.

Human factors

Accepting the diagnosis of a lost airway is a difficult mental process. As discussed above, anaesthetists are used to occasional difficulty with airway maintenance and are skilled in a variety of techniques to improve the situation (jaw thrust, four handed ventilation, the use of airways, laryngeal masks and tracheal intubation). The only thing that distinguishes the lost airway from other cases is that the anaesthetist's usual armamentarium of techniques do *not restore* ventilation. A common feature in deaths due to the lost airway is that time is lost in denial. The majority of anaesthetists will not have come across the situation before, and the diagnosis may only be accepted once the patient has become severely hypoxic and when an agonal rhythm appears on the ECG.

Whilst most anaesthetists can describe the Difficult Airway Society algorithm for failed ventilation it is not uncommon to find major deviations from optimal management (such as the anaesthetist making no attempt to perform a cricothyroidotomy) when reviewing cases where patients have died or suffered hypoxic brain injury secondary to an airway problem. The reason why well-trained, knowledgeable anaesthetists fail to perform as expected in a crisis such as this is increasingly being understood in the context of 'human factors'. These are well-described psychological and behavioural patterns observed when people are working under stress in a complex environment. Communication, decision making and practical skills all deteriorate.

By way of example, in several cases of lost airway due to breathing system blockage, anaesthetists have misdiagnosed the problem as upper airway obstruction and have persisted with repeated attempts following the DAS algorithm to no effect. They were doing everything right but for the wrong diagnosis. Training is needed in the decision-making processes to help anaesthetists identify a lost airway early and to help them choose the correct management strategy. Simulator-based training is safe and has been shown to be effective for this purpose. There is also some early evidence that team training in airway management may improve performance.

Key points

- The lost airway is an emergency, time is limited.
- A thorough machine/equipment check including all components of the breathing system should be performed prior to each anaesthetic.
- Equipment problems and distal airway problems should be rapidly excluded.
- Making the diagnosis of a lost airway is a difficult mental process and time is often lost in denial.
- Emergency cricothyroidotomy can be a difficult practical procedure, the sooner it is started, the

more likely is re-establishment of the airway before irreversible hypoxic brain injury occurs.
- The airway is only irrevocably lost after failed cricothyroidotomy (failure to try in time or failure to succeed in time).
- As it is rare, the necessary mental and practical skills for managing a lost airway cannot be learnt on routine operating lists. Mannikin/simulator training is required.

Further reading

Bell D. (2003). Avoiding adverse outcomes when faced with 'difficulty with ventilation'. *Anaesthesia*, **58**, 945–948.

Bennett JA, Abrams IT, Van Riper DF, Horrow JC. (1997). Difficult or impossible ventilation after sufentanil-induced anesthesia is caused primarily by vocal cord closure. *Anesthesiology*, **87**, 1070–1074.

Calder I, Yentis SM. (2008). Could 'safe practice' be compromising safe practice? Should anaesthetists have to demonstrate that face mask ventilation is possible before giving a neuromuscular blocker? *Anaesthesia*, **63**, 113–115.

Calder I, Yentis SM, Kheterpal S, Tremper KK. (2007). Impossible mask ventilation. *Anesthesiology*, **107**, 171.

Caplan RA, Posner KL, Ward RJ, Cheney FW. (1990). Adverse respiratory events in anesthesia: A closed claims analysis. *Anesthesiology*, **72**, 828–833.

Carter JA. (2004). Checking anaesthetic equipment and the Expert Group on Blocked Anaesthetic Tubing (EGBAT). *Anaesthesia*, **59**, 105–107.

Craven RM, Vanner RG. (2004). Ventilation of a model lung using various cricothyrotomy devices. *Anaesthesia*, **59**, 595–599.

Flin R, O'Connor P, Crichton M. (2009). *Safety At The Sharp End – A Guide to Non-Technical Skills*. Surrey, UK: Ashgate Publishing.

Goodwin MW, French GW. (2001). Simulation as a training and assessment tool in the management of failed intubation in obstetrics. *International Journal of Obstetric Anesthesia*, **10**, 273–277.

Kheterpal S, Han R, Tremper KK, et al. (2006). Incidence and predictors of difficult and impossible mask ventilation. *Anesthesiology*, **105**, 885–891.

Kheterpal S, Martin L, Shanks AM, Tremper KK. (2009). Prediction and outcomes of impossible mask ventilation. A review of 50,000 anesthetics. *Anesthesiology*, **110**, 891–897.

Kristensen MS. (2005). Tube tip in pharynx (TTIP) ventilation: Simple establishment of ventilation in case of failed mask ventilation. *Acta Anaesthesiologica Scandinavia*, **49**, 252–256.

Larson CP. (1998). Laryngospasm – the best treatment. *Anesthesiology*, **89**, 1293.

Patel B, Frerk C. (2008). Large-bore cricothyroidotomy devices. *Continuing Education in Anaesthesia, Critical Care & Pain*, **8**, 157–160.

Schober P, Hegemann MC, Schwarte LA, Loer SA, Noetges P. (2009). Emergency cricothyrotomy – a comparative study of different techniques in human cadavers. *Resuscitation*, **80**, 204–209.

Scrase I, Woollard M. (2006). Needle vs surgical cricothyroidotomy: A short cut to effective ventilation. *Anaesthesia*, **61**, 962.

Sulaiman L, Tighe SQ, Nelson RA. (2006). Surgical vs wire-guided cricothyroidotomy: A randomised crossover study of cuffed and uncuffed tracheal tube insertion. *Anaesthesia*, **61**, 565–570.

Vadodaria BS, Gandhi SD, McIndoe AK. (2004). Comparison of four different emergency airway access equipment sets on a human patient simulator. *Anaesthesia*, **59**, 73–79.

The airway in obstetrics

Steven M. Yentis

Introduction

Most anaesthetists are worried about the airway in obstetrics. This worry goes back over many years to the high number of cases of difficult and failed intubation and/or ventilation that regularly used to feature in the Reports on Confidential Enquiries into Maternal Deaths until about 20 years ago. Partly through better training and facilities, and partly through greater use of regional anaesthesia in obstetrics, the incidence of such problems in recent reports is low. However the risk of failed intubation remains (see below), and there is concern that recent changes in anaesthetic training in the UK have led to more limited exposure of trainees to clinical anaesthesia in general, and to general anaesthesia for caesarean section in particular.

The airway and pregnancy

There are several reasons why problems with the airway may be more common and serious in pregnant women than in other patients. First, technical aspects of airway management are more difficult; second, management is often particularly stressful because of the urgency of the case, increasing the importance of human factors; and third, the consequences of difficulty are more serious (Table 20.1).

Prediction of difficulty with the airway is notoriously inaccurate and is covered in detail in Chapter 7. Although there are many studies of prediction of difficulty, most have excluded pregnant women. The factors that might assist prediction of difficulty are thought, in general, to be the same as for non-pregnant patients.

Non-anaesthetic airway problems

Airway problems may occur as a result of pregnancy and labour alone, albeit rarely. Pre-eclampsia is common and results in oedema which may be marked, although airway obstruction in the absence of instrumentation would be rare. Airway obstruction associated with hypocalcaemia and tetany resulting from hyperventilation induced by labour pain has been described, as has surgical emphysema arising from excessive straining or pushing.

Regional anaesthesia

One advantage of regional anaesthesia, if not the main one, is the avoidance in most cases of the need for airway support. However although regional anaesthesia has a low *incidence* of high regional blocks, the large proportion of caesarean sections that are now done under regional anaesthesia means that the *number* of high regional blocks one would expect to see in routine practice is approximately equal to the number of failed intubations (see below). High blocks may develop insidiously and it is, therefore, important to observe the patient continuously during surgery. Even with a symptomatic high block, reassurance and oxygen may be sufficient treatment, but there should be a low threshold for tracheal intubation as outlined below.

General anaesthesia

Most authorities advocate that the routine technique of airway management used for general anaesthesia for obstetrics should be a standard rapid sequence induction (see Chapter 18), modified in the presence of pre-eclampsia to reduce the hypertensive response

---

Table 20.1. Technical and human factors contributing to difficulty with the airway in pregnancy, and reasons why the consequences of difficulty are greater

Technical factors	Human factors	Consequences of difficulty
• Relatively young age group; presence of a full set of teeth	• Inexperience of anaesthetist and assistant, related to low exposure to general anaesthesia for caesarean section	• Rapid hypoxaemia caused by reduced maternal functional residual capacity and increased oxygen consumption
• Increased weight-gain in pregnancy; deposition of fat and fluid around the head and neck	• Haste prompted by urgency of the case	• Increased risk of regurgitation of gastric contents and their aspiration
• Tendency for women to receive large amounts of intravenous fluid in labour, exacerbating oedema	• Knowledge that two patients are at risk	
• Risk of developing pre-eclampsia with further fluid retention/ overload	• Unfamiliarity with surroundings if staff are covering labour ward from another area	
• Worsening of facial/laryngeal oedema during labour and pushing	• Anxiety/panic of the patient, her partner and other staff	
• Hindrance of insertion of the laryngoscope blade into the mouth caused by enlarged breasts and the assistant's hand applying cricoid pressure		
• Distortion of laryngeal anatomy caused by cricoid pressure		
• Nasal venous dilatation, leading to bleeding upon instrumentation		

to intubation. More recently, a place for a non-depolarising neuromuscular blocking drug – rocuronium in particular – has been suggested as an alternative to suxamethonium, but this is not standard practice. Particular attention should be directed towards reducing the likelihood of difficulty, and reducing the severity of the consequences if difficulty occurs (Table 20.2).

Difficult and failed intubation

The incidence of these is uncertain since definitions vary (Chapter 7). The incidence of failed intubation in obstetrics is said to be approximately 1:300 to 1:800; there is general agreement however that the incidence is higher than in the non-pregnant population, for the reasons given in Table 20.1. Apart from the possible contribution of reduced training in airway

management and obstetric general anaesthesia, another factor that might lead to a higher reported incidence is that trainees are now taught to declare failure earlier rather than persist with attempts to intubate. The incidence of failed *ventilation* (by mask or other device) in obstetrics is unknown.

The value of a 'drill' in the management of difficult/failed intubation has long been recognised and a modern, simplified version is offered in Figure 20.1. Along with earlier declaration of 'failed intubation', noted above, is the modern emphasis on giving only a single dose of suxamethonium and performing a single laryngoscopy, rather than repeated doses/attempts that may lead to trauma and hypoxaemia (an exception might be when the vocal cords are seen fleetingly and the anaesthetist is confident that intubation is achievable at the

Table 20.2. Approach to airway management in the obstetric patient

	Comments
Reduce likelihood of difficulty	
Prediction before anaesthesia	Difficult
Avoiding need for general anaesthesia	Better communication; use of regional anaesthesia
Availability of and familiarity with a range of airways, intubation aids and laryngoscopes	Implications for resources and training. Smaller tracheal tubes than in non-pregnant patients (e.g., 6.0–7.0 mm) have been suggested as being easier to place and reducing trauma
Proper positioning of patient's head/neck	May be hindered by lateral tilt used to avoid aortocaval compression. Obese patients need pillows etc placed under the head, neck and upper shoulders. Head-up tilt has been recommended
Properly applied cricoid pressure	Can be assessed and practised immediately before induction using a weighing scales
Adequate dose of induction agent and neuromuscular blocking drug	To reduce awareness and improve intubating conditions respectively
Well-rehearsed 'drill'	To prevent repeated attempts and airway trauma that will hinder management of the airway even further
Reduce severity of consequences	
Use of antacids, H_2 antagonists and prokinetics	To reduce acidity and volume of gastric contents
Pre-oxygenation	To prolong the period of apnoea before hypoxaemia ensues. Either 2–3 minutes of normal breathing or 4–5 vital capacity breaths are considered adequate. Requires a tightly fitting facepiece and high fresh gas flow
Well-rehearsed 'drill'	To maintain oxygenation

second attempt). Although the ProSeal laryngeal mask airway is considered by some as being useful because of the ability to vent regurgitated material, most experience with salvage of potential disasters has been with the standard laryngeal mask airway. Similarly, though the intubating laryngeal mask airway may allow successful intubation, there is no evidence that it is more effective at saving life than the standard device in this situation.

The question of whether to proceed with an urgent case of fetal compromise without tracheal intubation (e.g., with a facemask or laryngeal mask airway), or to risk death of the fetus and allow the mother to wake, is a difficult one. In general, the primary duty of the anaesthetist to the mother should always be stressed – especially to trainees – and general anaesthesia continued only in exceptional circumstances and by an anaesthetist with adequate expertise of managing

difficult cases; usually this would be an experienced consultant. Once the mother is awake, she can be managed as for the known difficult case (below).

If a rescue device such as a laryngeal mask airway has been successfully inserted, it is unknown whether it is better to establish spontaneous breathing, or to paralyse the patient and ventilate the lungs. In either case, tipping the operating table head-up may reduce the risk of aspiration pneumonitis and improve respiratory excursions.

Care must also be taken with tracheal extubation, especially if there is a risk of laryngeal oedema, perhaps exacerbated by intubation, for example in pre-eclampsia. Deflating the cuff to ensure a gas leak around the tracheal tube when the proximal end is obstructed can be used for reassurance before the tube is removed. The risk of aspiration is ever-present and gastric emptying with a stomach tube should be

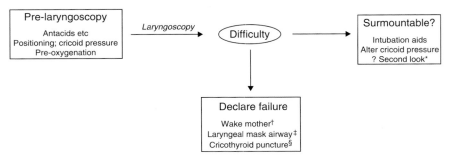

Figure 20.1. Simplified 'drill' suitable for difficult/failed intubation in obstetrics. *Standard teaching is that a second look is discouraged unless in exceptional circumstances. †Standard teaching is that the mother should always be woken unless her life is in immediate danger (e.g., haemorrhage), unless the fetus's life is at risk and the anaesthetist has sufficient expertise. ‡Some authorities advocate attempted ventilation via facepiece/oral or nasal airway before inserting the laryngeal mask airway. Insertion of the latter may be facilitated by temporary release of cricoid pressure. §some authorities advocate other devices, e.g., Combitube, before cricothyroid puncture.

considered in emergency cases. Needless to say, observation and monitoring of the patient should continue post-operatively.

Management of the known difficult case

There has been debate over whether a patient presenting for surgery with known airway difficulty should be managed with regional anaesthesia, thereby avoiding the need for intubation, or with awake fibreoptic intubation, thereby avoiding the possibility that control of the airway might be needed in an emergency. Advocates of the former point out the apparent absurdity of meeting a difficult problem head-on when it can be simply avoided, whereas those of the latter highlight the small but serious risk of high regional block. Awake intubation itself is along standard lines, bearing in mind that the mother may be terrified and require careful sedation, pregnancy is associated with increased nasal congestion, there may be difficulty with transtracheal injection due to oedema, aspiration may be more likely once the protective reflexes have been obtunded with local anaesthetic, and the systemic effects of vasoconstrictors are potentially hazardous in pre-eclampsia. If the mother has just been woken after failed intubation under general anaesthesia, she may be unable to cooperate fully.

Key points

- Airway management is more difficult and stressful in obstetrics, and the consequences of difficulty are more serious than in many other areas.
- Most problems involve general anaesthesia although airway management may be required in regional anaesthesia.
- It is important to practise a drill for difficult and failed intubation regularly.
- Problems may occur after tracheal extubation.

Further reading

Kuczkowski KM, Reisner LS, Benumof JL. (2003). Airway problems and new solutions for the obstetric patient. *Journal of Clinical Anesthesia*, **15**, 552–563.

McDonnell NJ, Paech MJ, Clavisi OM, Scott KL; ANZCA Trials Group. (2008). Difficult and failed intubation in obstetric anaesthesia: An observational study of airway management and complications associated with general anaesthesia for caesarean section. *International Journal of Obstetric Anesthesia*, **17**, 292–297.

Munnur U, de Boisblanc B, Suresh MS. (2005). Airway problems in pregnancy. *Critical Care Medicine*, **33**, S259–S268.

Russell R. (2007). Failed intubation in obstetrics: A self-fulfilling prophecy? *International Journal of Obstetric Anesthesia*, **16**, 1–3.

Chapter 21

The paediatric airway

Philippa Evans

Introduction

Paediatric patients range from the premature neonate to the adolescent child. There are a number of anatomical and physiological differences in the paediatric airway compared to that of the adult, which have implications for airway management especially in infants and young children. Airway-related problems are the most common critical incidents in paediatric anaesthesia and are four times more common in infants than in older children.

The neonate is defined as being less than 44 weeks post-conception age (PCA = gestational age + weeks after birth). An infant is any child of less than a year old.

Anatomical and physiological differences

Infants and small children have a disproportionately large head and short neck. Their tongues are relatively large with respect to the mandible, and their larynx is more anterior and cephalad in comparison to the adult. They are often described as obligate nasal breathers and find it more difficult to switch to mouth breathing when necessary. As a result blockage of the nasal passages, either congenital or acquired, can have serious consequences.

The epiglottis is relatively long and 'floppy' in nature. It is described as being U-shaped and projects posteriorly at an angle of 45 degrees above the glottic opening. The narrowest part of the airway is at the level of the cricoid cartilage, as opposed to the laryngeal inlet at the level of the vocal cords in adults. The trachea is approximately 5 cm long in the newborn, and this increases to about 8 cm in the first year of life. The carina initially is at the level of T2 (T4 in adults) and is also wider than in the adult. The angle between the left and right main bronchi is initially equal. However with time, the right main bronchus becomes relatively less angled than the left, and is also marginally larger in diameter. Therefore, if the tracheal tube is advanced too far, endobronchial intubation of the right side is more common.

In neonates and infants, the ribs tend to be horizontal, and the intercostal muscles relatively weak. As a result the tidal volume is fixed, and the only way in which minute ventilation can be increased is by an increase in respiratory rate. Breathing is predominantly diaphragmatic in this age group. In term neonates, about 30% of diaphragm muscles are type I (slow twitch; fatigue resistant). This will increase to the adult value of 55%, over the first year of life. Oxygen consumption in the neonate is approximately 5–6 ml/kg/min. This decreases during childhood to the adult value of 3.5 ml/kg/min. Neonates and infants exhibit a relatively small functional residual capacity (FRC), and more often than not the closing volume will exceed the FRC and encroach on the tidal volume. Thus, at the end of a normal tidal volume breath, small airways are prone to closure. Low FRC together with a high oxygen consumption rate mean that young children are prone to rapid desaturation in the presence of airway obstruction or apnoea.

Neonates and ex-premature infants of less than 60 weeks post-conception age are prone to apnoeas following anaesthesia, which has implications for their post-operative care. In addition to continuous saturation monitoring, they should be nursed on an apnoea mattress for the first post-operative night. This precludes these patients from being managed as day-cases.

Core Topics in Airway Management, Second Edition, ed. Ian Calder and Adrian Pearce. Published by Cambridge University Press.
© Cambridge University Press 2011.

Relevance to practice

Positioning

The large occiput generates a degree of spinal flexion. It is usual to keep the head in the neutral position (or even a slightly extended position in very small infants) while maintaining the airway in order to avoid airway obstruction due to excessive neck flexion.

Basic airway techniques

The relative macroglossia in infants and young children means that airway obstruction tends to occur early during induction of anaesthesia when there is loss of airway tone. This may be overcome with simple manoeuvres such as ensuring the mouth is open during ventilation, the early insertion of an oral airway or the application of CPAP via the breathing circuit.

Care must be taken when placing the facemask. Structures of the face are easily damaged with excessive pressure. Pressure on the soft tissues of the anterior neck in the infant may cause airway obstruction due to pushing the base of the tongue up against the palate, and due attention must be paid to the position of the fingertips when supporting the airway.

Inadvertent gastric insufflation is very common during mask ventilation in infants, and this can compromise ventilation due to splinting of the diaphragm. The stomach should be decompressed using a nasogastric tube when there has been prolonged or difficult mask ventilation or if the abdomen appears to be distended.

Laryngoscopy

Straight laryngoscope blades are useful in infants up to about the age of 3 to 6 months. Infants have relative macroglossia and a large floppy epiglottis that is angled into the lumen of the airway covering the laryngeal inlet. This together with the cephalad larynx makes it difficult to visualise the laryngeal inlet by conventional laryngoscopy (i.e., indirect elevation of the epiglottis with the tip of the laryngoscope blade placed between the epiglottis and the base of the tongue). The straight blade takes up less space in the mouth and allows the epiglottis to be lifted directly in order to reveal the glottic opening. One of two techniques can be employed: The epiglottis is visualised and the laryngoscope blade is then slid underneath it and the tip of the blade lifted so that the glottis is

Table 21.1. Tracheal tube sizes

Tube size	Internal diameter (mm) = age (years)/4 + 4.5
Tube length oral	Length (cm) = age/2 + 12
Tube length nasal	Length (cm) = age/2 + 15

These are commonly used formulae in children > 1 year. They are not absolute but should act as a guide. For children < 1 year the following is a useful guide:

Age	Internal diameter (mm)	Length (cm)
Neonate (3 kg)	3.0–3.5	10–10.5
6 months (6 kg)	4.0	11.5–12.5
1 year (10 kg)	4.5	13–13.5

exposed, or the laryngoscope blade is deliberately advanced into the oesophagus and then, with the tip lifted anteriorly, withdrawn slowly until the larynx drops into view. Both techniques bring the blade in to direct contact with the epiglottis which can cause intense vagal stimulation.

Tracheal tubes

The selection of the correct size and length for tracheal tubes (TTs) in children is based on age (see Table 21.1). The narrowest part of the airway in children is the cricoid cartilage, which forms a complete ring around the airway. The ideal size of TT is one that fits snugly at the level of the cricoid cartilage, allowing adequate ventilation at the same time as ensuring a small leak around the TT at 20 cmH$_2$O. For this reason it has been traditional to use uncuffed TT in children under the age of 8 years. The mucosa of the airway is very vulnerable to damage from an improperly positioned or sized TT. Damage to the underlying mucosa can result in airway oedema and post-extubation stridor or in the most serious cases acquired subglottic stenosis. The risk is greater in babies and small children.

There is increasing interest in using cuffed TTs in young patients. Proponents of their use would argue that a cuffed TT increases the likelihood of the selection of the correct size tube at the first intubation and avoids the potential trauma associated with multiple airway manipulations. Cuffed TTs certainly have a role in the intensive care setting in the management

Table 21.2. Laryngeal mask airway sizes

LMA size	Patient weight (kg)	Maximum cuff inflation (ml)
1	> 5	4
1.5	5–10	7
2	10–20	10
2.5	20–30	14
3	30–50	20

of patients with poorly compliant lungs in whom large airway leaks would seriously compromise ventilation. However there is a great variability in the design of cuffed paediatric TTs, especially with regards to the position of the cuff and its relationship to the laryngeal inlet when inflated. Studies with regards to the complications associated with the use of cuffed TTs have produced conflicting results. However a recent multi-centre, prospective, randomised trial found that cuffed tubes were associated with fewer tube exchanges and that there was no difference in the incidence of post-extubation stridor.

This remains a topic of debate among paediatric anaesthetists. It should be remembered that all TTs can be associated with airway trauma. Careful selection and placement of an appropriate TT, whether cuffed or not, is important in minimising airway injury.

Laryngeal mask airway (LMA)

In contrast to the TT, paediatric LMAs are sized according to patient weight (see Table 21.2).

The paediatric LMA was not specifically designed for use in children but is merely a scaled down version of the adult LMA, and this can have implications for its use in paediatric patients.

There exists a learning curve with regards to the use of the LMA in children. The complication rate with the use of the LMA is inversely proportional to patient size; displacement and airway obstruction occurring most frequently with size 1 and 1.5 LMAs. Airway obstruction develops if the LMA pushes the large and floppy epiglottis down, obstructing the laryngeal inlet. Difficulty can be encountered when using the traditional adult technique for LMA insertion in children. This may be due to the relative adenotonsillar hypertrophy present in children and

also secondary to the epiglottis impinging on the LMA grille. The LMA has been widely reported to provide an effective airway in infants and children with difficult airways. The size 1 LMA has a role in neonatal resuscitation.

The Pro-Seal LMA is available from size 1.5. It has an additional lumen running from its tip in parallel with the main airway that acts as an oesophageal drainage tube. This allows passive drainage of oropharyngeal contents and minimises gastric insufflation. The drainage tube also provides a route for nasogastric tube insertion and upper gastrointestinal endoscopy.

Different techniques of LMA insertion and removal have been described

The LMA can be inserted partially inflated lateral against the tongue and advanced until resistance is met (tonsil) and then rotated back into the midline. Alternatively, the LMA can be inserted 'back-to front' with the cuff facing the palate, and turned 180 degrees once the hypopharynx is reached.

There is no consensus for the optimal timing for removal of LMAs in children. However young children have reactive airways and may be more liable to the development of laryngospasm if removal is delayed until the return of airway reflexes. Many practitioners prefer to remove the LMA while the patient is still asleep.

Management of the difficult airway

Most difficult paediatric airways are predictable. A child who is unexpectedly difficult to manage with bag and mask ventilation is rare. There are a number of syndromes and pathologies that are known to be associated with difficult airway management (see Table 21.3). The overall incidence of difficult intubation in the paediatric population is unknown. Difficult laryngoscopy is reported at 4.7% in infants with cleft lip and palate, the incidence is higher in younger patients and when there is associated micrognathia. In children with mucopolysaccharidoses the overall incidence of difficult and failed intubation is 25% and 8% respectively. In the subgroup of children with Hurler syndrome (the classic phenotype) these figures rise to 54% and 23%.

Many of the techniques that are used in the management of the difficult paediatric airway have been

Table 21.3. Conditions associated with difficulties in intubation in paediatric practice

Congenital

Craniofacial

Pierre Robin syndrome – cleft palate, micrognathia, glossoptosis

Treacher-Collins syndrome – micrognathia, cleft palate, microstomia

Goldenhar's syndrome – hemifacial hypoplasia, mandibular hypoplasia,

Cervical spine anomalies

Lysosomal enzyme defects

Mucopolysaccharidoses – progressive tissue thickening due to depositions of cells in the upper airway, e.g., Hurler's

Congenital swellings

Cystic hygroma – can affect tongue, pharynx and neck. Distortion of anatomy

Cervical

Down's syndrome – atlanto-occipital instability, large tongue, small mouth

Acquired

Burns/Infection/Tumour

Post surgery/trauma, e.g., cervical spine fixation or maxillofacial surgery

Tracheal anomalies – subglottic stenosis (can be congenital)

adapted from adult practice. One of the main differences in paediatric practice is that awake techniques for securing the airway are not well tolerated in children. This presents a particular challenge to the paediatric anaesthetist. As with any difficult airway, preparation and planning are paramount for a successful outcome.

Recognition of the difficult airway

The presence of one of the conditions outlined in Table 21.3 will alert the anaesthetist to the potential difficult airway. A history of snoring or sleep apnoea may indicate a risk of early airway obstruction during induction of anaesthesia.

Signs of airway compromise include tachypnoea, use of accessory muscles and stridor. A formal examination of the airway should be performed; the extent of the examination will be limited by the degree of patient cooperation. As with adult practice, high Mallampati scores, poor mouth opening, decreased neck mobility, micrognathia, retrognathia and dysmorphic features are all predictors of a difficult airway, although formal validation of these parameters to identify the difficult airway is not found in paediatric practice.

A review of previous anaesthetic records can be invaluable. Due to their underlying condition, a number of these patients will present for repeated anaesthetics. However it should be remembered that the airway in these children might alter as they grow. For example, the airway in children with mucopolysaccharidoses will tend to worsen over time whereas it usually improves in those with Pierre Robin syndrome as the mandible grows.

Preparation

A pre-operative antisialogue such as atropine 20 μg/kg should be given either orally, intravenously or occasionally intramuscularly. A sedative premedication may be useful in the anxious child. However their use is best avoided if it is deemed that there is a risk of airway obstruction.

The anaesthetic room should be prepared and all the equipment checked. Ideally there should be two anaesthetists present; this is absolutely vital if a fibreoptic technique is planned.

Conduct of anaesthesia

A recent survey confirms inhalational induction with 100% oxygen and sevoflurane remains the technique of choice when managing difficult airways in infants and younger children. A carefully titrated dose of propofol is an alternative. Airway obstruction can occur as muscle tone is lost on induction. Airway obstruction can be managed by change in patient position or the insertion of an appropriately sized oral or nasopharyngeal airway. Guedel airways are available in sizes 000 through to size 4. They should be sized by measuring from the corner of the mouth to the angle of the jaw. Nasopharyngeal airways can be constructed from a cut TT as those that are commercially available are only manufactured in adult sizes. If airway obstruction occurs in the absence of intravenous access then intramuscular suxamethonium 5 mg/kg can be administered into the deltoid muscle.

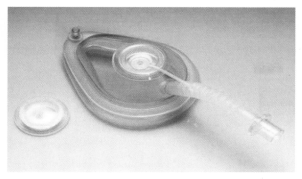

Figure 21.1. Endoscopic facemask. The central disposable silicone discs have holes of different sizes to allow the passage of different sized endoscopes and TT. The disc can be positioned for either nasal or oral intubation.

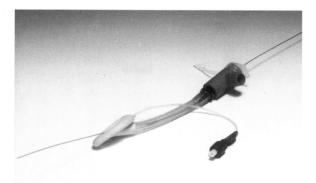

Figure 21.2. Rusch connector. The Rusch connector within the angle piece allows passage of the fibrescope and insertion of the wire without interruption to the supply of oxygen and volatile agent.

Table 21.4. Characteristics of paediatric fibrescopes

Scope external diameter	Tracheal tube internal diameter	Suction channel
2.2 mm	2.5 mm	No
2.5 mm	3.0 mm	Yes
3.8 mm	4.5 mm	Yes

Direct laryngoscopy

In addition to straight and curved laryngoscope blades, paediatric versions of the McCoy and polio blades are also available. The view at direct laryngoscopy is often aided by the application of cricoid pressure that brings the larynx into view. Bougies and stylets are available in paediatric sizes, but the smaller sized bougies are often difficult to manipulate. A well described technique in infants is a 'two person' technique, where the first operator obtains the best possible laryngeal view during laryngoscopy using external pressure to the larynx and a second anaesthetist passes the bougie.

Fibreoptic techniques

Performing an awake fibreoptic intubation in the paediatric population is challenging, if not impossible secondary to lack of cooperation and understanding on the part of the patient. The majority of fibreoptic procedures are performed on the anaesthetised child. There should always be two anaesthetists present if a fibreoptic technique is planned; one to induce and maintain anaesthesia, the second to secure the airway.

This immediately poses the question of how to maintain anaesthesia during manipulation of the airway. As stated above an inhalational induction preserving spontaneous ventilation is the technique of choice in the difficult paediatric airway. Oxygenation and anaesthesia need to be maintained during intubation. The method chosen to achieve this will depend upon the underlying airway pathology, the choice of route for intubation and the type of surgery that is planned. Anaesthesia can be maintained by use of a nasopharyngeal airway (cut TT) attached directly to the anaesthetic circuit; the use of a specifically designed endoscopic facemask; or an LMA with a Rusch connector (see Figures 21.1 and 21.2)

Paediatric fibreoptic bronchoscopes are available in three sizes. The smallest of these has an external diameter of 2.2 mm, which can hold a 2.5 mm TT. However it is described as 'whippy' in nature, can be difficult to manipulate and does not have a suction channel. The characteristics of the different sized 'scopes are summarised in Table 21.4.

The nasal route for fibreoptic intubation is indicated in patients with temporo-mandibular joint problems or limited mouth opening, or when surgery dictates the necessity of a nasal TT. Anaesthesia can be maintained either by placing a nasal airway in the contralateral airway and connecting this directly to the breathing circuit or through the use of the endoscopic facemask. The TT is mounted on the fibrescope which is then passed through the nose until a clear view of the vocal cords is achieved. Once this view has been optimised the fibrescope is advanced until the carina is identified. The TT is then railroaded over the fibrescope. It is necessary to suppress

197

the laryngeal reflexes in order that the TT can be advanced through the vocal cords. This can be achieved through topicalisation with lidocaine (3–4 mg/kg) via the suction channel, deepening anaesthesia with either an inhalational agent or small increments of propofol. If the airway is easy to maintain then a dose of a short acting opiate or a muscle relaxant can be administered at this point.

This method can also be used for oral intubation with or without the use of a guidewire. If a guidewire technique is used then the fibrescope does not have to be advanced into the trachea but can remain above the cords. A fine guidewire, such as those used by interventional radiologists is passed through the suction channel and manipulated into the trachea under direct vision. The scope is then removed and a TT passes over the wire. This technique is particularly useful if paediatric fibrescopes are not available. Due to the delicate and flimsy nature of these wires it is often useful to first feed a Cook exchange catheter over the wire in order to stiffen it. The TT is then passed over the exchange catheter.

The use of an LMA as a conduit for fibreoptic intubation in children is a well described technique. The LMA acts not only as a conduit for the fibrescope but also ensures adequate depth of anaesthesia by providing a patent airway during airway manipulation. If adequately controlled ventilation can be achieved using the LMA then some choose to administer a muscle relaxant in order to improve intubating conditions. Once an adequate depth of anaesthesia has been achieved, the fibrescope is introduced through the LMA until a view of the cords is achieved, it is then inserted into the trachea until the carina is visualised. The short length of paediatric TTs means that they tend to disappear inside the LMA if they are railroaded over the scope. This problem can be overcome by loading two TTs that are fixed together onto the scope and using the top one to push the lower one into position and hold it there as the LMA is removed. A very popular technique is the use of a guidewire and airway exchange catheter. The wire is fed via the suction channel into the trachea, the fibrescope is then removed and a stiffening device such as a Cook airway exchange catheter is passed over the wire through the LMA. The guidewire is then removed and the position of the airway exchange catheter confirmed by capnography. At this point the LMA is removed and a TT is railroaded over the catheter.

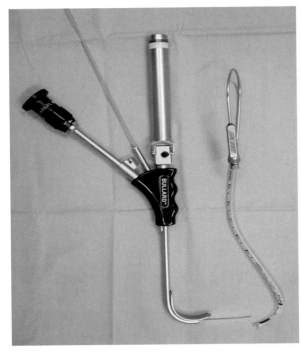

Figure 21.3. The Bullard.

The intubating LMA is available in size 3 and above. It can be a useful conduit for fibreoptic intubation in children over 25 kg and has a particular role in those patients with cervical pathology.

Other equipment is available for the management of the difficult paediatric airway.

Bullard laryngoscope

This is a rigid fibreoptic laryngoscope which is available in three sizes: newborns/infants, paediatric and adult. It aids in glottic visualisation when the oral, pharyngeal and laryngeal axes are poorly aligned. Once the larynx is visualised a TT can be advanced either over the Bullard intubating stylet or via a bougie. The Bullard can also assist in nasal intubation by providing visualisation of the vocal cords while the TT is introduced via the nasal route. It requires minimal neck movement for its use and can be used in patients with a mouth opening of just 6 mm (see Figure 21.3).

Video-laryngoscopes

Video-laryngoscopy describes the transmission of the view from the laryngoscope blade tip via a fibreoptic

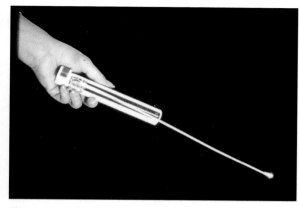

Figure 21.4. The Light Wand.

Table 21.5. Causes of airway obstruction in the child

Congenital	Acquired
Choanal atresia	Epiglottitis
Laryngomalacia	Foreign body
Subglottic stenosis	Laryngotracheobronchitis
Subglottic haemangioma	Bacterial tracheitis
Webs	Subglottic stenosis
Cysts	Burns
Tracheal stenosis	Peritonsillar abscess
Vascular rings or slings	Angioneurotic oedema
Bilateral vocal cord paralysis	Nerve palsies
	Mediastinal masses

endoscope to a video display. Video-laryngoscopes are useful teaching aids when learning the techniques of paediatric intubation, a supervising anaesthetist can follow exactly where the laryngoscope travels and monitor the passage of the TT. Video-laryngoscopes may prove useful in the difficult paediatric airway (see Chapter 15).

Light wand

This is a preformed stylet that has a lighted tip that trans-illuminates the soft tissues of the neck (see Chapter 14). It can be used with or without a laryngoscope and is of particular value when there is limited mouth opening or cervical instability. A TT is mounted on the wand, and the passage of the illuminated tip is monitored at the front of the neck as it is advanced midline towards the larynx. The Trachlight comes in two paediatric sizes, the infant version is compatible with a 2.5 mm tube and the child size will fit a 4 mm tube (see Figure 21.4).

Intubating the child with airway obstruction

There are a number of causes, both congenital and acquired, of airway obstruction in the child (see Table 21.5). The general principles of airway management are the same regardless of underlying cause, however, there are two scenarios that deserve special attention. In addition, practitioners should be aware that post-obstructive negative-pressure pulmonary oedema can occur, which may require a period of positive pressure ventilation.

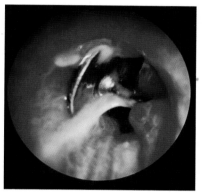

Figure 21.5. Inhaled foreign body.

Inhalation of a foreign body

This is the most common reason for a bronchoscopy in the 1–3 year old age group. Presentation may be as an acute emergency, with obstruction of the upper airway. Or in the case of lower airway obstruction, the history may be that of a cough or wheeze over a few days in conjunction with a plausible history. It is important to have early involvement of ENT and anaesthetic teams (Figure 21.5).

Pre-operative assessment

The airway should be assessed and the degree of any respiratory compromise determined. Important signs include the respiratory rate, degree of stridor, use of accessory muscles, sternal, subcostal and intercostal recession. If the child is tiring, that makes the situation even more urgent.

Peri-operatively

The child is transferred, with their parents, to an anaesthetic room. The child should be receiving high flow oxygen. The use of Heliox should be considered, as this reduces the resistance to turbulent airflow because of its relatively low density.

An inhalational induction, consisting of 100% oxygen and high inspired concentration of sevoflurane, should be performed. Spontaneous ventilation should be maintained. Intravenous access and full standard monitoring should be secured once a deep plane of anaesthesia has been achieved. Laryngoscopy can then be performed so that the epiglottis, larynx and vocal cords can be sprayed with 1% lidocaine. The surgeons should only insert the rigid broncho-scope once enough time has elapsed for the lidocaine to have its effect in order to avoid coughing and laryngospasm. The breathing circuit can then be attached to the side arm of the bronchoscope. Traditional teaching is that spontaneous ventilation should be maintained throughout, as positive pressure may push the foreign body further into the airway. However if the foreign body is fairly distal, the use of a muscle relaxant may in fact make removal less difficult.

A dose of dexamethasone 0.25 mg/kg may be given intraoperatively, especially if the removal proved to be particularly difficult.

Post-operative period

The child should be nil by mouth for at least 2 hours, in order to allow the effects of topical lidocaine to wear off. They should be nursed in an area where they can be monitored for stridor and commenced on humidified oxygen therapy. Adrenaline nebulisers (400 µg/kg) should be prescribed for the management of stridor.

Acute epiglottitis

This is an acute life-threatening emergency. Historically this was commonly due to an underlying *Haemophilus influenza* B (HiB) infection. However the introduction of the HiB vaccination in childhood now means that the most common causative agent is streptococcus. Infections with non-B serotypes of *Haemophilus* carry with them significant morbidity

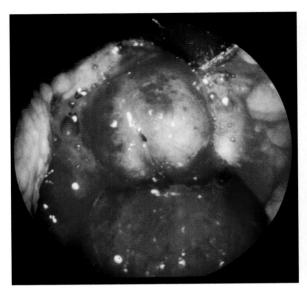

Figure 21.6. Epiglottitis.

and mortality. The peak incidence is at age 2–3 years, and it involves the rapid onset of oedema around the epiglottis. Approximately, 60% of children with epiglottitis will require intubation. Again it is vital to have early input from a senior anaesthetist and ENT surgeon (see Chapter 25) (Figure 21.6).

Pre-operative assessment

The child looks unwell. They have a high fever and drool because they are unable to swallow. They have signs of respiratory compromise and present with rapid onset inspiratory and expiratory stridor. They adopt a position that provides them with a patent airway; typically they lean forwards or lie prone.

Peri-operatively

The child and parents should be transferred swiftly to the anaesthetic room. Distress to the child should be kept to a minimum, as there is a risk of precipitating complete airway obstruction.

Anaesthesia should only be induced in the presence of a senior ENT surgeon, and all the equipment to perform a cricothyroidotomy or rapid tracheostomy should be readily available. An inhalational induction using oxygen and sevoflurane should be performed. Induction may be slow because of the degree of airway obstruction. Intravenous access should only be obtained once a deep plane of anaesthesia has been achieved. Various sizes of TT must be available. Laryngoscopy may be extremely difficult, the laryngeal inlet may be very difficult to identify and bubbles of air may be the only clue to the position of the opening. In this instance it is useful to use a bougie and railroad a TT over it. Muscle relaxants should only be administered once the airway has been secured – but see Chapter 25.

The child should then be transferred to the intensive care unit and remain intubated until there is an audible leak around the TT (usually 24–36 hours after starting treatment with antibiotics).

Rapid sequence induction in neonates and young children

The risk of aspiration of gastric contents in children ranges from 1 to 9 cases per 10 000 anaesthetics and the risk of serious morbidity following aspiration is very rare.

Pre-operative fasting prior to elective surgery maximises gastric emptying and reduces the risk of aspiration. However it should be kept to the minimum in order to prevent patient discomfort and in the neonate and young infant to avoid the risk of hypoglycaemia and significant dehydration. Current fasting recommendations are 2 hours for clear fluids, 4 hours for breast milk and 6 hours for formula milk or solids.

In the emergency setting the gold standard for the management of a patient with a 'full stomach' is rapid sequence induction (RSI). However the practicalities and potential risks of delivering an RSI in a neonate or young child need careful consideration.

Reliable intravenous access may be difficult to achieve in a small, awake, dehydrated patient.

Adequate pre-oxygenation can be difficult to achieve in the non-compliant, distressed child. Struggling with a crying child may in fact increase oxygen consumption and reduce oxygen reserves.

During the period of apnoea following administration of the muscle relaxant, the combination of a low FRC and high oxygen consumption can lead to rapid oxygen desaturation, particularly in the neonate or small child. To avoid hypoxia it is common to inflate the lungs of the neonate or small infant gently with cricoid pressure in place in order to maintain oxygen saturations prior to intubation.

The cricoid cartilage is higher at the level of C4 at birth. Excessive or incorrect cricoid pressure applied by an inexperience assistant can lead to distortion of

the airway and subsequent difficulty in intubation. Surveys have found that 50–60% of experienced paediatric anaesthetists do not use cricoid pressure in children – even those at risk of aspiration.

The incidence of aspiration in children reported in the USA where RSI is widely used, although very low, is in fact higher than that reported in France, where cricoid pressure is less frequently used. It seems reasonable, in view of the practical limitations of RSI, that it should be reserved for the cooperative or sick child with gross abdominal distension or active upper gastrointestinal bleeding and that in others, a modified technique can be employed.

Key points

- Desaturation is very rapid in children.
- Overinflation easily causes gastric distension.
- The small size and active reflexes of children's airways make them particularly prone to obstruction.
- Tracheal intubation is typically easy in children, except in some well known syndromes and diseases, when it demands the highest levels of skill and equipment.
- Cuffed tubes are becoming more popular.
- Rapid sequence induction is not a standard in paediatric practice.

Further reading

Bingham R, Patel P. (2009). Laryngeal mask airway & other supraglottic airway devices in paediatric practice. *Continuing Education in Anaesthesia, Critical Care & Pain*, **9**(1).

Black A. (2008). Management of the difficult airway. In: Bingham R, Lloyd-Thomas AR, Sury MRJ (Eds.), *Hatch & Sumner's Textbook of Paediatric Anaesthesia*. 3rd ed. London: Hodder Arnold. pp. 315–331.

Borland LM, Sereika SM, Woelfel SK, et al. (1998). Pulmonary aspiration in pediatric patients during general anesthesia: incidence and outcome. *Journal of Clinical Anaesthesia*, **10**, 95–102.

Brady M, Kinn S, O'Rourke K, et al. (2005). Preoperarive fasting for preventing perioperative complications in children. *Cochrane Database Systematic Reviews*, **2**, CD005285.

Brooks P, Ree R, Rosen D, Anserimo M. (2005). Canadian pediatric anesthesiologists prefer inhalational anesthesia to manage difficult airways. *Canadian Journal of Anesthesia* **52**, 285–290.

Caldwell M, Walker RWM. (2003). Management of the difficult paediatric airway. *British Journal of Anaesthesia, CEPD Review*, **3**, 167–169.

Faden H. (2006). The dramatic change in the epidemiology of pediatric epiglottitis. *Pediatric Emergency Care*, **22**, 443–444.

James I. (2001). Cuffed tubes in children. Editorial. *Paediatric Anaesthesia*, **11**, 259–263.

Jenkins IA, Saunders M. (2009). Infections of the airway. *Paediatric Anaesthesia*, **19**(Suppl 1), 118–130.

Katz J, Steward DJ. (1993). *Anesthesia and Uncommon Pediatric Diseases*. 2nd ed. Philadelphia: WB Saunders.

Lang SA, Duncan PG, Shephard DA, Ha HC. (1990). Pulmonary oedema associated with airway obstruction. *Canadian Journal of Anaesthesia*, **37**, 210–218.

Marcus RJ, Thompson JP. (2000). Anaesthesia for manipulation of forearm fractures in children: A survey of current practice. *Pediatric Anaesthesia*, **10**, 273–277.

Roberts S, Thornington R. (2005). Paediatric bronchoscopy. *Continuing Education in Anaesthesia, Critical Care & Pain*, **5**, 41–44.

Seidel J, Dorman T. (2006). Anesthetic management of preschool children with penetrating eye injuries: postal survey of pediatric anesthetists and review of the available evidence. *Pediatric Anesthesia*, **16**, 769–776.

Steward D, Lerman J. (2001). *Manual of Pediatric Anaesthesia*. 5th ed. New York: Churchill Livingstone.

Stoddart PA, Brennan L, Hatch DJ, Bingham R. (1994). Postal survey of paediatric practice and training among consultant anaesthetists in the UK. *British Journal of Anaesthesia*, **73**, 559–563.

Tiret L, Nivoche Y, Hatton F, et al. (1988). Complications related to anaesthesia in infants and children. A prospective survey of 40240 anaesthetics. *British Journal of Anaesthesia*, **61**, 263–269.

Walker R. (2000). The Laryngeal Mask Airway in the difficult airway: An assessment of positioning and use in fibreoptic intubation. *Paediatric Anaesthesia*, **10**, 53–58.

Warner MA, Warner ME, Warner DO, et al. (1999). Perioperative pulmonary aspiration in infants and young children. *Anesthesiology*, **90**, 66–71.

Weiss M, Dullenkopf A, Fischer JE, Keller C, Gerber AC. (2009). Prospective randomized controlled multi-centre trial of cuffed endotracheal tubes in small children. *British Journal of Anaesthesia*, **103**, 867–873.

Weiss M, Schwartz U, Dillier CM, Gerber AC. (2001). Teaching and supervising tracheal intubation in paediatric patients using videolaryngoscopy. *Paediatric Anaesthesia*, **11**, 343–348.

Chapter

22

Bariatrics

Will Peat and Mark C. Bellamy

General

With the recent and dramatic increase in the prevalence of obesity – now affecting up to 30% of the adult population – every anaesthetist is likely to encounter the associated airway management problems. Elective surgery allows time for fuller assessment and investigation, but such patients may present at more challenging times and places.

There are many definitions of obesity in clinical practice. Perhaps the most widely adopted in European practice is the set of definitions based on body mass index. The body mass index is calculated by dividing the weight of the patient (in kilograms) by the square of the height in metres. A body mass index (BMI) between 20 and 25 kg per square metre represents a normal or 'ideal' body weight. A cut-off point (depending on the definition used) at 25 or 27 kilograms per square metre marks the beginning of the overweight range; this continues until a body mass index of 30. Above this, the patient is said to be obese. A body mass index exceeding 40 kilograms per square metre, or greater than 35 kilograms per square metre in the presence of obesity related co-morbidity (such as type 2 diabetes, hypertension or obstructive sleep apnoea), signals morbid obesity.

Obesity was the commonest factor identified in the first 2000 incidents reported to the Australian Incident Monitoring Study.

Obstructive sleep apnoea (OSA) and diabetes mellitus, diseases closely associated with obesity, are also associated with difficult intubation and airway control. Reliable intravenous access can also be difficult to achieve in obese subjects, which has considerable consequence for airway control.

It is therefore surprising that the level of difficult intubation in obese patients is disputed. Obesity per se was not associated with difficult intubation in one study, whilst another reported an incidence of difficult intubation of up to 25%.

Perhaps more important to recognise are the problems of airway assessment and difficulty in mask ventilation. A BMI of greater than 26 kg/m^2 is an independent risk factor for, but a weak predictor of, difficult mask ventilation (see Chapter 7).

Airway anatomy and physiology are altered in obesity, and an understanding of these changes is key to appropriate airway management.

Anatomy of the airway
Fat deposition

Magnetic resonance imaging (MRI) demonstrates that the tongue, soft palate, parapharyngeal fat pads and lateral pharyngeal walls (between medial and lateral pterygoids), are all important in the calibre and compliance of the upper airway of obese patients.

Airway shape

The airway shape may also play a factor in airway collapse. The long axis of the airway in patients with obesity and sleep apnoea is directed anterior–posterior rather than laterally. It is hypothesised that this places the anteriorly found pharyngeal dilator muscles at a mechanical disadvantage and so leaves the pharynx at increased risk of collapse.

Body fat distribution

The fat distribution has a significant effect on airway anatomy and ease of intubation. The classical male type of fat distribution is known as android, and the classical female distribution is known as gynaecoid.

Core Topics in Airway Management, Second Edition, ed. Ian Calder and Adrian Pearce. Published by Cambridge University Press. © Cambridge University Press 2011.

In the android fat distribution, the arms and legs are thin, but there is excessive intra-peritoneal fat and fatty involvement in the neck and airway. In the gynaecoid distribution, abdominal fat is predominantly extraperitoneal, and additionally fat is distributed to the limbs and buttocks. The airway tends to be less commonly involved. These fat distributions are sometimes known as 'apples and pears'. Of course, while the android fat distribution is predominantly seen in men, it is occasionally also seen in women; likewise, men can display the gynaecoid fat distribution. The android fat distribution is more commonly associated with the metabolic syndrome (hypertension, diabetes, dyslipidaemia, airway involvement, and in women, polycystic ovaries and hirsutism) than the gynaecoid distribution. Hence, with an android fat distribution there is a greater central fat distribution that may lead to difficult airway control compared to the gynaecoid fat distribution.

Gender differences

Compared with men, women have a greater frequency of obesity and a greater amount of body fat, but the prevalence of obstructive sleep apnoea is far greater in men. Although women have a significantly smaller oropharyngeal junction and pharynx they have milder obstructive symptoms as defined by respiratory disturbance index. This may indicate that there is an inherent structural and functional difference between the airway in males and females.

Posture

The effects of posture change on airway dimensions differ between the sexes. Men have a larger decrease in upper airway area at the oropharyngeal junction than women on change of posture from sitting to supine. In addition to this women have larger supine upper airway area at the oropharyngeal junction with increasing neck circumference, suggesting that women are able to maintain their upper airways better in response to mass loading.

Weight loss

Weight loss can significantly alter the airway anatomy. Ross et al reported that a patient had a change in Cormack and Lehane grade from IV to II resulting from the loss of 38 kg.

Studies of the upper airway using MRI before and after weight loss surgery indicated significant reductions of the lateral pharyngeal wall and parapharyngeal fat pads but not the tongue or soft palate.

Respiratory physiology
Pulmonary function tests

Longitudinal studies of pulmonary function have shown reduction in pulmonary tests with obesity. A Canadian study showed that BMI at baseline and subsequent weight gain were significantly related to decline in pulmonary function.

Functional residual capacity (FRC) and the rate of desaturation

Computer modelled figures suggest that after pre-oxygenation the time to SaO_2 of 85% is reduced from 502 seconds for a 70 kg adult to only 171 seconds for a 127 kg adult. This is less time than expected in a 20 kg child.

The FRC is reduced further by the conduct of general anaesthesia. Damia et al. showed that in morbidly obese patients there was a reduction of the FRC to approximately 50% of pre-anaesthetic values.

The other factor that influences rate of desaturation is the rate of oxygen consumption. In the obese, the resting metabolic rate, oxygen consumption and also carbon dioxide production are all increased, compounding the reduction in FRC.

V/Q mismatch

In addition to acting as an oxygen store FRC is important in splinting small airways. Closing capacity (CC) is the sum of the closing volume and residual volume. If CC exceeds FRC there is closure of small airways leading to shunted blood and arterial hypoxaemia. In lean patients the CC exceeds FRC in the supine position at 45 years, and 65 years in the erect position. As FRC is reduced, these changes occur earlier in life in the obese, and may occur at normal tidal breathing in the supine position.

Respiratory mechanics

Respiratory mechanics are affected even in moderate obesity. This is mostly related to reduced chest wall compliance but also increased airway resistance. Work of breathing increases to such an extent as body mass increases that it is close to commonly reported limits of muscle fatigue in most overweight patients during 'normal' breathing. This means that spontaneously breathing obese patients can rapidly progress to respiratory failure.

Predictors of airway difficulty

Maybe the most feared situation for an anaesthetist is 'can't intubate, can't ventilate'.

This is an even greater concern in obesity because of the speed of desaturation. Evaluation of the airway to predict potential 'difficult intubation' is standard pre-operative practice; however the evaluation of the ease (or difficulty) of mask ventilation is difficult and not routine. Arguably, the emphasis of airway assessment should shift to ease of facemask ventilation rather than the difficulty of intubation, as profound desaturation can occur even when the intubation is straightforward. This factor alone in some cases is a sufficient indication for an awake intubation.

Predictors of difficult mask ventilation

Kheterpal et al graded mask ventilation (MV) in a similar fashion to Cormack and Lehane's classification of view at laryngoscopy.

Grade 3 MV was defined as MV that was inadequate to maintain oxygenation, or MV requiring two providers. Grade 4 MV was impossible MV.

The incidence of grade 3 or grade 4 MV was 1.5% (1.4% grade 3 and 0.16% grade 4).

Several characteristics commonly seen in the obese population were independent risk factors for grade 3 MV: BMI of 30 kg/m^2 or greater, a beard, Mallampati classification of 3 or 4 and snoring.

More disturbingly, Yildiz's group reported an incidence of difficult MV of 7.8%, and the incidence of difficult MV among patients with difficult intubation was 15.5%.

Predictors of difficult intubation

The incidence of difficult intubation in the obese patient is disputed. Accurate prediction of difficult intubation in normal weight patients is not without problems. This is not helped by the fact that studies have not adopted one standard definition of a difficult intubation. When the prevalence of difficult intubation is so rare, unless the tests are highly sensitive

and specific, positive and negative predictive values are low.

Brodsky et al showed that neither absolute obesity nor BMI were associated with problems at intubation. Logistic regression identified neck circumference as the single best indicator of difficult intubation in obese patients. Nelligan et al did not find a relationship between difficult intubation and BMI or obstructive sleep apnoea in a study of 180 patients where the mean BMI was 49.4 kg/m^2, and the prevalence of OSA was 68%.

A French study set out to look further at neck circumference as a predictor. Their 'difficult to intubate' group had a significant preponderance of patients with raised BMI, neck circumference, and Mallampati score over 3.

Voyagis et al looked more specifically at Mallampati score in the obese. Although, in contrast to many other studies, obesity alone was a predictor of difficult intubation, it yielded a high false positive rate.

Ultrasound has been used to assess the role of soft tissue in the neck. There are relatively few data, but there is a suggestion that there is increased tissue at the level of the vocal cords in patients who are difficult to intubate.

The factors that appear to have an association with difficult intubation in the obese across several studies are increased Mallampati score and increased neck circumference.

Airway techniques

As with any anaesthetic, correct and thorough preparation is required. The theatre table should be of adequate size and able to accommodate the weight of the obese patient. The anaesthetist should have a clear plan as to the route of securing the airway and back-up plans in case of difficulty. There should be adequate provision for management of difficult ventilation and intubation, including equipment for fibreoptic intubation and cricothyroid puncture. Laryngoscopes of various sizes and geometries should be available. An adequately trained operating department practitioner is required and a sufficient number of circulating staff to assist in turning or moving the patient in case of difficulties.

Positioning

In the obese patient the 'ramped' or 'stacked' position has been described as the position best suited to guide

(a)

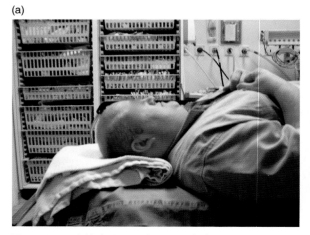

(b)

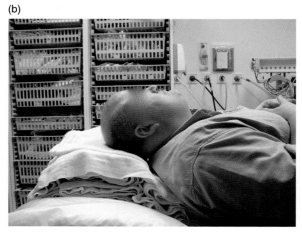

Figure 22.1. (a,b) The 'ramped' position for laryngoscopy. The patient's upper body and head are elevated to create a horizontal alignment between the external auditory meatus and the sternal notch.

laryngoscopy. This is when the patient's upper body and head are elevated to create a horizontal alignment between the external auditory meatus and the sternal notch (Figure 22.1).

Collins et al investigated the difference between the two positions. The 'ramped' position provided a statistically significant improvement in the laryngeal grade (Cormack and Lehane) when compared to a standard 'sniff' position.

Body position may also affect pre-oxygenation. A head-up or reverse Trendelenburg position is thought to increase the FRC and provide a greater oxygen store and prolonged time to desaturation.

In obese patients where pre-oxygenation occurred in either a sitting or supine position before being laid supine for intubation, the mean time to desaturation was significantly longer in the sitting group despite the change to the supine position for the intubation.

Techniques for pre-oxygenation

Novel techniques have been described for pre-oxygenation in addition to traditional methods. Nasal insufflation of oxygen has been described as a means of prolonging time to desaturation. Following adequate pre-oxygenation, when 5 litres/min of oxygen was insufflated into the nasopharynx, 16 of 17 morbidly obese patients had 100% SpO_2 at 4 minutes. If no oxygen was used 17 control patients desaturated. The exact mechanism for this effect is yet to be fully elucidated.

Adjuncts to securing the airway

Although awake intubation is occasionally performed in the morbidly obese patient population, the vast majority of obese patients are intubated following direct laryngoscopy. Consequently, there has been considerable enthusiasm in developing airway adjuncts for improving the facility, speed and safety of 'asleep' intubation in this patient group. The combination of enthusiastic inventors and commercial developers has led to a burgeoning number of airway devices described to assist securing the airway.

Several airway devices have been described as adjuncts to securing the airway.

The use of the intubating laryngeal mask airway (ILMA) has been described. There is an obvious disadvantage with the laryngeal mask that the airway is not 'secure' and there is a risk of aspiration. Although they aided intubation in the majority of patients, using these devices failed to prevent desaturations and the intubations took a significantly longer time to complete.

In another study the use of the Airtraq™ was compared to the performance of the standard Macintosh laryngoscope. The study showed that tracheal intubation was successfully carried out in all patients within 2 minutes in the Airtraq™ group. Six patients in the Macintosh group could not be intubated within 2 minutes but were subsequently intubated within a mean of 27 seconds with the Airtraq™.

Awake fibreoptic intubation

If there is any doubt whether the anaesthetist will be able to intubate and/or ventilate the obese patient then awake fibreoptic intubation should be considered.

There are a great number of 'recipes' described for awake fibreoptic intubation. Adequate topical anaesthesia of the airway together with conscious sedation with remifentanil are the cornerstones to our local practice. The techniques chosen will depend to a great extent on the anaesthetist's own personal experience. Specific techniques are discussed in Chapter 13. Interestingly, patients most frequently viewed as requiring 'awake intubation' (male, BMI greater than 35, sleep apnoea and collar size over 17.5 inches) often have relatively attenuated upper airway reflexes. The serendipity of a reduced gag or cough reflex can be very helpful to the anaesthetist during an awake fibreoptic intubation.

Extubation

PEEP should be used intraoperatively to negate atelectasis formation and minimise ventilation perfusion mismatch. Extubation should occur only when the patient is fully awake, sitting up and following a recruitment manoeuvre. If the patient has a history of OSA it is important to recommence their CPAP soon after extubation.

Current UK practice

As an indication of current practice a recent national survey has been performed surveying anaesthetists who regularly performed bariatric surgical lists (Moore J. National UK Bariatric Anaesthesia Survey – Personal Communication). Most anaesthetists surveyed reported that in their experience difficult intubation was rare in obese patients. As described in the techniques earlier, the majority of UK anaesthetists intubate patients in approximately 20–30 degrees reverse Trendelenburg and combine this with a ramping position to aid intubation. Indications for fibreoptic intubation in this population were perceived as similar to the general population and suxamethonium was used routinely in 29% of cases.

Most anaesthetists in UK bariatric practice administer induction drugs according to body weights other than the actual body weight. This is an area of considerable variation in practice because of the paucity of data in subjects with a BMI exceeding 50. The ideal body weight (based on height) is often used. Another approach is to use ideal body weight plus a fixed fraction of the difference between this and the actual weight, typically 20–30%.

A similar strategy is employed for calculating the dose of neuromuscular blocking agents, where ideal body weight is appropriate. The major exception to this is suxamethonium, the dose of which is based on actual body weight. An interesting paradox concerns the reversal of rocuronium by sugammadex. The dose of the relaxant is based on ideal body weight, but that of the cyclodextrin on actual weight, reflecting the radically different volumes of distribution of these agents.

Key points

- Prediction of difficulty: Mallampati score and neck circumference are better predictors than BMI and a history of OSA, but their predictive value is not strong.
- Difficult mask ventilation and difficult intubation are uncommon.
- Desaturation is swift if ventilation is interrupted.
- Pre-oxygenation should be thorough and a semi-sitting posture with pharyngeal insufflations of oxygenation during apnoea is helpful.
- Awake intubation is worthwhile if difficulty is expected, because of the rapid desaturation problem.

Further reading

Altermatt FR, Munoz HR, Delfino AE, Cortinez LI. (2005). Pre-oxygenation in the obese patient: Effects of position on the tolerance to apnoea. *British Journal of Anaesthesia*, **95**, 706–709.

Baraka AS, Taha SK, Siddik-Sayyid SM, et al. (2007) Supplementation of pre-oxygenation in the morbidly obese patients using nasopharyngeal oxygen insufflation. *Anaesthesia*, **62**, 769–773.

Brodsky JB, Lemmens HJM, Brock-Utne JG, et al. (2002). Morbid obesity and tracheal intubation. *Anesthesia and Analgesia*, **94**, 732–736.

Chen Y, Horne SL, Dosman JA. (1993). Body weight and weight gain related to pulmonary function decline in adults: A six year follow up study. *Thorax*, **48**, 375–380.

Chung F, Yegneswaran B, Herrera F, Shenderey A, Shapiro CM. (2008). Patients with difficult intubation may need referral to sleep clinics. *Anesthesia and Analgesia*, **107**, 915–920.

Collins J, Lemmens H, Brodsky JB, et al. (2004). Laryngoscopy and morbid obesity: A comparison of the 'sniff' and 'ramped' position. *Obesity Surgery*, **14**, 1171–1175.

Dmia G, Mascheroni D, Croci M, Tarenzi T. (1998). Perioperative changes in functional residual capacity in morbidly obese patients. *British Journal of Anaesthesia*, **60**, 574–578.

Ezri T, Gewurtz G, Sessler D, et al. (2003). Prediction of difficult laryngoscopy in obese patients by ultrasound quantification of anterior neck soft tissue. *Anaesthesia*, **58**, 1101–1118.

Ezri T, Medalion B, Weisenberg M, et al. (2003). Increased body mass index *per se* is not a predictor of difficult laryngoscopy. *Canadian Journal of Anesthesia*, **50**, 179–183.

Frappier J, Guenoun T, Journois D, et al. (2003). Airway management using the intubating laryngeal mask airway for the morbidly obese patient. *Anesthesia and Analgesia*, **96**, 1510–1515.

Gonzales H, Minville V, Delanoue K, et al. (2008). The importance of increased neck circumference to intubation difficulties in obese patients. *Anesthesia and Analgesia*, **106**, 1132–1136.

Horner RL, Mohiaddin RH, Lowell DG, et al. (1989). Sites and sizes of fat deposits around the pharynx in obese patients with obstructive sleep apnoea and weight matched controls. *The European Respiratory Journal*, **2**, 613–622.

Juvin P, Lavaut E, Dupont H, et al. (2003). Difficult tracheal intubation is more common in obese than in lean patients. *Anesthesia and Analgesia*, **97**, 595–600.

Kheterpal S, Han R, Tremper KK, et al. (2006). Incidence and predictors of difficult and impossible mask ventilation. *Anesthesiology*, **105**, 885–891.

Langeron O, Masso E, Huraux C, et al. (2000). Prediction of difficult mask ventilation. *Anesthesiology*, **92**, 1226–1236.

Leiter JC. (1996). Upper airway shape: Is it important in the pathogenesis of obstructive sleep apnea? *American Journal of Respiratory and Critical Care Medicine*, **153**, 894–898.

Lemmens HJ, Brodsky JB. (2006). Anesthetic drugs and bariatric surgery. *Expert Review of Neurotherapy*, **6**, 1107–1113.

Leykin Y, Pellis T, Lucca M, Lomangino G, Marzano B, Gullo A. (2004). The pharmacodynamic effects of rocuronium when dosed according to real body weight or ideal body weight in morbidly obese patients. *Anesthesia and Analgesia*, **99**, 1086–1089.

Lundstrøm LH, Møller AM, Rosenstock C, Astrup G, Wetterslev J. (2009). High body mass index is a weak predictor for difficult and failed tracheal intubation: A cohort study of 91,332 consecutive patients scheduled for direct laryngoscopy registered in the Danish Anesthesia Database. *Anesthesiology*, **110**, 266–274.

Martin SE, Mathur R, Marshall I, Douglas NJ. (1997). The effect of age, sex, obesity and posture on airway size. *European Respiratory Journal*, **10**, 2087–2090.

Mashour GA, Kheterpal S, Vanaharam V, Shanks A, et al. (2008). The extended Mallampati score and a diagnosis of diabetes mellitus are predictors of difficult laryngoscopy in the morbidly obese. *Anesthesia and Analgesia*, **107**, 1919–1923.

Mohsenin V. (2001). Gender differences in the expression of sleep-disordered breathing: Role of upper airway dimensions. *Chest*, **120**, 1442–1447.

Mortimore IL, Marshall I, Wraith PK, et al. (1998). Neck and total body fat deposition in non-obese and obese patients with sleep apnea compared with that in control subjects. *American Journal of Respiratory and Critical Care Medicine*, **157**, 280–283.

Ndoko SK, Amathieu R, Tual L, et al. (2008). Tracheal intubation of morbidly obese patients: A randomised trial comparing performance of Macintosh and Airtraq laryngoscopes. *British Journal of Anaesthesia*, **100**, 263–268.

Nelligan PJ, Porter S, Max B, et al. (2009). Obstructive sleep apnea is not a risk factor for difficult intubation in morbidly obese patients. *Anesthesia and Analgesia*, **109**, 1182–1186.

Pelosi P, Croci M, Ravagnan I, Tredici S. (1998). The effects of body mass on lung volumes, respiratory mechanics, and gas exchange during general anesthesia. *Anesthesia and Analgesia*, **87**, 654–660.

Ravussin E, Burnand B, Schutz Y, Jequier E. (1982). Twenty-four-hour energy expenditure and resting metabolic rate in obese, moderately obese and control subjects. *American Journal of Clinical Nutrition*, **35**, 566–573.

Ross AK, Jefferson P, Ball DR. (2008). Improvement in laryngoscopy grade with dramatic weight loss. *Anaesthesia*, **63**, 1022.

Voyagis GS, Kyriakis KP, Dimitriou V, Vrettou I. (1998). Value of oropharyngeal Mallampati classification in predicting difficult laryngoscopy among obese patients. *European Journal of Anaesthesiology*, **15**, 330–334.

Welch K, Foster G, Rittler C, et al. (2002). A novel volumetric magnetic resonance imaging paradigm to study upper airway anatomy. *Sleep*, **25**, 530–540.

Williamson JA, Webb RK, Szekely S, Gillies ER, Dreosti AV. (1993). Difficult intubation: An analysis of 2000 incident reports. *Anaesthesia and Intensive Care*, **21**, 602–607.

Yentis S. (2006). Predicting trouble in airway management. *Anesthesiology*, **105**, 871–872.

Yildiz TS, Solak M, Toker K. (2005). The incidence and risk factors of difficult mask ventilation. *Journal of Anesthesia*, **19**, 7–11.

Chapter 23

Maxillofacial surgery

Joy E. Curran and James Nicholson

Maxillofacial surgery has a large case mix, from paediatric exodontia to 10 hour intra-oral tumour resection and free tissue flap reconstruction. This chapter will look at airway assessment specific to maxillofacial work and airway management in dento-alveolar surgery, upper airway tumours (intra-oral), orthognathic surgery, maxillofacial trauma and infections.

The relationship between the surgeon and anaesthetist is never more crucial than in maxillofacial surgery. It can be likened to a co-habiting couple squabbling over living space. The anaesthetist and surgeon must agree on the most appropriate method of airway management.

Airway assessment

A detailed section on airway assessment appears elsewhere in this book (Chapter 7). There are a higher proportion of difficult airways in this group of patients. Standard airway examinations may pick up on the following issues:

- Poor mouth opening due to either temporo-mandibular joint (TMJ) dysfunction, trismus due to pain or infection, restriction by previous surgery or radiotherapy (curative radiotherapy to area(s) of the masticatory muscles and /or ligaments of the TMJ resulted in trismus in 45% of patients in one study)
- Increased tongue volume if the floor of mouth is raised
- Decreased tongue mobility
- Retrognathia.

But may not pick up

- Posterior tongue tumours or pharyngeal wall tumours

- Increased rigidity of neck structures following radiotherapy or chronic infection
- Airway displacement due to abscess or tumour.

Nasal route of intubation

Nasal intubation is often the most appropriate technique, but can have significant complications. Historically, nasal intubation was introduced by Kuhn in 1902, and nasal and oral intubation was popularised by Magill and Gilles in the post-World War one era.

Nasendoscopy and/or intubation can be traumatic because the nasal mucosa is extremely vascular and the cavity contains the nasal turbinates (Figure 23.1). However there are both anaesthetic and surgical reasons for opting for the nasal route. Limited mouth opening may make the nasal route the obvious choice, and although mouth opening will often improve after induction of anaesthesia, it is important to make a considered assessment of how likely this is. In general chronic problems will NOT resolve with anaesthesia. Heard et al have suggested the use of pre-anaesthetic mandibular nerve blockade to clarify which patients will improve after induction.

The additional space afforded for surgery by a nasal tube facilitates minor surgery, is almost essential for complex intra-oral procedures, and nasal tubes are less likely to be obstructed by surgical manoeuvres. Nasal tubes permit intra-operative dental occlusion for correct alignment of the mandible with maxilla in facial fracture repair or elective jaw realignment.

Epistaxis is the commonest complication of nasal intubation, but although a prevalence as high as 80% with some tubes has been reported, it is usually minor and self-limiting. Patients with coagulopathies are at risk from more serious haemorrhage and the need for

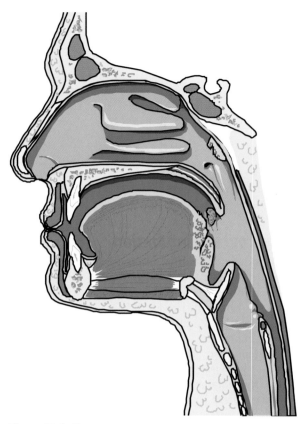

Figure 23.1. Nose anatomy.

a nasal intubation must therefore be justified, and pre-operative correction considered. Patients on low dose aspirin may also be at risk although there is little in the literature about this group. Aspirin combined with another antiplatelet drug such as clopidogrel will certainly raise the risk of haemorrhage.

Nasal intubation can cause a bacteraemia (2 out of 175 anaesthetists who had a nasal intubation as part of a fibreoptic intubation training course developed rigors and one a chest infection, whilst 20% had nasal bleeding). NICE guidelines do not recommend prophylactic antibiotics for patients undergoing ear, nose and throat procedures who are at risk of endocarditis, but suggest that the risks are discussed. Nasal application of Mupirocin cream 10 hours pre-operatively may reduce transfer of nasal bacteria to the trachea.

Fracture of the turbinate bones can occur during nasal intubation and complete avulsion of turbinates has been reported. A narrow nasal passage may cause pinching of the tracheal tube restricting its diameter.

Very rarely perforation of the mucosa of the posterior nasal space can lead to deep cervical infection or mediastinitis so undue force should never be used if a nasal tube impacts in the nasopharynx. Nasal tubes can obstruct the ostia of the paranasal sinuses and infection is common if the tube is left in situ for more than 24 hours.

Although this is a long list of potential complications, in practice nasal intubation is usually straightforward and significantly aids intra-oral surgery. A tube is, first, well lubricated, directed down along the floor of the nose and never placed with undue force. Rotation of the tube as it is passed helps to prevent the bevel obstructing on turbinates or the arytenoids.

Some of this trauma can be avoided by passing nasal tubes over an introducer such as a suction catheter or fibreoptic endoscope.

Throat packs

A pack is often inserted during maxillofacial surgery to limit the spread of blood or other material down the oesophagus or trachea. Deaths have occurred after extubation when the pack has not been removed.

The UK National Patient Safety Agency has produced a 'safer practice notice', which recommends that a pack is only used when specifically required, and both a visual check and a documentary check are carried out. Our practice is to use a surgical swab as the pack and this is placed by either the surgeon or anaesthetist in theatre. The throat pack is then part of the surgical swab count. The presence of a throat pack is also written on the whiteboard and entered into the theatre computer record. It remains a joint responsibility to confirm that the airway is clear at the end of a case with the added safety of a swab count by the scrub team.

Dento-alveolar surgery

Minor surgery involving the teeth and teeth bearing portions of the jaws is known collectively as dento-alveolar surgery and is the most common form of maxillofacial surgery (see Chapter 24). Options for airway management include: simple facemask anaesthesia (for quick extractions in children), the nasal mask (again for rapid extractions in children), a supraglottic airway device (and the flexible version of the classic LMA is probably the best of these, an oral tube or a nasal tube. In general the more posterior and/or impacted the teeth to be removed the more difficult the extractions. Thus the more likely it is that the use of an LMA will be problematic in terms of airway obstruction during surgery. A surgeon's ability to work around an LMA varies considerably! A nasotracheal tube has considerable advantages in terms of space for the surgeon to work and with practice is easier to insert than an oral tube. With good technique a nasal tube can be passed with either a bolus of alfentanil, remifentanil or small dose of a short-acting muscle relaxant such as mivacurium. This is beneficial in a high volume, rapid turnover list.

Tumours of the upper airway

The vast majority of tumours within the oral cavity are squamous cell carcinomas. There is a slight male to female predominance. A high proportion of patients are cigarette smokers (85% in a New Zealand series). Smoking and high alcohol consumption have been shown to be independent factors for poorer prognosis. Clinical staging and tumour size have significant influences on prognosis.

Chemoradiotherapy is used for patients who have advanced stage disease or are deemed unfit for major surgery. All head and neck cancer patients are seen at a multidisciplinary team clinic to discuss and plan treatment. Anaesthetic input at this point is useful to allow thorough pre-operative assessment and to help determine which patients are not medically suitable for a long (8 to 12 hour) surgical procedure.

Assessment and planning

Eighty percent of intra-oral tumours are on the tongue, and it is these which have the most potential to cause difficult direct laryngoscopy. The further back and the larger the tumour, the more the view at direct laryngoscopy is degraded due to the loss of space at the base of the tongue. All patients with diagnosed head and neck cancer will have had a CT or MRI scan which enables the anaesthetist to gain an understanding of tumour site, size and anatomical distortion. The use of 3-D modelling software further enhances the scans. Patients undergoing diagnostic examination and biopsies should be approached with caution, since they may not have been as thoroughly investigated. Nasendoscopy carried out as outpatients can give very good information, it is however not always undertaken and the written description varies in its usefulness. Important clinical features to look out for are difficulty in swallowing, change in voice,

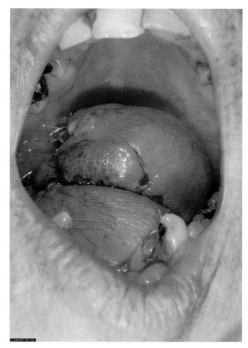

Figure 23.2. Intra-oral flap. This patient needed to return to theatre a few days after the primary surgery for debridement of an area of the flap which had become necrotic.

rigidity of the neck tissues and a swollen or fixed tongue. Previous anaesthetic records, whilst useful, can be misleading as tumour growth occurs and the soft tissues are affected by previous surgery, radiation and lymph nodes. Stridor is much more common with laryngeal tumours (see Chapter 25) but can occur with very large upper airway masses. Stridor may also only be present in certain positions or on exercise.

Secondary surgery

One of the most challenging groups of patients with maxillofacial surgery is those returning to theatre after head and neck reconstruction. A common technique is to place a free tissue graft (this can be skin and muscle – usually a radial forearm flap, or include bone – such as fibula or iliac crest), which fills the deficit from the resected tumour and surrounding soft tissue, but may distort the oropharynx. Patients with posterior tongue grafts have a tracheostomy formed at the primary surgery, but this is usually removed by day 5 to 7. Patients returning to theatre after this time can be particularly difficult due to oedema and distorted anatomy (Figure 23.2).

Other types of reconstruction such as a local flap using the pectoralis muscle are used, which give a more robust flap within a shorter time period (particularly used with frail patients, those with poor vessel quality or when the initial operation of free tissue transfer has failed). This flap results in a fixed cervical flexion deformity of varying severity.

Another possible complication is that of fistula formation, and a fistula between the oropharynx and neck skin makes facemask ventilation difficult as a part of the tidal volume escapes via the fistula. Simple packing of the fistula may be enough to overcome this, but is unpredictable.

Key points

- High risk of medical co-morbidity.
- Large proportion of smokers.
- Thorough pre-op assessment before accepting a very lengthy surgical option.
- Airway assessment using available history, patient examination, patient CT/MRI scans and surgical input.
- Patients returning to theatre with complications (both as emergency and electively) are the most challenging.

Induction and intubation

There is no 'one size fits all' approach. Patient factors, in particular their ability to cooperate, disease factors, co-morbidities and operator expertise will produce varying solutions.

For intra-oral cancer, if difficulties in direct laryngoscopy are anticipated we will plan for a fibreoptic intubation and avoid blind nasal intubation. If there is an issue with the airway which *might* make ventilation difficult (such as trismus, posterior tongue tumour, difficulty swallowing, high BMI, reflux, bull neck, intra-oral oedema) then we will plan for an awake technique. This is normally an awake fibreoptic intubation aided by local anaesthesia and large doses of alfentanil (not sedation) but can also be a transtracheal jet ventilation (TTJV) cannula method followed by asleep fibreoptic intubation. If there is only a suspicion that direct laryngoscopy could be difficult then an asleep fibreoptic technique can be used.

Tracheostomy

The formation of a tracheostomy is covered elsewhere (Chapter 28). In maxillofacial surgery it is used where

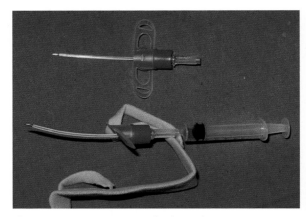

Figure 23.3. Ravussin trans-tracheal cannula.

there is concern that the upper airway may be obstructed post-operatively by soft tissue oedema such as after a bilateral neck dissection or posterior tongue resection and reconstruction, also for management of significant facial fractures (see later). A tracheostomy has its pros and cons, but following reconstructive surgery is better tolerated than a nasal tube and allows more rapid awakening of the patient without excessive movement of the delicate anastamotic site of the reconstruction (Figure 23.3).

Key points

- Thorough pre-operative assessment leads on to careful planning.
- Use an awake technique if there is doubt regarding pathology and patient factors which predispose the patient to the 'can't ventilate' scenario.

Orthognathic surgery

Dentofacial deformity can affect up to 20% of the population and results in a varying amount of functional and aesthetic problems. As a broad generalisation, orthognathic surgery corrects the relationship between maxilla and mandible to give normal mastication and speech. It is also used sometimes if a short jaw is implicated in sleep apnoea. It is usually preceded by some years of orthodontic treatment. Ideally, the operation is carried out after the main growth spurt in the teenage years.

A whole spectrum of growth abnormalities can present for orthognathic surgery; retrognathia, prognathia, hypo- and hyperplasia of the maxilla. These can also be unilateral giving rise to asymmetry and midline shifts which can affect TMJ function limiting mouth opening. Congenital problems such as cleft lip and palate give rise to poor growth development in the maxilla. Previous trauma may also need further correction by using these techniques. From this it can be seen that difficult intubation can occur.

Dental occlusion is mandatory for this type of surgical procedure so a nasal endotracheal tube is essential. Intra-operative fixation is used to check for correct occlusion and bite. Either both jaws (bimaxillary osteotomy) or just the upper (Le Fort I osteotomy) or lower (sagittal split sliding osteotomy) are planned to be operated on. The chin position is sometimes adjusted at the same time (genioplasty).

With unilateral cleft lip and palate patients the endotracheal tube should preferably be passed on the opposite side to the cleft and care must be taken to avoid damaging the pharyngeal tissues around the soft palate.

Distraction techniques

In some patients there is insufficient bone to allow for the desired movements and distraction is used. For the upper jaw a Le Fort I cut is made and the lower segment attached to rigid wires which protrude anteriorly to attach to a halo frame arrangement (Figure 23.4).

Over a period of weeks the wires are slowly pulled forward to encourage bone formation and plating is carried out when this has occurred. These patients represent a challenge on their return to theatre for the final plating. Where tolerated an awake fibreoptic approach can be used, but often these patients are children and then a nasal mask can be used to provide oxygenation before asleep fibreoptic intubation. If the surgeon permits cutting the wires then a facemask can usually be fitted over the protruding maxillary fixings. If not, wire cutters should be to hand in case of an emergency. For the lower jaw an external fixator type arrangement is placed on either side of the mandibular split and then slowly winched apart. These can also get in the way of facemask ventilation but not to the same extent.

Intra-operative problems

Accidental damage to the tracheal tube can be caused by the surgeons during down fracture of the maxilla

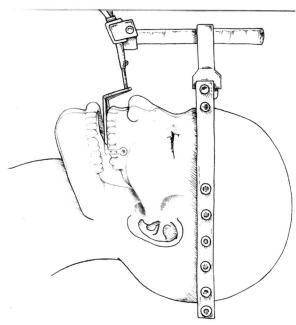

Figure 23.4. Halo frame attachment for maxillary distraction technique.

during a Le Fort I osteotomy (Figures 23.5 and 23.6). Complete transection is fortunately very unlikely. There may be a small manageable leak or the tube might need changing. This is best done with a tube exchanger such as the Cook Airway Catheter. There can be a considerable amount of haemorrhage at this time and a wide bore sucker must be available. Muscle relaxation used for intubation will have worn off by this point, so unless using a remifentanil technique, a further dose should be given. A throat pack will normally be in place so it will need removing and replacing.

Surgical cuts

Cutting through the highly vascular maxilla will create a reasonable amount of haemorrhage, and to both decrease blood loss and aid surgical techniques head-up tilt and deliberate hypotension are usually used. It is an occasion when a throat pack is required. Occlusion of bronchi by blood clot and lobe collapse has occurred in the past in the writer's institution.

Post-operative care

The main risks are of swelling and haemorrhage, both of these are more significant to the airway after a

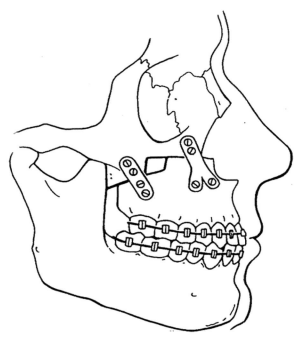

Figure 23.5. Le Fort I osteotomy cuts with plate.

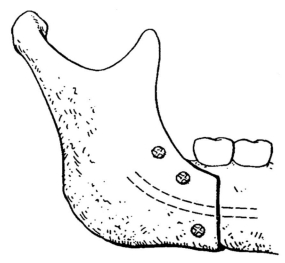

Figure 23.6. Sagittal split osteotomy cuts with screws.

lower jaw procedure. Bleeding into the floor of the mouth after a genioplasty can lead to rapid tongue swelling. Patients are nursed as upright as possible, ice packs hung around the face may help, and patients should be observed in HDU for the next 12 hours. Major haemorrhage post-op is rare but may need anterior and posterior nasal packing. If this fails then surgical re-exploration is necessary.

Key points

- Orthognathic surgery is carried out to correct growth deformity or secondary to trauma.
- Intra-operative inter-maxillary fixation (IMF) means that nasal intubation is mandatory.
- The considerable haemorrhage following the Le Fort I cuts means that both a throat pack and hypotension are required.
- Surgical damage to the tracheal tube can occasionally occur intra-operatively. The potential for post-operative swelling and haemorrhage means that HDU care is required over night.

Airway management for maxillofacial trauma

Facial trauma is clearly of particular concern to anaesthetists as it involves the upper airway which can lead to acute airway obstruction. This may occur as a result of tissue disruption, blood, oedema, foreign bodies, vomiting, or coexisting head injury causing a lowered conscious level. The nature of the injury will determine the choice and timing of the definitive airway management. The options available are discussed below. Definitive management of facial injuries is often delayed for days while other more pressing injuries are treated. However a relatively small number of maxillofacial injuries pose a formidable challenge during resuscitation due to difficult airway management and massive haemorrhage.

Trauma in this region has other unique implications as it commonly affects vital structures associated with four of the five senses, and may have significant cosmetic and psychological implications.

Aetiology

The majority of maxillofacial trauma occurs in young males. Inter-personal violence accounts for a progressively larger proportion of maxillofacial trauma (with alcohol and drugs increasingly involved). Motor accidents are the second largest group, however, these injuries have decreased over recent decades with improvements in road safety legislation, car design, and use of seat belts. Sports injuries and falls are also significant causes.

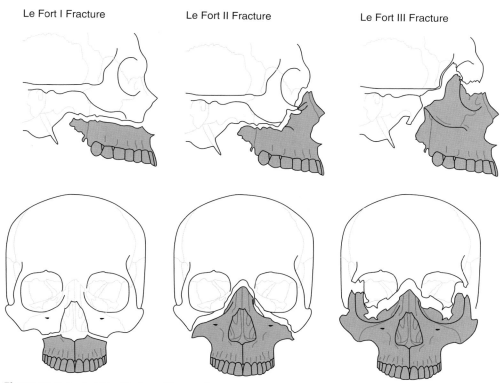

Figure 23.7. Le Fort Classification of fracture lines.

Associations with other injuries

When a high-velocity injury occurs, almost any form of accompanying injury may co-exist, and indeed supersede the craniofacial damage in terms of treatment priority. The mechanism of significant craniofacial injury is often associated with potential cervical spine damage. Patients involved in high-velocity trauma should be treated as having cervical spine injury until 'cleared' by appropriately trained personnel.

A retrospective study in the US showed that cervical spine injury co-existed in 9.4% of maxillofacial trauma cases. The mechanism was most commonly motor vehicle accident (45%) or falls (36%). Similar retrospective data demonstrates 45% of patients with facial trauma have associated head injury.

Classification and types of injury
Bony injuries Le Fort classification

Facial fractures tend to cause airway compromise either due to posterior displacement of midface structures, or severe haemorrhage. The classification of the fracture is of relevance to anaesthetists as they not only delineate severity of injury, but also give an indication of the likelihood of airway compromise, and the need for a tracheostomy (Figure 23.7). It has been demonstrated that 43.5% of those with a Le Fort III injury require tracheostomy compared with 9.1% of patients with a Le Fort I or II fracture. Le Fort III injuries have a 26% chance of acute airway compromise. Overall, around a third of patients with facial fractures require intubation.

Laryngotracheal injuries/laryngeal fractures

Laryngotracheal injury occurs in around 1:5000 of maxillofacial trauma cases, but can be life-threatening. The mechanism is more likely to be blunt trauma – particularly motor vehicle accidents. Assault and sports injuries are also recognised causes.

Findings on presentation are most commonly dyspnoea and dysphonia, but also include dysphagia, odynophagia, and haemoptysis. Examination may

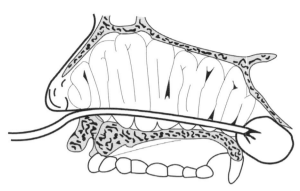

Figure 23.8. Nasal packing showing a balloon posterior nasal pack and anterior ribbon gauze pack.

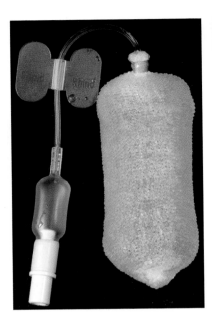

Figure 23.9. Rapid Rhino pack for nasal haemorrhage.

reveal subcutaneous emphysema, tenderness, oedema and haematoma. Management in all but mild cases (where there is only slight dysphonia, dyspnoea and no airway compromise) is definitive airway control with a tracheostomy performed under local anaesthesia. Cricothroidotomy can be carried out as a temporary measure in emergencies. The larynx should be visualised wherever possible by fibreoptic laryngoscopy to evaluate the injury, and CT imaging performed (after the tracheostomy if there is airway compromise).

Penetrating injuries

Penetrating injuries to the face will often require emergency airway management. A retrospective review of 86 patients concluded that gunshot wounds (GSW) were more susceptible to airway compromise than shotgun or stab wounds, and that mandibular injuries required intubation in 53% of cases compared to 25% of midface injuries. The implication from this review based on a post-hoc analysis of airway requirements for different injury types, was that even when the airway was not compromised, a definitive airway should be sought in the following scenarios: GSW to mandible, intra-oral bleeding or oedema and close-range shotgun injuries to the face. These injuries have shown themselves to be the most likely to require emergency airways if initially treated conservatively.

Initial management
Airway
Initial assessment and management

Initial management should be according to the ABCDE approach advocated by the ATLS® guidelines. Where maxillofacial trauma has occurred or is suspected,

particular attention should be paid to the nasal and oral airway for compromise due to fractured bones, blood, loose teeth, foreign bodies or evidence of laryngeal injury. Airway bleeding should be addressed: in the case of anterior nasal bleeding, nasal packing may be appropriate, or for posterior nasal bleeding a Foley catheter (see Figure 23.8) or a specialised 'rapid rhino' (Figure 23.9) may be employed. If severe bleeding occurs fracture reduction is normally effective. If not embolisation or ligation of the arterial supply may be required.

The indications for intubation may be divided into absolute, urgent and relative, as shown below. They should be balanced against the resultant loss of contact with the patient that will prohibit continued clinical evaluation of neurological or eye function making diagnosis of intracranial bleeding or dangerous eye swelling difficult.

Other recommendations from the AAGBI include that maxillofacial trauma patients who require transfer to another site are intubated and ventilated in the following circumstances: copious bleeding into mouth, loss of protective laryngeal reflexes, a GCS of under 9, or that has dropped by 2 or more points, seizures and deteriorating arterial blood gases. Difficulties are most likely to occur when oro-pharyngeal masses, obesity and polytrauma are involved. Intoxication with drugs and/or alcohol may decrease conscious level, increase the risk of vomiting and create a combatative or confused patient.

Indications for intubation	
Absolute	Unrelieved airway obstruction
	Apnoea
	Respiratory distress
	Severe neurological deficit
	Depressed consciousness
Urgent	Penetrating neck injury
	Persistent refractory hypotension
	Chest wall injuries with respiratory dysfunction
Relative	Oro-maxillary injury
	Impending respiratory failure
	Risk of impending deterioration with diagnostic procedures
	Risk of respiratory depression with sedatives/analgesics

Intubation may also be necessary when immediate resuscitation or emergency surgery is required.

Methods of intubation

In the majority of cases that require airway support, intubation will be necessary. However there are times when airway adjuncts may be appropriate as a temporising measure. Oral Guedel airways are poorly tolerated and can induce vomiting. A nasal airway may be better tolerated, but can exacerbate epistaxis. Suspected base of skull fractures are not necessarily a contraindication to nasal airways when sited by an experienced anaesthetist. The perceived risk of intracranial tube placement is somewhat overstated, and further discussed below.

Definitive options and indications
Tracheal intubation

Emergency definitive airway control is normally best provided with oral tracheal intubation. Other options include nasal tracheal intubation, cricothyrotomy and tracheostomy. Any hard collar or other cervical fixation devices should be loosened or removed if required to permit intubation (see Chapter 26). Intubation may be more straightforward than anticipated, due to mobile facial bones, which can be gently displaced during laryngoscopy. Difficulties obtaining a useful view of the anatomy occur when blood or oedema in the oropharynx obscure the view. For this reason, alternative plans, with the necessary personnel and equipment, should be in place should the first attempt fail. This should include a difficult intubation trolley, an experienced assistant and a surgeon standing by should an emergency surgical airway be required. The difficult airway trolley should include a supra glottic airway, a 'gum-elastic' type bougie, a Cook exchange catheter, a method for cricothyroidotomy and jet ventilation equipment.

Alternative emergency strategies

Cricothyroidotomy can be performed as a life-saving manoeuvre when oral or nasal tracheal intubation are impossible due to an inability to visualise of the vocal cords, or oro-nasal bleeding. It is quicker than a formal tracheostomy, however it can only serve as a short-term measure. A horizontal incision is made through skin and cricothyroid membrane, and dilators used to aid passage of the tube. Complications include stomal stenosis and subglottic obstruction.

Tracheostomy

Tracheostomies can be of use in the emergency situation where time allows. A survey of surgeons and anaesthetists found that tracheostomies were used in 11.6% of mandibular, pan-facial and Le Fort fractures. Their benefits include clearance of the nasal and oral passages of tubes (if present) and allowing maxillo-mandibular closure. Whilst complications include stomal infection or haemorrhage, and surgical emphysema, a recent review ($n = 125$) of tracheostomy use in maxillofacial trauma in a US trauma centre reported no major complications. Percutaneous tracheostomy has also been shown to be a safe alternative.

Nasal intubation

Broadly speaking nasal intubation is less appropriate in the emergency situation, but is occasionally a useful alternative. Blind nasal intubation is generally not recommended. Fibreoptically assisted intubation may be particularly difficult in the presence of blood and oedema.

Definitive surgical repair of facial fractures will normally be a semi-elective procedure (unless the fracture is being reduced to aid haemorrhage control). In this situation, the nasal route is often essential, as the surgeon will require good surgical access to the mouth and

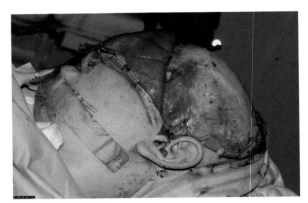

Figure 23.10. Reflection of anterior facial tissues via a coronal flap to allow fixation of supra-orbital fractures.

temporary dental occlusion. The exception being zygomatic and orbital surgery, where a south facing oral tube is probably best. Occasionally supra-orbital fractures will require access via a coronal flap which allows the scalp to be reflected over the face (Figure 23.10).

Particularly complex or pan facial fractures may require access to the nose *and* dental closure, which may necessitate an intra-operative change from a nasal to oral tube. Alternatively, a tracheostomy or submental intubation avoids this intra-operative disruption (see below).

The method of intubation will depend on the airway assessment. 'Blind nasal' intubation, direct laryngoscopy, or fibreoptically assisted intubation are all viable options. Limited mouth opening is a relatively common finding in patients with facial injuries. Trismus may commonly be as a result of pain, muscle spasm or occasionally the fracture itself will impinge on the TMJ causing a mechanical obstruction to mouth opening. Pain will clearly resolve on induction of anaesthesia, however, if (after discussion with the surgeon), a mechanical cause is felt to be likely, then a fibreoptically assisted intubation technique may be appropriate. Persistent trismus occurs when there is a late presentation with an infected fracture with sub-masseteric pus or rarely if there is central dislocation of the TMJ into the temporal fossa or a fractured zygoma which obstructs the coronoid process of the mandible. If there is any concern regarding the ease with which intubation or airway maintenance may be performed – a patient with a large neck, or history of obstructive sleep apnoea, difficulty swallowing, or swelling for instance – then an 'awake' technique is warranted.

A long held tenet of trauma anaesthesia has been to avoid nasal intubation if a base of skull fracture is suspected (the Le Fort II or III fractures). Looking critically at the anatomy it is apparent that it would be a very poorly directed nasal tube that would pass via the cribiform plate and only if there is a midline fracture of the body of the sphenoid bones would there be any risk of an anaesthetic tube penetrating the middle cranial fossa.

Thus only with midline compound fractures of the middle cranial fossa would it be prudent to avoid any form of 'blind' nasal technique. A fibreoptic nasotracheal intubation allows safe passage through the nasopharynx in the elective situation.

There has been concern regarding the increased risk of meningitis associated with nasal intubation in the presence of base of skull fractures. Studies reviewing cases of base of skull fractures found no difference in the complication rates between orally and nasally intubated patients. Other theoretical concerns regarding the perceived risk of intracranial intubation in the presence of skull base fractures are largely unfounded and based on anecdotal evidence. Base of skull fractures are present in 2–4% of maxillofacial fractures. A study comparing complications of oral and nasal intubations in 160 patients with these co-existing injuries found no difference. Interestingly, there are more reports of intracranial insertion of nasogastric tubes than tracheal tubes.

Nasal packing from the haemorrhage at the time of injury may mean that the nasal route is not possible.

Other intubation options

Submental intubation is an alternative technique to tracheostomy for airway management during definitive surgical repair of cranio-maxillofacial trauma (Figure 23.11). Originally described in 1986, it provides a secure airway with an unobstructed intra-oral surgical field, and allows maxillo-mandibular closure during the reconstruction of complex mid-facial or pan-facial fractures. It also avoids changing the tracheal tube from a nasal to an oral tube mid-operation as is sometimes required in fractures involving the naso-orbital-ethmoid (NOE) complex. The technique requires a reinforced tracheal tube, which can either be used for the initial intubation, or be introduced over an exchange catheter in theatre. The surgeon makes a 1.5-cm incision parallel to the inferior border

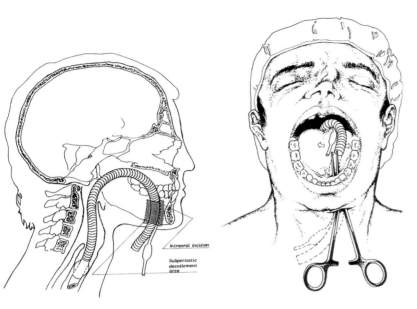

Figure 23.11. Submental intubation. (Taken from Altemir's original paper 1987 with permission: Altemir FH. (1986) *Journal of Maxillofacial Surgery.* 14;64–65. The publisher then was Georg Thieme Verla Stuttgart – New York.)

of the mandible, and forms a passage through mylohyoid to the floor of the mouth by blunt dissection. Having been disconnected from the breathing circuit, first the pilot balloon, then the ETT (with tube connector temporarily removed) is pulled through the passage with forceps. Due to the more acute angle of the ETT passage it is preferable to use a reinforced tracheal tube. However not all of these come apart (the ILMA is one that does) so this element of equipment must be checked beforehand. The patient is then reconnected to the circuit, and the tube position confirmed by capnography and auscultation prior to being secured by suturing. It should be borne in mind that flexion and extension of the neck will alter the tube tip position in the trachea to a greater extent than with oral or nasal tube. Inadvertent extubation and bronchial intubation have been reported. It is therefore important to ensure the placement of the tube tip is midway between the carina and cords. Although not commonly performed it is usually technically straightforward. However a recent series of 25 consecutive cases reported 2 subsequent floor of mouth infections.

Bleeding

Haemorrhage is responsible for 30–40% of trauma mortality. Life-threatening bleeding as a result of facial fractures has a reported incidence around 1%. This increases to around 5% in the subset of mid-face fractures.

The main sources of arterial bleeding associated with mid-facial trauma are the internal maxillary, facial, and superficial temporal branches of the external carotid arteries and the ethmoid and ophthalmic branches of the internal carotid arteries.

In most cases the bleeding is clearly evident, however, occipital bleeding may be missed in the immobilised supine patient, and mid-face fractures can cause significant concealed blood loss due to bilateral collateral blood supply. This should be borne in mind if the more common sites for occult blood loss have been excluded, and the patient is failing to respond to resuscitation. Bleeding as a result of facial injury can also result in unexpected vomiting, which can further endanger the airway.

Haemorrhage control

Procedures available to control life-threatening haemorrhage after maxillofacial trauma include anterior nasal packing, posterior nasal packing or balloon tamponade, emergent intermaxillary fixation (IMF), trans-arterial embolisation (TAE), and operative control of bleeding by direct arterial ligation or 'blind' ligation of the external carotid arteries. A recent review of experience from nine trauma centres in the United States developed two algorithms

Suggested treatment plan for maxillofacial injuries with severe oronasal bleeding (modified from Cogbill)

Figure 23.12. Algorithm for massive oronasal bleeding.

Airway/Breathing:	Endotracheal intubation Cricothyroidotomy Tracheostomy
Circulation:	IV Fluids Blood transfusion Correct coagulopathy
Haemorrhage control:	Anterior / posterior packing if amenable If blunt trauma – consider temporary fracture reduction If this fails – Transarterial embolisation If this fails – To theatre for direct arterial ligation

Delayed maxillofacial repair once bleeding under control

(see Figure 23.12) for the management of massive oronasal bleeding dependent on whether the mechanism of injury was either blunt or penetrating.

Key points – trauma

- Follow the ATLS guidelines.
- Watch for associated head and cervical injuries.
- Intubate orally in the acute situation with manual in line stabilisation, RSI, good assistance (at least two assistants) and surgical back-up. Intubate early if there is high energy gunshot wound to the face.
- If a nasotracheal tube is required, intracranial placement is only a serious possibility in midline fractures of the sphenoid bone.
- Consider a submental intubation as an alternative to tracheostomy if the nasal route is not possible.
- Control haemorrhage by anterior and posterior nasal packing, and reducing fractures.

Airway management for maxillofacial sepsis

Head and neck infection is a common presenting problem in maxillofacial surgery, the majority of which is odontogenic in origin. A recent national review of admissions to maxillofacial units with severe cervicofacial infection showed that the incidence is increasing: 81% of patients required admission, and 46% required a surgical procedure under general anaesthesia.

Infection can spread rapidly from the source, through the anatomical spaces of the head and neck along the path of least resistance. The airway management of these cases for surgery varies according to the severity of infection, and the extent of involvement of local tissues. The spectrum of disease ranges from the localised dental abscess with no airway compromise, through more severe infection causing local swelling and trismus, and at the extreme, Ludwig's angina – a fulminant bilateral sub-mandibular infection with woody neck cellulitis resulting in asphyxiation.

Most patients with sub-mandibular space infections are young, healthy adults who present with mouth pain, dysphagia, drooling and a stiff neck. In the case of Ludwig's angina, massive tongue and floor of mouth oedema can rapidly lead to posterior and superior displacement of the tongue as well as anterior displacement out of the mouth (see Figure 23.13). The patient often maintains the neck in an extended position and may have a muffled or characteristic 'hot potato' voice. The neck shows a characteristic erythematous woody swelling but fluctuance is usually absent. Trismus, which indicates lateral pharyngeal or masticator space involvement, should be absent in isolated sub-mandibular space infections.

The priority in the management of such cases is airway control, followed by IV antibiotics and surgical drainage. Airway control may in some cases be achieved by close observation on an ICU; however, definitive control is often required in the form of tracheostomy, fibreoptic intubation or cricothyroidotomy. Intubation is made difficult not only by the tissue distortion described above, but also because

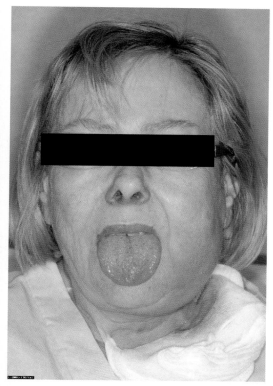

Figure 23.13. Bilateral submandibular abscess with floor of mouth swelling.

neck oedema causes venous congestion resulting in vocal cord oedema, reduced neck mobility and limited mouth opening. Attempts at oral or blind nasal intubation with muscle relaxation are contra-indicated as they may precipitate a 'can't intubate, can't ventilate' scenario. The authors prefer an awake fibreoptic intubation technique. If possible tracheos-tomy or cricothyrotomy should be avoided as the stoma will be in close proximity to open infected wounds, with increased risk of mediastinal infection.

Lateral pharyngeal space infection also poses problems to the anaesthetist. It presents with pain, fever, sub-mandibular swelling and trismus. Airway impingement due to medial bulging of the pharyngeal wall and supraglottic oedema can occasionally occur but is much less likely than in Ludwig's angina. Treat-ment is similar to that of Ludwig's angina, except that surgical drainage is usually required and frank purulence commonly encountered.

Extubation should not be allowed until it is clear that tissue swelling is decreasing. In patients with Ludwig's type infections there is often little pus to actually drain, improvement is slow, and swelling may briefly become worse after surgery. There is also a risk of infection tracking down to the mediastinum following which, significantly generalised sepsis can occur.

Key points – sepsis

- Chronic infection may cause trismus which does not resolve with anaesthesia.
- Treatment with intra venous antibiotics may improve oedema and swelling but surgical treatment should not be delayed for this reason.
- For Ludwig's angina type infections, awake fibreoptic intubation is advised.
- Observation pre- and post-operatively should be in the HDU or ITU setting. Do not extubate until the swelling is definitely subsiding.

Further reading

Cogbill TH, Cothren CC, Ahearn MK, et al. (2008). Management of maxillofacial injuries with severe oronasal hemorrhage: A multicenter perspective. *The Journal of Trauma*, **65**(5), 994–999.

Goodisson DW, Shaw GM, Snape L. (2001). Intracranial intubation in patients with maxillofacial injuries associated with base of skull fractures? *Journal of Trauma*, **50**, 363–366.

Gudziol V, Mewes T, Mann WJ. (2005). Rapid rhino: A new pneumatic nasal tamponade for posterior epistaxis. *Otolaryngology–Head and Neck Surgery*, **132**(1), 152–155.

Hall CE, Shutt LE. (2003). Nasotracheal intubation for head and neck surgery. *Anaesthesia*, **58**, 249–256.

Heard AM, Green RJ, Lacquiere DA, Sillifant P. (2009). The use of mandibular nerve block to predict safe anaesthetic induction in patients with acute trismus. *Anaesthesia*, **64**, 1196–1198.

Jamal BT, Diecidue R, Qutub A, Cohen M. (2009). The pattern of combined maxillofacial and cervical spine fractures. *Journal of Oral and Maxillofacial Surgery*, **67**(3), 559–562.

Latto IP, Vaughan RS. (1996). *Anatomy of the Airways. Difficulties in Tracheal intubation.* 2nd ed. Philadelphia: Saunders.

Matzelle SJ, Heard MM, Khong GL, Riley RH, Eakins PD. (2009). A retrospective analysis of deep neck infections at Royal Perth Hospital. *Anaesthesia and Intensive Care*, **37**, 604–607.

McLeod AD, Calder I. (2000). Spinal cord injury and direct laryngoscopy – the legend lives on. *British Journal of Anaesthesia*, **84**, 705–709.

221

Mithani SK, St-Hilaire H, Brooke BS, Smith IM, Bluebond-Langner R, Rodriguez ED. (2009). Predictable patterns of intracranial and cervical spine injury in craniomaxillofacial trauma: Analysis of 4786 patients. *Plastic and Reconstructive Surgery*, **123**(4), 1293–1301.

Mohan R, Iyer R, Thaller S. (2009). Airway management in patients with facial trauma. *The Journal of Craniofacial Surgery*, **20**(1), 21–23.

National Patient Safety Agency. (2009). *Reducing the Risk of Retained Throat Packs After Surgery*. Issued April 28, 2009. Gateway ref: 11700. Available at: www.nrls.npsa.nhs.uk/resources/?entryid45=59853.

O'Connell JE, Stevenson DS, Stokes MA. (1996). Pathological changes associated with short-term nasal intubation. *Anaesthesia*, **51**, 347–350.

Perry M, Morris C. (2008). Advanced trauma life support (ATLS) and facial trauma: Can one size fit all? Part 2: ATLS, maxillofacial injuries and airway management dilemmas. *International Journal of Oral and Maxillofacial Surgery*, **37**(4), 309–320.

Schütz P, Hamed HH. (2008). Submental intubation versus tracheostomy in maxillofacial trauma patients. *Journal of Oral and Maxillofacial Surgery*, **66**(7), 1404–1409.

Shaw IH, Kumar C, Dodds C. (in press). *Anaesthesia for Oral and Maxillofacial Surgery*. New York: Oxford University Press.

Wolford LM. (2007). Surgical planning in orthognathic surgery. In: Ward-Booth P, Schendel SA, Hausamen JE (Eds.), *Maxillofacial Surgery*. 2nd ed. Chapter 60. St. Louis: Churchill Livingstone. pp 1155–1210.

Woodall NM, Harwood RJ, Barker GL. (2008). Complications of awake fibreoptic intubation without sedation in 200 healthy anaesthetists attending a training course. *British Journal of Anaesthesia*, **100**, 850–855.

Dental caries were common in our ancestors. In contrast to the gleaming incisors of the stars of today, in historical portraits the nobility have tightly shut mouths which hide teeth that were often black. Pain drove them to have dental extractions without effective analgesia, so it is small wonder that the first anaesthetic in Britain was given for dental surgery. The extraction in 1846 of a molar tooth by Mr Boot in London set the pattern of dental anaesthesia for over a century. Many of the techniques used were taboo in other fields and only recently has anaesthesia for dentistry re-joined the mainstream in terms of techniques and practices.

For example, Mr Boot was an operator anaesthetist, a practice which was certainly not allowed in other fields, although it continued in dentistry until 1981. The patient was often in the sitting position, which is controversial in other specialties. The first anaesthetic was also for a procedure which involved the shared airway, which is among the most anaesthetically challenging situations. Given all these risk factors, it is fortunate for the development of anaesthesia that the patient survived unscathed.

Dental operations

Dental surgery comprises operations on teeth or to remove teeth and is distinct from maxillofacial surgery which involves surgery to the mouth as a whole and often includes major bone and soft tissue surgery.

Dentists perform two sorts of procedure: *conservation* and *exodontia*.

Conservation comprises all the procedures carried out to preserve teeth, for example, filling, crowning and root canal treatment.

Exodontia is removing teeth: either primary dentition, labelled A to E, or secondary dentition, labelled

1 to 8, both starting from midline to each side. Extraction sometimes involves raising gum flaps or removing bone. General anaesthetic for straightforward extractions is rare but it is necessary for some patient groups.

Indications for general anaesthesia (GA)

There is still a huge demand for dental treatment under GA in the United Kingdom. Elsewhere in Europe for unexplained reasons it seems to be less common. Anaesthesia in dental surgeries was stopped in 2002 and since then dental anaesthesia has been hospital-based. There are some definite indications for GA:

- For young children who would be unable to tolerate treatment under local anaesthesia. Some patients present after failure to treat successfully using local anaesthesia and nitrous oxide/oxygen mixture ('relative analgesia').
- Where the dentistry is likely to be prolonged and extensive so that it is not suitable to have the patient awake.
- For patients with physical or mental disabilities which make cooperation with the surgeon difficult.
- Allergy to local anaesthetics (rare).
- Where there is acute infection which may make local anaesthesia ineffective.
- For some dental-phobics.

Anaesthetic technique

It is vital to liaise with the dental surgeon before embarking on anaesthesia. Unlike all other branches of anaesthesia, in dental surgery the anaesthetist is involved in the surgery itself, and is not merely giving the anaesthetic and monitoring the patient remotely. In practice, much dental anaesthesia is for operations on children and therefore experience in paediatric anaesthetic techniques is also needed.

For exodontia, it is important to establish the anticipated degree of difficulty in extracting the teeth because that will dictate the technique. First-dentition teeth are usually easy to remove unless they are broken down, but adult teeth are more difficult, and in general, the further back they are, the greater the difficulty.

Induction

In practice, this may be the most challenging part of the anaesthetic especially in children and adults with co-morbidities. Anaesthetists have a lot to learn from paediatric dentists on patient management, and it is often easier to keep children as happy as possible by, for example, allowing parents to be present and allowing the child to choose how to go to sleep. It is unusual for a child to select an injection and such a choice is often the result of parental pressure. Should an intravenous induction be performed, the pre-application of local anaesthetic cream is important, and it is also necessary to ensure that administration of propofol does not hurt. Additives such as lignocaine can help with this but are not 100% reliable, and using a large vein in the antecubital fossa is often the easiest way of ensuring a calm and pain-free induction. It is important to realise that an appreciable number of adults in this country fail to have routine dental care because of a fear of dental treatment, and it is extremely important not to terrify children during early contacts with the dental profession because it will affect their perception of dentistry for the rest of their lives. Surveys have shown that most parents are not against restraint of children during induction of anaesthesia for dental treatment but they prefer to do it themselves. Sometimes they ask for help, and it is then permissible to assist. However restraining a child without the request of the parent is not acceptable.

Gaseous induction with sevoflurane is quick and pleasant. Measures such as challenging the patient to breathe deeply to increase the oxygen saturation above 100% (one anaesthetist describes offering a £20 bribe to any child who could do this) or single breath induction, where the child's competitive instinct is

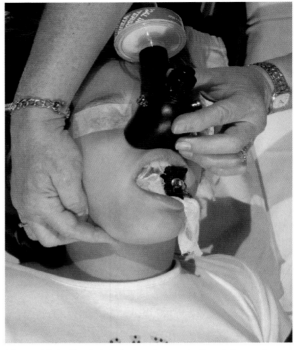

Figure 24.1. Classical chair dental anaesthesia – sitting patient, Goldman nasal mask.

used in timing their ability to breath-hold after a single vital capacity breath of anaesthetic gases, are quick and effective.

In the case of patients with learning difficulties or severe behavioural problems it is usually best to take the advice of the parent or escort on management.

In all cases an ECG and pulse oximeter should be placed pre-induction. Whatever the mode of induction, an intravenous cannula should be placed once the child is asleep for anything but the briefest operation, for example removal of one A.

Choice of airway in exodontia

Historically a special Goldman dental mask was used for extraction procedures. It fitted over the nose and with a high gas flow would provide sufficient anaesthesia to allow the teeth to be removed with the patient asleep. The sitting position was common, and the head was positioned so that the chin sloped down by means of a support behind the occiput. This also tended to prevent aspiration as blood fell out of the mouth forwards (Figure 24.1). The surgeon packed the mouth from buccal sulcus to buccal sulcus to prevent aspiration of tooth fragments and also to

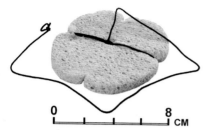

Figure 24.2. 'Butterfly' sponge pack.

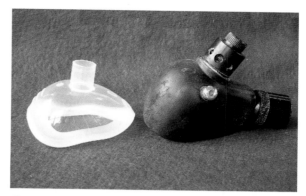

Figure 24.3. Neonatal mask used as nasal mask, and Goldman nasal mask.

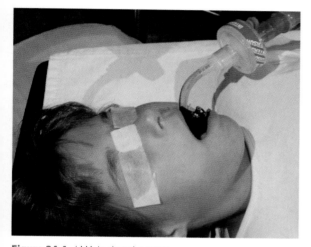

Figure 24.4. LMA in dental surgery.

limit the inflow of room air. This can also be done with gauze or a 'butterfly' sponge (Figure 24.2). This technique is still used for straightforward extractions although commonly patients are now supine. A dental prop is inserted on the side which is not being operated on, and the anaesthetist holds the bottom jaw forward to keep a clear airway through the nose and via the pharynx. A certain amount of experience is needed on the part of both parties, but in particular the dentist must not pack too far back or the airway will be obstructed. A transparent neonatal mask used to fit over the nose is easier to use than the traditional Goldman mask, because it is possible to make sure that the external nares are not obstructed and also it will mist with respiration (Figure 24.3).

Whatever the patient position, it is important to realise that extracting teeth is sometimes difficult and involves the dental surgeon first pushing to release the tooth and then pulling hard. It is part of the anaesthetist's job to counteract these movements, both to limit

damage to the patient's neck and also to provide counter-pressure so that the tooth can be removed.

Constant vigilance is necessary when using a nasal mask as the usual indicators of adequate airway may be absent. In the presence of a large leak through the mouth there will be no end-tidal CO_2 trace, and the circuit bag may not move.

Many anaesthetists are happier to use a laryngeal mask airway (LMA) for all but the quickest and easiest extractions. This provides a satisfactory barrier to aspiration of tooth fragments and blood and saliva. The armoured variety often has a narrower tube and leaves more room for the dentist and is more flexible. It is important to hold on to the LMA throughout the operation as there is a tendency for it to twist or come out during dental surgery with the extreme head movements which accompany the procedure. The LMA may also be obstructed by heavy downward pressure applied during extractions from the lower jaw, so the anaesthetist must also support the jaw throughout and watch the end-tidal CO_2 trace constantly (Figure 24.4).

Choice of airway in conservation

Operations for dental conservation tend to take longer than extractions and involve the use of the drill, which sprays water into the mouth, and a sucker to aspirate the water. There is little room for an LMA tube in all but the most trivial conservation operations, and endotracheal intubation, preferably by the nasal route, is the technique of choice. It is sometimes possible for the dentist to work around an oral tube in a small child having minor fillings, and the avoidance of nasal intubation is obviously preferable

225

where possible. A pack should also be used as sometimes considerable quantities of water are poured into the mouth and not all is sucked up by the surgical assistant.

Maintenance

For extractions of one or two teeth, the extraction takes place during recovery from induction. For longer operations consultation with the surgeon is important. Any technique which allows rapid return to consciousness is suitable. Long operations may necessitate controlled ventilation, but for shorter procedures a technique using spontaneous respiration allows flexibility and rapid recovery.

Recovery

A study of deaths related to dental anaesthesia found that more than half of them occurred during recovery. Many were attributed to airway obstruction. These are difficult patients to recover and need to be looked after by a nurse experienced in dental recovery. Dental sockets continue to bleed for some time after extractions and infected tooth sockets bleed heavily. Once the operation is over, therefore, it cannot be expected that bleeding will stop. For this reason, the patient should be turned on the side with the head tipping down and any airway must be left in place until the protective reflexes have returned. Removal of the LMA while the patient is still deeply asleep has been associated with lower oxygen saturations in dental patients, and it is common sense that leaving an unprotected airway in the presence of a mouthful of blood and possibly bits of tooth is not safe.

Specific airway problems

Many of the genetic conditions which lead to abnormal cranial anatomy, such as Pierre Robin, may be associated with learning difficulties which mean that carers have problems in maintaining dental hygiene thus necessitating dental treatment. The dental anaesthetist is wise to seek the help of a specialist colleague in cases where major airway difficulties are anticipated. Patients with Down's syndrome are at risk of cervical instability. However there is no screening procedure which reliably predicts those at risk, and

the best practice is to take great care in manipulating the head.

Key points

- Anaesthesia for dentistry demands great cooperation between the anaesthetist and surgeon both in choice of technique and in carrying out the surgery.
- Dental anaesthesia is all about the airway.
- A technique allowing rapid return to consciousness is desirable.

Further reading

Brimacombe J, Berry A. (1995). The laryngeal mask for dental surgery – A review. *Australian Dental Journal*, **40**, 10–14.

Coplans MP, Curson I. (1982). Deaths associated with dentistry. *British Dental Journal*, **153**, 357–362.

Department of Health. (2000). *A Conscious Decision: A Review of the Use of General Anaesthesia in Primary Dental Care*. London: Department of Health.

Dolling S, Anders NR, Rolfe SE. (2003). A comparison of deep vs. awake removal of the laryngeal mask airway in paediatric dental day-case surgery. A randomised controlled trial. *Anaesthesia*, **58**, 1224–1228.

Jhamatt A. (2008). *Restraint During Induction Of Chair Anaesthesia: What do Parents Think?* Proceedings of 2007–2008 Annual Conference Association of Dental Anaesthetists, Manchester, UK.

Morton RE, Khan MA, Murray-Leslie C, et al. (1995). Atlantoaxial instability in Down's syndrome: A five year follow-up study. *Archives of Disease in Children*, **72**, 115–119.

Quinn AC, Samaan A, McAteer EM, et al. (1996). The reinforced laryngeal mask airway for dento-alveolar surgery. *British Journal of Anaesthesia*, **77**, 185–188.

Royal College of Anaesthetists. (1999). *Standards and Guidelines for Anaesthesia in Dentistry*. London: Royal College of Anaesthetists.

Standing Committee on Sedation in Dentistry. (2007). *Standards for Conscious Sedation in Dentistry: Alternative Techniques*. Royal College of Surgeons of England and Royal College of Anaesthetists.

Standing Dental Advisory Committee. (1990). *General Anaesthesia Sedation and Resuscitation in Dentistry. Report of an Expert Working Party*. London: Department of Health.

Ear, nose and throat (ENT) patients probably present more airway management problems than any other branch of surgery. ENT procedures encompass a range of operations varying in duration, severity and complexity from high-volume cases such as myringotomy, tonsillectomy and simple nasal procedures through to complex head and neck cancer patients. For a successful outcome these shared airway procedures require close cooperation between anaesthetist and surgeon, an understanding of each other's problems, knowledge of specialist equipment, and a thorough pre-operative evaluation to identify potential problems.

Airway safety and maintenance

Factors affecting airway safety and maintenance during ENT surgery may be classified into eight groups.

1. Patient factors. Patients may present with distorted upper airway anatomy or airway obstruction.
2. Remote surgery. After surgery has begun the anaesthetist is remote from the airway, making adjustments more difficult and disruptive.
3. Surgical factors. Significant lateral rotation of the head may be required for ear procedures and head extension for neck procedures. During intra-oral procedures instruments to keep the mouth open may obstruct the airway. Occasionally a tracheal tube may be damaged or inadvertently sutured during surgery. Surgery may result in a narrowed or oedematous airway making extubation/ emergence more difficult.
4. Shared airway. Shared airway procedures involving surgery of the glottis, subglottis and

trachea require an understanding of specialist equipment, techniques and laser safety.
5. Throat packs. Oropharyngeal and nasopharyngeal packs should be specifically recorded and accounted for at the end of the procedure. A recent communication from the National Patient Safety Agency on throat packs suggests a procedure involving a visual check *and* a procedure involving documented evidence should be used (Table 25.1).
6. Airway soiling. For nasal and intraoral surgery the airway requires protection from blood and debris.
7. Coroner's clot. Direct inspection and suction clearance of blood and debris from the oronasopharynx should be undertaken at the end of the procedure to prevent possibly fatal aspiration of blood clot on emergence.
8. Recovery. ENT operations particularly intra-oral, laryngeal, subglottic and tracheal procedures have an inferior recovery profile compared to the general surgical population with a higher incidence of coughing, laryngospasm and desaturation following tracheal tube extubation.

Facemask

Historically a facemask was used for simple, short ear procedures such as myringotomy and tube insertion. The patient retained spontaneous ventilation but this required the anaesthetist to hold the facemask and the surgeon to 'work around' the anaesthetist's hands and facemask. Most of these short duration procedures are now undertaken with a laryngeal mask airway. The quality of airway management with the laryngeal mask airway is superior to a facemask with better oxygenation, improved seal with less oropharyngeal

Core Topics in Airway Management, Second Edition, ed. Ian Calder and Adrian Pearce. Published by Cambridge University Press. © Cambridge University Press 2011.

Table 25.1. National Patient Safety Agency: reducing risk of retained throat packs

Procedures involving visual checks

- Label or mark patient
  - either on head or other part of body
  - use an adherent sticker or marker
- Label tracheal tube or supraglottic airway
- Attach pack securely to airway
- Leave part of pack protruding

Procedures involving documentary checks

- Formalised, recorded two-person check of insertion and removal
- Record insertion and removal of throat pack on swab board

air leaks, better monitoring of tidal gases particularly at low flow, and with less pollution. Surgical conditions are superior for ear surgery in children with a laryngeal mask airway because there is less movement of the surgical field.

Flexible laryngeal mask airway (FLMA)

The FLMA is also used in ear, nose and throat procedures including tonsillectomy. The cuff of the device is identical to a standard Classic LMA^{TM} but the flexible shaft is better suited and tolerant to head rotation, flexion and extension during surgery. The successful use of the FLMA requires the acquisition of new skills for the anaesthetist, surgeon and recovery room staff. The FLMA requires training and experience for successful use and this is probably the main limitation. An understanding of the device, in particular sizing, insertion, placement and recognition of misplacement is necessary.

During recovery the FLMA is tolerated better than a tracheal tube during emergence and can be left in place until return of protective reflexes. The improved recovery profile leads to a smoother recovery with a reduced incidence of respiratory complications, including coughing, bucking, straining, airway obstruction, laryngospasm and desaturation.

FLMA: nasal surgery

Using a FLMA during nasal surgery is an advanced use of the device and if there is incorrect sizing or

insertion, malposition, dislodgement or suboptimal recovery there is the potential for airway obstruction and blood contamination of the airway.

It seems intuitive that a tracheal tube would protect the airway more effectively than a FLMA because of the seal offered by contact of the tracheal tube cuff on the tracheal wall; however, this may not be true. The tracheal cuff is below the glottic and subglottic airway and blood can pass down from the nasopharynx, past a throat pack, along the outer surface of the tracheal tube to the level of the vocal cords, subglottis and upper trachea. In contrast, a correctly sited FLMA covers and protects the supraglottic and glottic airway and blood is diverted laterally to the pyriform sinus and postcricoid region.

Direct comparisons of airway contamination by fibreoptic examination at the end of nasal surgery show patients managed with a FLMA are significantly less likely to have blood staining the airway (glottis and trachea) than patients managed with a tracheal tube. The FLMA effectively and satisfactorily protects the glottic and tracheobronchial airway from blood exposure during nasal and sinus surgery and can offer *better* protection of the tracheobronchial airway than a tracheal tube in many instances (Figures 25.1–25.3).

Both emergence quality and overall airway protection following nasal surgery appear to be *better* for a FLMA than a tracheal tube.

FLMA – tonsillectomy

The use of a FLMA for tonsillectomy is an advanced technique and requires an experienced anaesthetist who is familiar with the insertion and maintenance of the device and a surgeon who is competent at working around a FLMA. In small children the inexperienced should not use a FLMA for tonsillectomy.

The use of a FLMA for tonsillectomy requires close cooperation and meticulous attention to detail by both the anaesthetist and surgeon. Particularly care is required by the surgeon on placement and opening of the mouth gag and intraoperative manipulation of the gag. Mechanical obstruction during the use of a tonsillar gag varies from 2% to 20%, and for the majority of these cases the obstruction is correctable. Access to the inferior pole of the tonsil has been documented as being more difficult.

The advantages of using a FLMA for tonsillectomy are (i) the superior recovery profile with fewer

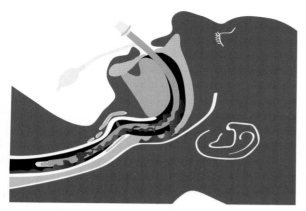

Figure 25.1. Uncuffed tube – note blood can pass tube.

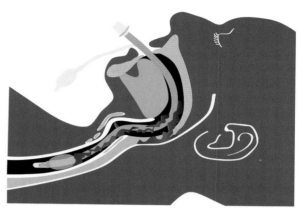

Figure 25.2. Cuffed tube – note blood can pass down to cuff.

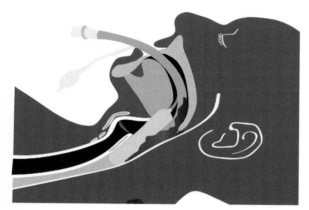

Figure 25.3. Correctly placed LMA protects laryngeal inlet from soiling.

episodes of bronchospasm, laryngospasm, and desaturation, (ii) less aspiration of blood when compared to an uncuffed tracheal tube and (iii) better protection of the lower away from blood and secretions until awake.

The FLMA is removed when patients open their eyes to command. The cuff should remain inflated allowing blood and secretions on the backplate to be suctioned out as the FLMA is removed from the mouth.

Oral tracheal tube

Tracheal tubes are commonly used in ENT surgery. Reinforced tubes are useful for procedures where head and neck movements and positioning are anticipated for surgery. South facing oral tubes are particularly suitable for surgery involving the pharynx where

a gag is used. The advantages of using an oral tracheal tube are (i) familiarity with its use, (ii) relative resistance to compression and (iii) the ability to secure and protect the *lower airway – distal to tube cuff* from above (blood and debris in the oropharynx) and below (regurgitated gastric contents) during spontaneous and positive pressure ventilation.

Extubation and recovery

Extubation of a tracheal tube is usually undertaken with the patient either 'awake' or 'deep' (see Chapter 17 for more detail). Awake extubation is preferred when the priority is airway maintenance or protection in the presence of blood, secretions or difficult airway management. The disadvantage is the higher incidence of laryngospasm, coughing, bucking, oxyhaemoglobin desaturation and increased risk of bleeding. Deep extubation is used in an attempt to improve the recovery profile. Recovery with a laryngeal mask airway will provide protection of the lower airway from blood from the pharynx and a superior recovery profile compared to awake or deep extubation.

Laryngeal surgery

Operations on the airway are unique in that both anaesthetist and surgeon are working in the same anatomical field. The anaesthetist is concerned with adequate oxygenation, removal of carbon dioxide, maintenance of an adequate airway and the prevention of soiling of the tracheobronchial tree, while the surgeon requires an adequate view of a clear motionless operating field. Close cooperation and

Table 25.2. The ideal anaesthetic technique would be

- Simple to use
- Provide complete control of the airway
- No risk of aspiration
- Control ventilation with adequate oxygenation and carbon dioxide removal
- Provide smooth induction and maintenance of anaesthesia
- Provide a clear motionless surgical field, free of secretions
- No time restrictions on the surgeon
- No risk of airway fire
- No cardiovascular instability
- Allow safe emergence with no coughing, bucking, breath-holding or laryngospasm
- Produce a pain-free, comfortable, alert patient with minimum hangover effects

communication between anaesthetist and surgeon are essential for success. Patients presenting for laryngeal surgery vary from young healthy individuals, with voice changes secondary to benign vocal cord pathology (e.g., small nodules and polyps), to elderly, heavy smokers with chronic obstructive pulmonary disease presenting with stridor caused by glottic carcinoma.

The ideal anaesthetic technique for laryngeal surgery

The ideal anaesthetic technique (Table 25.2) for all laryngoscopy procedures does not exist. The technique chosen will be dependent on (i) the patient's general condition, (ii) the size, mobility and location of the lesion and (iii) surgical requirements including the use of a laser.

The presence of a cuffed tracheal tube whilst providing control of the airway and preventing aspiration, may obscure a glottic lesion and is not laser safe. A cuffed laser tube provides some protection against laser-induced airway fires but has a greater external diameter to internal diameter ratio and may obscure laryngeal lesions. Jet ventilation techniques require specialist equipment and knowledge, an understanding of their limitations and do not protect the airway from soiling.

Pre-operative assessment

At the end of the pre-operative assessment, the anaesthetist should have some idea of the size, mobility, vascularity and location of the lesion. Standard airway assessments to predict the ease of ventilation, visualisation of the laryngeal inlet and tracheal intubation should be performed. Airway pathology and its impact on airway management should be assessed.

The severity and size of lesions at the glottic level are assessed by direct or indirect laryngoscopy undertaken by ENT surgeons in an outpatient setting and a photograph of the findings is often recorded in the notes. Information about subglottic and tracheal lesions is provided by chest radiography, CT and MRI.

Size – lesion size gives an indication of potential airflow obstruction. Stridor indicates a significantly narrowed airway. In the adult, stridor implies an airway diameter of less than 4–5 mm, but the absence of stridor does not exclude a narrowed airway.

Mobility – very mobile lesions (e.g., multiple large vocal cord polyps or papillomas) may cause *partial* airway obstruction following induction of anaesthesia but *total* airway obstruction is extremely uncommon. Obstruction is worse during anaesthesia with spontaneous ventilation because of the loss of supporting tone in the oropharynx and laryngo-hypopharynx collapsing the airway.

Location – supraglottic lesions, if mobile, can obstruct the airway or make visualisation of the laryngeal inlet difficult. Subglottic lesions may allow a good view of the laryngeal inlet but cause difficulty during the passage of a tracheal tube.

Figures 25.4–25.7 accompany Tables 25.3 and 25.4 to illustrate some of the conditions.

Anaesthetic techniques for laryngoscopy

For the majority of benign vocal cord lesions and early malignant lesions, airway obstruction is not a feature. Where airway obstruction is anticipated the anaesthetic plan will change, but for non-obstructing lesions a number of anaesthetic techniques are suitable.

Anaesthetic techniques can be broadly classified into two groups. *'Closed'* systems in which a cuffed tracheal tube is employed with protection of the lower airway and *'Open'* systems in which no tube is used

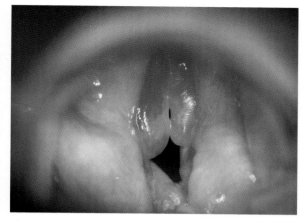

Figure 25.4. Bilateral Reinke's oedema on vocal cords.

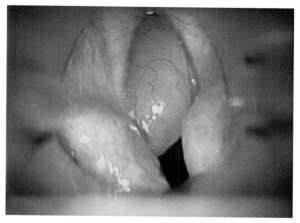

Figure 25.5. Large vocal cord cyst occluding the majority of the airway.

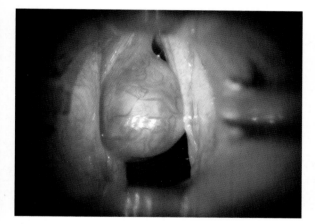

Figure 25.6. Vocal cord polyp.

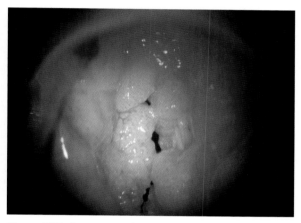

Figure 25.7. Extensive vocal cord papilloma.

leaving the airway 'open'. Open systems use spontaneous ventilation or jet ventilation techniques.

The decision to use a 'closed' or 'open' technique will be dependent upon the experience of the anaesthetist, the experience of the surgeon, the equipment available, the requirements for surgical access, the size, mobility and location of the lesion and its vascularity. The technique chosen for any given procedure is not absolute and may have to change as surgical and anaesthetic requirements change. For example, an open system utilising jet ventilation on a lesion thought to be relatively avascular may change to a closed system employing a cuffed tracheal tube if the lesion is bleeding with the risk of soiling of the tracheobronchial tree. Conversely a system employing a cuffed tracheal tube may have to change during surgery to an open system if the

tracheal tube overlies a lesion making surgery very difficult or impossible.

Induction technique for laryngoscopy

An intravenous induction technique is suitable for the vast majority of benign and early malignant glottic lesions where airway obstruction is not anticipated. After intravenous induction of anaesthesia and administration of muscle relaxants appropriate to the length of surgery laryngoscopy is undertaken to visualise the larynx, establish laryngoscopy grade and administer topical local anaesthetic (lidocaine). This helps cardiovascular stability, reduction of airway reflexes and smooth recovery. Confirmation of pathology is important because the disease may have progressed since the last outpatient visit and the anaesthetic plan may have to change.

231

Table 25.3. Vocal cord pathology

1. Cysts
2. Polyps
3. Nodules
4. Sulcus
5. Granulomas
6. Papillomas
7. Haemangiomas
8. Reinke's oedema
9. Microweb
10. Post-operative scarring or stenosis
11. Congenital lesions
12. Malignant tumours

Closed systems

Closed systems employ a tracheal tube with an inflatable cuff and include microlaryngoscopy tubes and laser tubes (see Table 25.5 and Chapter 10).

Open systems

Open systems include spontaneous/insufflation techniques, intermittent apnoea techniques and jet ventilation techniques (Table 25.6).

Spontaneous/insufflation ventilation technique

Spontaneous ventilation and insufflation techniques are useful in the removal of foreign bodies, evaluation of airway dynamics (tracheomalacia) and paediatric

Table 25.4. Pre-operative assessment

Assessment	Implication
History of endoscopic procedures	Previous difficulty, severity, vascularity and site of obstruction. Anaesthetic technique used previously
Hoarse voice	Non-specific symptom. Can occur without airway compromise
Voice changes	Non-specific symptom. Minor lesions can change the voice
Dysphagia	Significant and suggests supraglottic obstruction. If associated with carcinoma implies upper oesophageal extension
Altered breathing position	Significant. Patients with partially obstructing lesions will compensate by changing their body positioning to limit airway obstruction
Unable to lie flat	Significant. Suggests severe airway obstruction and patients may need to sleep upright
Difficulty breathing during sleep	Significant. Difficulty in breathing at night or waking up at night in a panic suggests severe obstruction
Stridor	Significant and indicates critical airway obstruction with over 50% reduction in airway diameter and in adults an airway diameter of 4–5 mm
Stridor on exertion	Significant. Suggests airway obstruction is becoming critical. Patients may have no stridor at rest
Stridor at rest	Significant. Critical airway obstruction is present
Inspiratory stridor	Significant. Suggests extrathoracic airway obstruction
Expiratory stridor	Significant. Suggests intrathoracic airway obstruction
Absence of stridor	Generally reassuring BUT in exhausted adults and children there are limited chest movements and insufficient airflow to generate enough turbulent flow for stridor. These circumstances suggest life-threatening compromise
Fibreoptic awake flexible laryngoscopy	All adult patients should have this to visualise the vocal cords. In patients with symptoms and signs of severe airway obstruction great care must be taken to avoid local anaesthetic and fibrescope contact with the vocal cords precipitating total airway obstruction
CXR/CT/MRI scans	Can identify severity and depth of glottic, subglottic, tracheal and intrathoracic lesions

Table 25.5. Closed anaesthetic systems

Advantages

1. Protection of the lower airway

2. Control of the airway

3. Control of ventilation

4. Minimal pollution by volatile agents

5. Routine technique for all anaesthetists

Disadvantages

1. Limitation of visibility and surgical access

2. Risk of laser airway fire

3. Risk of air entrapment and pneumothorax/ hypotension with small tubes

4. Risk of high inflation pressures and inadequate ventilation

Table 25.6. Open anaesthetic systems

Advantages

1. Complete laryngeal visualisation

2. Minimal risk of tube-related trauma to the glottis

3. Laser safety

Disadvantages

1. Unprotected lower airway

2. Require specialist equipment, knowledge and experience

Table 25.7. Limitations of spontaneously breathing/insufflation techniques

Advantages

1. Complete laryngeal visualisation

2. Laser safe

3. No tube-related trauma

Disadvantages

1. No control over ventilation

2. Loss of protective airway reflexes and the potential for airway soiling

3. Theatre pollution when volatile agents are used

Insufflation of anaesthetic gases and agents can be via a number of routes:

- Small catheter introduced into the nasopharynx and placed above the laryngeal opening
- Tracheal tube cut short and placed through the nasopharynx emerging just beyond the soft palate
- Nasopharyngeal airway
- Side arm or channel of a laryngoscope or bronchoscope.

Movements of the vocal cords are minimal or absent despite a spontaneously breathing technique provided an adequate level of anaesthesia is maintained. For satisfactory spontaneously breathing/insufflation techniques an adequate depth of anaesthesia is vital before any instrumentation of the airway takes place. If the depth of anaesthesia is too light, the vocal cords may move, the patient may cough or laryngospasm occur. If the depth of anaesthesia is too great the patient may become apnoeic with cardiovascular instability. Careful observations throughout the procedure, noting movements, respiratory rate and depth, cardiovascular stability and constant observation for unobstructed breathing are vital, with the concentration of volatile anaesthetic or intravenous anaesthetic adjusted accordingly.

Intermittent apnoea technique

Intermittent apnoea techniques have been described for the laser resection of juvenile laryngeal papillomatosis when the presence of a tracheal tube obstructs surgery (Table 25.8). Following induction of general anaesthesia muscle relaxants are administered

airways (Table 25.7). Both techniques require a spontaneously breathing patient and allow a clear view of an unobstructed glottis.

Inhalational induction is commenced with sevoflurane or halothane in 100% oxygen. At a suitable depth of anaesthesia as assessed by clinical observations on the rate and depth of respiration, pupil size, eye reflexes, blood pressure and heart rate changes, laryngoscopy is undertaken and topical local anaesthetic (lidocaine) is administered above, below and at the level of the vocal cords. Then 100% oxygen is administered by facemask with spontaneous ventilation and anaesthesia continued with inhalational (insufflation) or an intravenous anaesthetic technique (propofol infusion). At a suitable depth of anaesthesia, again assessed by clinical observations, the surgeon undertakes rigid laryngoscopy or bronchoscopy.

Table 25.8. Intermittent apnoea technique

Advantages

1. Immobile, unobstructed surgical field

2. Laser safe (No tracheal tube to act as fuel source)

Disadvantages

1. Variable levels of anaesthesia

2. Interruption to surgery for re-intubation

3. Potential trauma through multiple re-intubation

4. The risk of aspiration of blood and debris with the tracheal tube removed

followed by tracheal intubation. The patient is hyperventilated with a volatile anaesthetic agent in 100% oxygen. The tracheal tube is then removed, leaving the surgeon a clear, unobstructed, immobile surgical field. After an apnoeic period of typically 2–3 minutes, surgery is stopped, the tracheal tube is re-inserted and the patient hyperventilated once more.

Jet ventilation

Jet ventilation techniques involve the intermittent administration of high-pressure jets of air, oxygen or air-oxygen mixtures with entrainment of room air. In 1967 Sanders first described a jet ventilation technique using a 16-gauge jet placed down the side arm of a rigid bronchoscope relying on air entrainment to continue ventilation with an open bronchoscope. Sanders used intermittent jets of oxygen (rate 8/min, 3.5 bar driving pressure) to entrain air and showed the technique maintained supranormal oxygen pressure with no rise in the carbon dioxide pressure.

Since 1967, modifications to Sanders original jet ventilation technique have been made for endoscopic airway surgery. These modifications include the *site* at which the jet of gas emerges (supraglottic, subglottic, transtracheal) and the *frequency* of jet ventilation (low frequency <1 Hz, <60 breaths/min or high frequency >1 Hz, >60 breaths/min). In 1971 Spoerel demonstrated transtracheal jet ventilation and in 1983 Layman reported the use of transtracheal jet ventilation in 60 patients with difficult airways. In 1985, Ravussin designed a dedicated transtracheal catheter, and the Difficult Airway Society included it in techniques for the difficult airway in 1998.

High frequency jet ventilation

High frequency jet ventilation techniques typically use rates around 100–150/min. This allows:

- A continuous expiratory flow of air, enhancing the removal of fragments of blood and debris from the airway
- Reduced peak and mean airway pressures (compared with low frequency) with improved cardiovascular stability
- Enhanced diffusion and interregional mixing (compared with low frequency) within the lungs resulting in more efficient ventilation.

These advantages are of particular importance in patients with significant lung disease and obesity. High frequencies are achieved by automated high frequency jet ventilators, which have alarms and automatic interruption of jet flow when preset pause pressure limits have been reached (i.e., blockage of entrainment or exhalation have occurred).

Jet ventilation techniques

Jet ventilation techniques are suitable for the vast majority of benign glottic pathology and early malignancy where airway obstruction is not anticipated. A typical jet ventilation technique will include pre-oxygenation followed by intravenous induction and administration of muscle relaxants. Laryngoscopy is undertaken and topical local anaesthetic (lidocaine) administered. A laryngeal mask airway is inserted, and ventilation is continued with 100% oxygen until the surgeon is ready to site the rigid (suspension) laryngoscope onto which a jetting needle has been attached in preparation for supraglottic jet ventilation. Alternatively, facemask ventilation is continued until the surgeon is ready to site the laryngoscope. Anaesthesia is maintained with an infusion of propofol, supplemented by bolus administration or infusion of alfentanil or remifentanil. At the end of surgery, the laryngeal mask airway is re-inserted before antagonism of residual muscle relaxation and cessation of intravenous anaesthesia, to facilitate smooth emergence.

During the procedure the adequacy of jet ventilation should be continuously assessed by observation of chest movements, oxygen saturation readings and by listening for changes to the sound during air entrainment and exhalation. The patency of the airway and any surgical obstruction can also be

(a)

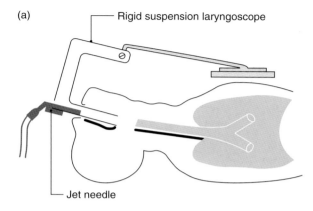

Rigid suspension laryngoscope

Jet needle

(b)

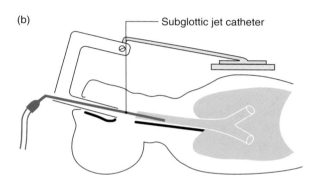

Subglottic jet catheter

(c)

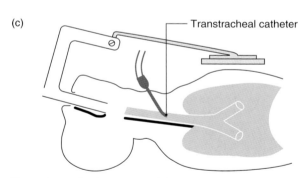

Transtracheal catheter

Figure 25.8. The three sites used for jet ventilation:
(a) supraglottic, (b) subglottic and (c) transtracheal.

assessed by watching the endoscopic image on a television screen.

Jet ventilation techniques are categorised by the site of catheter into supraglottic, subglottic and transtracheal (Figure 25.8).

Supraglottic jet ventilation

Supraglottic jet ventilation describes a technique in which the jet of gas emerges in the supraglottis by

Table 25.9. Supraglottic jet ventilation

Advantages

1. Clear, unobstructed view for the surgeon

2. No risk of a laser-induced airway fire

Disadvantages

1. Risk of barotrauma with pneumomediastinum, pneumothorax and subcutaneous emphysema

2. Gastric distension with entrained air

3. Misalignment of the suspension laryngoscope or jetting needle resulting in poor ventilation

4. Blood and debris or fragments being blown into the distal trachea

5. Vibration and movement of the vocal cords

6. Inability to monitor end tidal CO_2 concentration

attachment of a jetting needle to the rigid suspension laryngoscope (Table 25.9). High or low frequency ventilation can be employed (Figure 25.8a).

Subglottic jet ventilation

Subglottic jet ventilation allows delivery of a jet of gas directly into the trachea by the placement of a small (2–3 mm) catheter or specifically designed tube (Benjet, Hunsaker) through the glottis and into the trachea (Figure 25.8b and Table 25.10)

Transtracheal jet ventilation

Transtracheal jet ventilation has a vital role in the management of the 'can't intubate – can't ventilate' emergency scenario (Figure 25.8c). Transtracheal catheter placement under local anaesthetic in individuals with significant airway pathology or under general anaesthesia for elective laryngeal surgery has been described. Compared with supraglottic and subglottic jet techniques, transtracheal techniques carry the greatest risk of barotrauma and a high risk of subcutaneous emphysema. Its use for benign glottic pathology should be questioned with a careful evaluation of the potential risks and benefits made. Other potential problems include misplacement, blockage, kinking, infection, bleeding and failure to site the catheter.

235

Table 25.10. Subglottic jet ventilation

Advantages

1. Greater minute ventilation at any given driving pressure (compared to supraglottic)

2. Greater minute ventilation at any given frequency (compared to supraglottic)

3. Minimal influence on ventilation of laryngoscope alignment to the laryngotracheal axis

4. No vocal cord movements

5. No time constraints for the surgeon in the placement of the rigid laryngoscope

Disadvantages

1. Potential for a laser-induced airway fire (laser-resistant tubes are available, e.g., Hunsaker)

2. Greater risk of barotrauma compared with supraglottic jet techniques

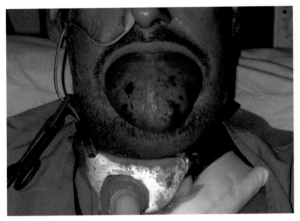

Figure 25.9. Massive tongue swelling causing airway compromise.

Head and neck surgery

Head and neck surgery involves the treatment of patients with diseases of the upper airway, larynx and pharynx. When airway compromise is not an issue most procedures are largely uneventful. When airway compromise is a feature the anaesthetic plan needs to change according to the severity and site of obstruction.

Major head and neck procedures include laryngectomy, pharyngolaryngectomy, radical neck dissection and the resection of large thyroid lesions. A laryngectomy involves the resection of the larynx and the creation of an end-tracheal stoma, a pharyngolaryngectomy also resects structures within the pharynx, including part or all of the tongue and oesophagus. A radical neck dissection resects sternomastoid, internal and external jugular veins and cervical lymph nodes.

The treatment of upper airway tumours depends on the staging (Tumor, Node, Metastasis – TNM classification) and site. Chemotherapy, radiotherapy, laser endoscopic resection, transoral laser surgery, major soft tissue and organ excision, radical neck dissection and flap reconstruction, alone or in combination, are the principal treatment options.

All patients with airway compromise should be considered as a possible difficult intubation, whereas not all patients with a difficult intubation have airway compromise.

No airway compromise

Laryngeal pathology without symptoms or signs of airway compromise, such as early T1 and some T2 tumours, can be managed by a number of anaesthetic techniques including intravenous induction of general anaesthesia and placement of a cuffed tracheal or laser tube. Alternatively, a supraglottic or subglottic jet ventilation technique can be employed for biopsy and laser resection.

Airway compromise

The recognition of a compromised or anatomically distorted upper airway is paramount in the preoperative assessment of head and neck patients (Figure 25.9). For elective procedures a detailed history, examination and investigations can be undertaken, but for more urgent procedures with severe airway compromise investigations may not be possible. Anaesthetic management will depend on the urgency of the intervention, site of the lesion, size of the lesion, level of obstruction, extension of the lesion, and degree of airway compromise.

Symptoms and signs of airway compromise include respiratory distress, tachypnoea, accessory muscle use, sternal retraction, tracheal tug, stridor, hypoxia, tachycardia, and exhaustion.

Airway compromise – level of obstruction

Difficult airways can be divided according to the level at which a problem exists (Figures 25.10–25.14).

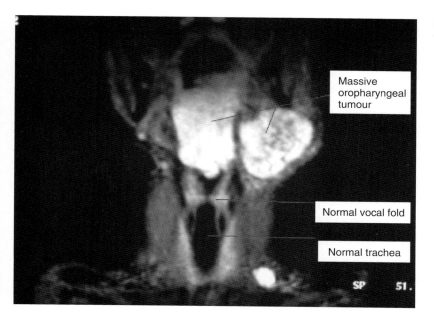

Figure 25.10. Level of obstruction: oropharyngeal tumour.

Massive oropharyngeal tumour

Normal vocal fold

Normal trachea

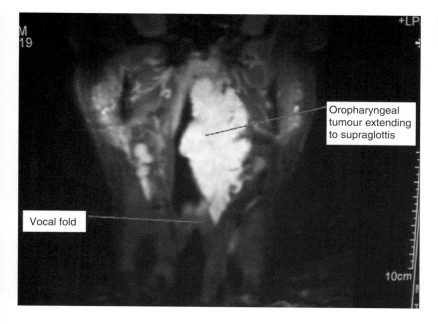

Figure 25.11. Level of obstruction: oropharyngeal tumour extending to supraglottis.

Oropharyngeal tumour extending to supraglottis

Vocal fold

Disease states are not confined to these anatomical areas and can pass through many levels (Table 25.11).

Airway compromise – management options

Whatever technique is chosen as the primary anaesthetic technique, a back-up plan should be thought through, discussed with the surgeon and instituted when difficulties arise (Table 25.12).

Airway compromise – oral cavity/oropharyngeal lesions

An intravenous induction in these patients may result in airway obstruction and an inability to ventilate or

237

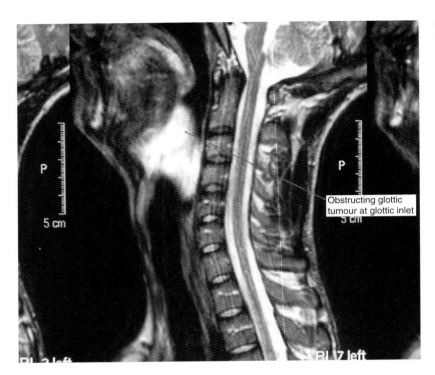

Figure 25.12. Level of obstruction: glottic inlet.

Obstructing glottic tumour at glottic inlet

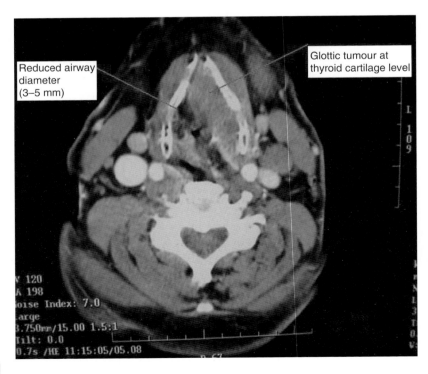

Figure 25.13. Level of obstruction: glottic tumour with grossly narrowed airway.

Reduced airway diameter (3–5 mm)

Glottic tumour at thyroid cartilage level

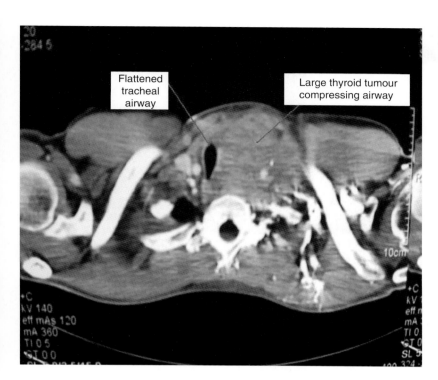

Figure 25.14. Level of obstruction: compressed trachea.

Flattened tracheal airway

Large thyroid tumour compressing airway

Table 25.11. Level of obstruction

Oral cavity

Oropharynx

Tongue base and supraglottic

Glottic

Subglottic and upper tracheal

Midtracheal

Lower tracheal and bronchial

Table 25.12. Potential management options for airway compromise

Intravenous induction of general anaesthesia +/− relaxants

Inhalational induction with maintenance of spontaneous ventilation

Inhalational induction with 'take over' of ventilation

Awake fibreoptic intubation

Asleep fibreoptic intubation

Awake transtracheal catheter placement and jet ventilation

Awake tracheostomy under local anaesthesia

Asleep tracheostomy under general anaesthesia

oxygenate (Figures 25.15 and 25.16). The normal techniques to prevent this such as facemask ventilation with oral or nasal airways may not be effective. The glottis and lower airway are often normal in these patients, and the principal problem around intubation is one of bypassing a large obstructing mass without traumatising it whilst maintaining a patent airway. An awake fibreoptic intubation technique is often used in this group of patients. Other anaesthetic techniques include awake transtracheal

catheter placement with jet ventilation, and awake tracheostomy.

Airway compromise – tongue base/supraglottic lesions

Even small lesions at the tongue base and supraglottis can have significant effects on the airway because of their location at the entrance to the glottis, and their

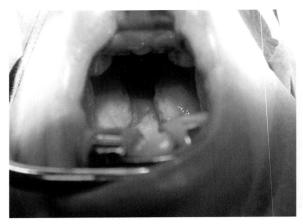

Figure 25.15. Oral cavity with normal, large tonsils.

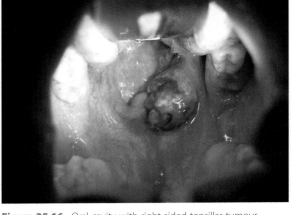

Figure 25.16. Oral cavity with right sided tonsillar tumour.

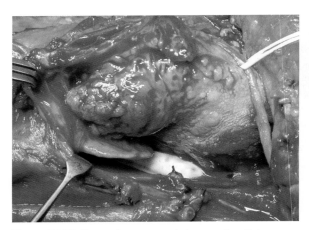

Figure 25.17. Tongue-base cancer during resection. Note endotracheal tube and downward displacement of the epiglottis.

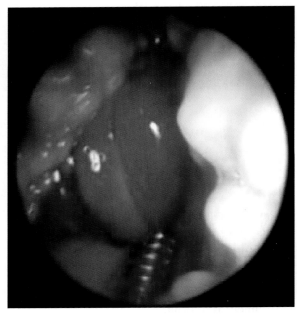

Figure 25.18. Acute epiglottitis with cherry red appearance.

effect on the epiglottiss (Figures 25.17–25.19). As a tongue base lesion expands it fills the space in the valleculae and directs the epiglottis downwards increasing airway obstruction at the glottic inlet. A large epiglottic or vallecular cyst results in airway obstruction and compromise in a similar manner to epiglottitis. The danger of an intravenous induction in these patients is airway obstruction following the loss of supportive tone from the soft tissues. An oral or nasal airway may be ineffective in relieving the obstruction, and a strong jaw thrust manoeuvre displacing the mandible and tongue base forwards creating an airspace at the supraglottic inlet may be required.

Standard curved blade laryngoscopy can traumatise any lesion at the tongue base and valleculae, causing bleeding and swelling with the potential for complete airway obstruction. Although straight blade laryngoscopy aims to pass below the epiglottic tip and lift the epiglottis upwards this can be difficult with a distorted epiglottis. Great care and attention needs to be taken during attempted laryngoscopy with these lesions.

Any patient in which there is concern about a lesion at the tongue base or supraglottis, or in which there is evidence of significant airway obstruction, an

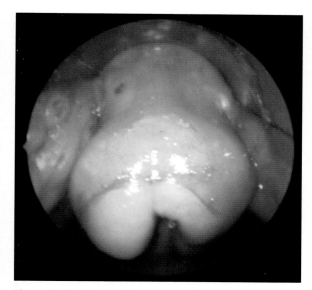

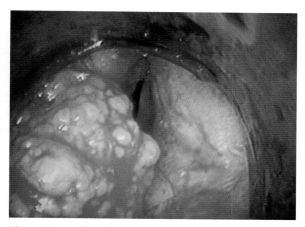

Figure 25.20. Glottic lesion, extensive carcinoma.

Figure 25.19. Chronic inflammatory epiglottitis.

awake fibreoptic intubation, awake transtracheal catheter, or an awake local anaesthetic tracheostomy should be considered.

Airway compromise – glottic lesions

Awake fibreoptic techniques are suitable for oral cavity, oropharyngeal and tongue base lesions because they *pass around* the mass, but are unsuitable for advanced obstructing laryngeal disease in which the fibrescope has to *pass through* the mass, resulting in complete airway occlusion (Figure 25.20). Good topical anaesthesia is also difficult to achieve in this group, and technically fibreoptic intubation through an anatomically distorted, large, vascular, friable, necrotic tumour is difficult.

Some investigators advocate inhalational induction techniques for the obstructed airway in which spontaneous ventilation is maintained throughout. Inhalational induction for advanced laryngeal tumours with airway obstruction is difficult, slow, extremely challenging and often fails.

Physiological problems include a reduction in airflow with spontaneous ventilation, an increased collapsibility of the airway, increased work of breathing, critical instability at points of narrowing leading to further airway collapse and a reduction in functional residual capacity. Induction is slow with apnoeic periods and episodes of obstruction are common.

Patients often become more hypoxic and hypercarbic with long periods of instability, arrhythmias and apnoea.

The traditional view is that the technique is safe because if the patient obstructs, the volatile agent will no longer be taken up, and the patient will lighten up. This frequently does not happen and the technique is often unreliable.

Controversy exists as to the suitability of 'taking over' the patient's own spontaneous ventilation with bag-mask ventilation. Taking over ventilation allows a suitable depth of anaesthesia for laryngoscopy to be achieved more easily. This avoids the long periods of spontaneous ventilation waiting for an adequate depth of anaesthesia in which the patient may become unstable.

The administration of a muscle relaxant will provide optimum ventilation and intubating conditions for any airway and should be considered if tracheal intubation is thought possible.

At a suitable depth of anaesthesia laryngoscopy is undertaken and the best chance of success is usually at the first attempt when bleeding, trauma and swelling are minimal. A gum elastic bougie or stylet may be useful. Failure to intubate requires an urgent tracheostomy and the surgeon should be gowned and immediately ready.

Transtracheal catheter placement under local anaesthesia at a level below the distal margin of the tumour is a recognised technique for the difficult airway. The catheter is placed usually at the level of the second or third tracheal rings, avoiding the tumour and the risk of bleeding and tumour seeding.

241

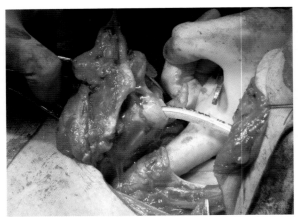

Figure 25.21. During laryngectomy showing tube through glottis and finger in upper oesophagus.

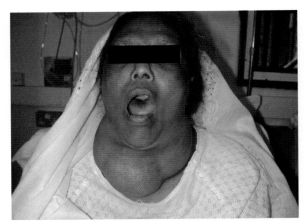

Figure 25.22. Large thyroid mass: awake fibreoptic intubation needed.

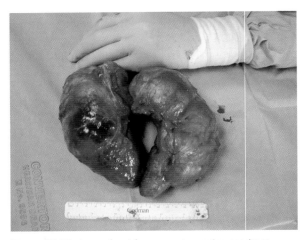

Figure 25.23. Large thyroid mass: post-resection specimen.

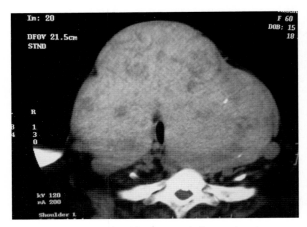

Figure 25.24. Large thyroid mass: grossly flattened trachea.

Once catheter placement has been confirmed in an awake patient by an end-tidal capnography trace, intravenous induction is started. After induction jet ventilation through the transtracheal catheter is commenced, ideally with a high-frequency ventilator with automated cut-off at a preset pause pressure limit to reduce the incidence of barotrauma. An experienced anaesthetist should remain at the head end of the patient ensuring a patent and adequate upper airway by chin lift, jaw thrust, oral or nasal airway.

Airway compromise – subglottic and upper tracheal lesions

Patients with advanced laryngotracheal stenosis may have airway diameters of 2–4 mm and airway management usually involves a supraglottic jet ventilation technique.

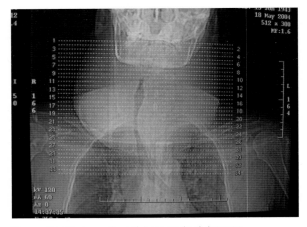

Figure 25.25. Large thyroid mass: tracheal distortion.

Airway compromise – mid and lower tracheal

Tracheal obstruction can be caused by lesions arising within the trachea itself or by compression from surrounding structures or tumours (Figures 25.22–25.25). The upper airway is usually normal at laryngoscopy and the problems are secondary to an inability to pass a tracheal tube and difficulties placing a surgical airway below the obstruction. Awake fibreoptic intubation should be considered but may not be possible. A rigid bronchoscope may be required to secure the airway. Lower tracheal lesions and large mediastinal masses should be managed in specialist centres.

Key points

- Anaesthesia for ENT surgery requires specialised equipment and techniques.
- Shared airway cases require careful planning between surgeon and anaesthetist.
- Use of the laser adds another hazard.
- Thorough airway evaluation includes review of CT and MR scans.
- Review recent flexible nasendoscopy findings.
- The site of airway obstruction determines the most appropriate strategy.
- Take great care when employing high-pressure oxygen.

Further reading

Ahmed ZM, Vohra A. (2002). The reinforced laryngeal mask airway (RLMA) protects the airway in patients undergoing nasal surgery – an observational study of 200 patients. *Canadian Journal of Anaesthesia*, **49**, 863–866.

Boisson-Bertrand D. (1995). Tonsillectomies and the reinforced laryngeal mask. *Canadian Journal of Anaesthesia*, **42**, 857–861.

Brimacombe JR. (2005). Flexible LMA for shared airway. In: Brimacombe JR (Ed.), *Laryngeal Mask Airway Principles and Practise*. Philadelphia, Elsevier. pp 445–467.

Clarke MB, Forster P, Cook TM. (2007). Airway management for tonsillectomy: A national survey of UK practise. *British Journal of Anaesthesia*, **99**, 425–428.

Cohen D, Dor M. (2008). Morbidity and mortality of post-tonsillectomy bleeding: Analysis of cases. *The Journal of Laryngology and Otology*, **122**, 88–92.

Crosby ET, Cooper RM, Douglas MJ, et al. (1998). The unanticipated difficult airway with recommendations for management. *Canadian Journal of Anaesthesia*, **45**, 757–776.

Latto IP, Vaughn RS. (1997). *Difficulties in Tracheal Intubation*. 2nd ed. London: WB Saunders.

Mason RA, Fielder CP. (1999). The obstructed airway in head and neck surgery. *Anaesthesia*, **54**, 625–628.

National Patient Safety Agency. Reducing the risk of retained throat packs after surgery. www.nrls.npsa.nhs.uk

Nouraei SA, Giussani DA, Howard DJ, Sandhu GS, Ferguson C, Patel A. (2008). Physiological comparison of spontaneous and positive-pressure ventilation in laryngotracheal stenosis. *British Journal of Anaesthesia*, **101**, 419–423.

Ovassapian A. (1996). Management of the difficult airway. In: Ovassapian A (Ed.), *Fibreoptic Endoscopy and the Difficult Airway*. 2nd ed. New York: Lippincott-Raven.

Peterson GN, Domino KB, Caplan RA, et al. (2005). Management of the difficult airway: A closed claims analysis. *Anesthesiology*, **103**, 33–39.

Royal College of Surgeons. (2005). *National Prospective Tonsillectomy Audit*. London: Royal College of Surgeons. ISBN 1–904096–02–6.

Webster AC, Morley-Forster PK, Dain S, et al. (1993). Anaesthesia for adenotonsillectomy: A comparison between tracheal intubation and the armoured laryngeal mask airway. *Canadian Journal of Anaesthesia*, **40**, 1171–1177.

Webster AC, Morley-Forster PK, Janzen V, et al. (1999). Anesthesia for intranasal surgery: A comparison between tracheal intubation and the flexible reinforced laryngeal mask airway. *Anesthesia and Analgesia*, **88**, 421–425.

Williams PJ, Bailey PM. (1993). Comparison of the reinforced laryngeal mask airway and tracheal intubation for adenotonsillectomy. *British Journal of Anaesthesia*, **70**, 30–33.

Williams PJ, Thompsett C, Bailey PM. (1995). Comparison of the reinforced laryngeal mask airway and tracheal intubation for nasal surgery. *Anaesthesia*, **50**, 987–989.

Chapter 26

Airway management in cervical spine disease

Ian Calder

There are three areas of concern

- Difficult intubation
- Post-operative airway obstruction
- Spinal cord injury during anaesthesia

Difficult intubation in cervical spine disease

Difficulty with mask ventilation is rare in patients with cervical spine disease, but flexion deformity may prevent mask application.

Difficulty with intubation is more likely in patients with cervical disease because

- Mobility, particularly in extension, of the cranio-cervical junction and to a lesser extent the cervical spine below C2 is required.
- Mouth opening and jaw protrusion may be affected, because of temporo-mandibular joint dysfunction and because cervical stiffness in itself impedes mouth opening (see Chapter 7).

Identifying difficult patients

Most seriously difficult patients look sufficiently abnormal to alert a sensible practitioner. Internal or external fixator devices and gross flexion deformity are examples.

However it is not easy to identify all difficult patients. Reduced cranio-cervical movement can be compensated for by increased movement at lower levels and is difficult to detect clinically. Poor pharyngeal visibility (Mallampati score) is probably still the best alert. When patients with poor cervical movement are asked to open their mouths their chin seems

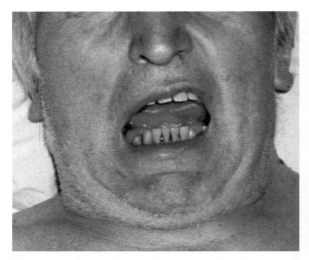

Figure 26.1. Poor cranio-cervical extension and mouth opening in cervical rheumatoid arthritis. Note the sub-mental folds.

to recede into their neck and submental folds are seen (Figure 26.1).

Radiological abnormalities of the cranio-cervical junction are good predictors of difficult laryngoscopy. Poor separation of the occiput, atlas and axis on lateral radiographs or sagittal CT scans is a good predictor of difficulty (Figure 26.2).

Some cervical diseases are notorious for difficulty in laryngoscopy, such as rheumatoid arthritis (which affects the temporo-mandibular joints and larynx as well), ankylosing spondylitis, and Klippel-Feil syndrome (Figures 26.3 and 26.4).

Intubating methods: developments in video-laryngoscopy may allow intubation in patients who would have been difficult with a direct laryngoscope. However a better view at laryngoscopy does not

Core Topics in Airway Management, Second Edition, ed. Ian Calder and Adrian Pearce. Published by Cambridge University Press.
© Cambridge University Press 2011.

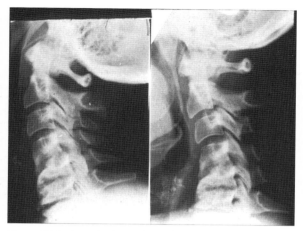

Figure 26.2. Lateral radiographs in flexion and extension. The patient has degenerative changes at the C4/5/6 joints but the posterior atlanto-occipital and atlanto-axial gaps open and close indicating that there is movement at the cranio-cervical junction.

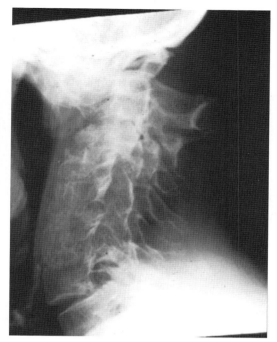

Figure 26.3. Severe cervical rheumatoid arthritis. There is loss of joint space at all levels and gross anterior atlanto-axial subluxation.

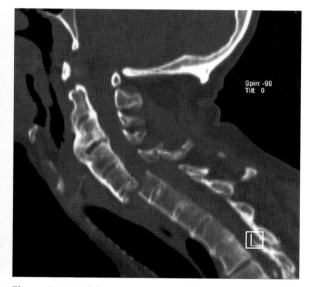

Figure 26.4. Ankylosing spondylitis. There is a displaced fracture at C6.

always mean easier intubation, and the overall superiority of video-laryngoscopy is not yet proven. The flexible fibreoptic laryngoscope remains the instrument of choice in severe cervical disease.

Post-operative airway obstruction
Causation

- Prolonged (5 hours) anterior cervical operations, especially at higher levels. The obstruction is caused by peri-glottic pharyngeal tissue swelling due to venous and lymphatic obstruction or haematoma. The obstruction is not due to tracheal compression, and the presence of a drain does not reduce the incidence. It is particularly likely to occur after combined anterior and posterior surgery. If the anterior procedure precedes the posterior surgery and/or surgery is prolonged it is safer to leave the tube in overnight (see Figure 26.5).

- Maxillotomy or mandibular and tongue splitting approaches to the cranio-cervical junction. Serious tissue swelling is common after these procedures and a preliminary tracheostomy and percutaneous gastrostomy is advisable.

- Laryngeal oedema or haematoma due to traumatic intubation. This is particularly likely in patients with rheumatoid arthritis (see Chapter 7, Figure 7.9). Recurrent laryngeal nerve palsy can occur after anterior surgery and causes a weak cough and voice, but does not cause obstruction.

- Cranio-cervical fixation in an excessively flexed posture can cause airway obstruction.

245

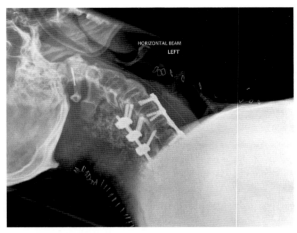

HORIZONTAL BEAM
LEFT

Figure 26.5. Anterior and posterior fixation of the fracture seen on Figure 26.4.

Presentation

- Usually within 6 hours.
- Patients complain of not being able to breathe, want to sit up and have difficulty in swallowing and talking.
- Stridor is not always present.
- SpO_2 may be above 90% until there is complete obstruction if extra oxygen is being given.

Management

Management will depend on the clinical situation. Decision making is easier when the situation is critical. In extremis, one does what one does best, quickly, which is likely to be direct laryngoscopy and 'gum-elastic' bougie or a supraglottic airway. Inhalational induction has been traditionally advised when the upper airway is obstructed. There can be no doubt that this situation is a very hazardous one, and in the author's opinion nothing should be ruled in or out.

Traditional teaching has emphasised the safety inherent in maintaining spontaneous ventilation if possible, but it has been shown that intravenous induction, paralysis and positive pressure ventilation with a supraglottic airway is effective in cases of laryngo-tracheal obstruction, and the author has used that technique successfully in this situation (see Chapter 25). The SGA can then be used as a conduit for fibreoptic intubation. The tube should not be removed until it is clear that tissue swelling is decreasing (typically 24 hours). There are some general points:

- Open the wound. This may reduce tissue pressure sufficiently to relieve a critical level of obstruction, even if there is no haematoma. The patient should then be transferred to theatre. Concerns about bleeding are of minor importance compared with airway obstruction.
- Helium or epinephrine inhalation may buy some time but re-intubation is required in the majority of cases. The ease or difficulty of intubation at the initial operation should be established, and consideration given to whether the surgery will have radically altered the situation (a cranio-cervical fixation will almost certainly prevent direct laryngoscopy).
- Assemble appropriate staff and equipment for surgical tracheostomy.
- Flexible fibreoptic intubation may be the best option, especially if the patient is a known difficult direct laryngoscopy. Vision will be difficult as secretions will be abundant and there will be pharyngeal tissue swelling. The patient should be kept sitting and the endoscope advanced during expiration (vision is usually impossible during inspiration). It may be simplest to give a dose of propofol to facilitate intubation after the endoscope has been placed in the trachea, as secretions may make topical anaesthesia less effective and lidocaine can produce airway obstruction due to irritation.
- A gum-elastic or similar bougie is often *the* vital piece of equipment.

Spinal cord injury during anaesthesia – for details of causation, types and treatment of SCI – see the Appendix

Neurological injury occurs during anaesthesia, both to peripheral nerves (the ulnar nerve being the most reported) and the neuraxis. The suspicion that airway management and direct laryngoscopy in particular can cause spinal cord injury (SCI) is deeply entrenched, but may be mythical. It is unlikely that there will ever be proof either that it is a real phenomenon or that it is not. Intubation is inevitably followed by a procession of other possible causes so that trying to establish that intubation caused or did

Table 26.1. The MRC motor power grades

Grade 5. Normal movement

Grade 4. Movement against resistance, but weaker than the other side

Grade 3. Movement against gravity, but not against resistance

Grade 2. Movement only with gravity eliminated

Grade 1. Palpable contraction but no visible movement

Grade 0. No movement

Table 26.2. Criteria for stability following cervical trauma

Conscious patient	Unconscious patient
a. Alert, no distracting injuries b. No midline pain c. Normal movement d. No neurology	a. Plain radiographs are inadequate b. The combination of plain films and CT scans is adequate to diagnose bony injuries *and* ligamentous instability c. MR scans are not required for the exclusion of instability

not cause a neurological deterioration is rather like trying to establish whether failure of a marriage is due to an event at the wedding.

The possibility of SCI occurring during anaesthesia certainly does not cease when airway management has been completed. It may be that attention to spinal cord perfusion is as or more important than how the patient is intubated.

- **Pre-anaesthetic neurological condition:** It is useful to establish and record the neurological findings, and the motor power in particular. Motor power can be classified according to the MRC grades (Table 26.1). If sensory or motor changes are established it is sensible to avoid suxamethonium in case denervation hyperkalaemia occurs.

- **'Clearing' the cervical spine in suspected injury:** 25 to 50% of patients with a traumatic cervical spine injury have an associated head injury, so that the need to confirm or exclude a cervical injury in an unconscious patient is a common problem. There is local variation in practice, but Table 2 summarizes the current position in the UK (Table 26.2).

- **Spinal instability versus spinal stenosis:** Reports of SCI during anaesthesia nearly all involve patients with spinal stenosis rather than instability. This does not mean that we should be less concerned about a diagnosis of instability, both because stenosis will occur if instability progresses, and vertebral instability may mean vascular instability. In the author's view anaesthetists have been rather over-concerned about spinal instability and under-concerned about stenosis. In addition the wide spectrum of meaning of the term instability should be

appreciated (see the Appendix for definitions of instability) (Figure 26.6).

- **Airway management:** The concept of airway management, and direct laryngoscopy in particular causing SCI has been described as a 'legend of anesthesia'. There is neither a case report that satisfactorily demonstrates the issue, nor any evidence of outcome difference with a particular technique. However absence of evidence cannot prove that the phenomenon does not exist. In two studies of the effect of airway management in cadavers rendered grossly unstable, basic life support techniques (head tilt, jaw thrust) produced more disturbance at the unstable sites than direct laryngoscopy. If this is true in vivo, it might be an argument for 'awake' intubation. However the quantity of vertebral displacement or angulation that occurs in a truly unstable spine during an awake intubation is not known, and could be greater than during intubation under general anaesthesia.

- **Awake flexible fibreoptic intubation:** Surveys of anaesthetists have indicated that this technique is regarded as a good option in patients with suspected cervical instability, but the procedure is by no means always straightforward and has resulted in laryngeal damage and even complete airway obstruction, necessitating an emergency surgical airway. In this author's view it would not be in a patient's interests for an anaesthetist inexperienced in awake endoscopy to attempt an awake intubation on the grounds of suspected or actual

(a)

(b)

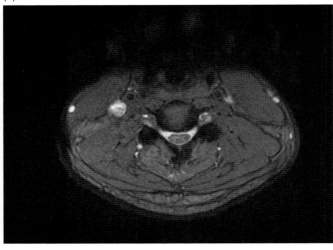

(c)

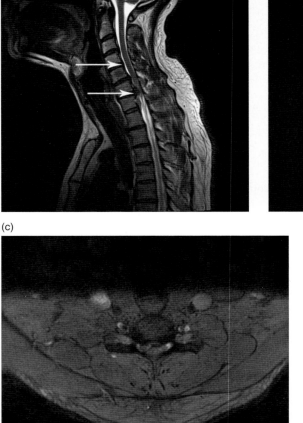

Figure 26.6. (a, b and c) MR scans showing spinal stenosis due to disc or osteophyte at C6/7. (b) An axial section at the level of the upper arrow in panel a. The cord is surrounded by CSF (white). (c) An axial section at the level of the lower arrow in panel a. No CSF is seen and the cord is compressed.

cervical instability. Instability is a vague term and the clinical import is very variable – see the Appendix.

- **Laryngoscopy:** Whether or not video-laryngoscopy is clinically superior to direct laryngoscopy is unknown. Robitaille et al found no significant difference in cervical spine movement between Glidescope® video-laryngoscopy and direct laryngoscopy, despite not using the sensible tactic suggested by Nolan and Wilson in 1993, which involves only exposing the glottis sufficiently to allow the introduction of a gum-elastic bougie. Direct laryngoscopy with the Macintosh laryngoscope remains an accepted method of intubation for anaesthetists and emergency physicians; the use of a bougie is to be encouraged. Manual in-line stabilisation (MILS) is an accepted practice, but there is no evidence that it affects outcome. MILS can make laryngoscopy more difficult and like cricoid pressure during rapid-sequence intubation should not be allowed to jeopardise successful intubation (see Chapter 18). The anterior portion of rigid cervical collars should be removed during airway interventions. Cricoid pressure should be applied if necessary, but suxamethonium should be avoided if spinal cord damage is suspected (risk of hyperkalaemia).

- **'Awake' positioning:** Prolonged abnormal spine positioning carries a small risk of neuraxial damage even in patients with normal spines, and this risk is compounded in patients with spinal disease. The majority of reports of SCI during anaesthesia have involved patients with spinal stenosis, not instability.

- It would be marvellous to be able to tell whether a position will be tolerable for whatever the duration of anaesthesia turns out to be. Spinal cord monitoring techniques offer a guide to positional adequacy (see the Appendix). 'Awake' positioning has been suggested as a sensible tactic, but unsurprisingly, damage can still occur, since not even the patient can predict whether a position will still be tolerable some hours later. If awake positioning is undertaken, consideration must be given as to:

  - Where the dividing line between sedation and anaesthesia is to be drawn. In practice, this is not always clear-cut, and what is intended to be sedation can more closely resemble anaesthesia. Disinhibition and withdrawal of cooperation are possible, although unusual if the patient is properly prepared.

  - Some thought should be devoted to what will be done if a problem is suspected, since false positives have been described, and the patient may not be advantaged by postponement.

Key points

- Difficult intubation is most likely when the disease affects the cranio-cervical junction.
- Mouth opening ability and cranio-cervical movement are related.
- Post-operative airway obstruction is most likely after anterior surgery combined with posterior surgery, or anterior surgery lasting more than 5 hours.
- Stridor and desaturation may not occur until obstruction is nearly complete, and drains make no difference.
- Opening the wound may relieve obstruction.
- Instability is hard to define and has a wide spectrum of significance.

- Most reports of spinal cord injury during anaesthesia involve spinal stenosis.
- No method of airway management has been shown to produce a better outcome after cervical trauma.

Further reading

Bhardwaj A, Long DM, Ducker TB, Toung TJ. (2001). Neurologic deficits after cervical laminectomy in the prone position. *Journal of Neurosurgical Anesthesiology*, **13**, 314–319.

Blumenthal S, Nadig M, Gerber C, Borgeat A. (2003). Severe airway obstruction during arthroscopic shoulder surgery. *Anesthesiology*, **99**, 1455–1456.

Calder I, Calder J, Crockard HA. (1995). Difficult direct laryngoscopy and cervical spine disease. *Anaesthesia*, **50**, 756–763.

Combes X, Dumerat M, Dhonneur G. (2004). Emergency gum elastic bougie-assisted tracheal intubation in four patients with upper airway distortion. *Canadian Journal of Anaesthesia*, **51**, 1022–1024.

Crosby ET. (2006). Airway management in adults after cervical spine trauma. *Anesthesiology*, **104**, 1293–1318.

Dickerman RD, Mittler MA, Warshaw C, Epstein JA. (2006). Spinal cord injury in a 14-year-old male secondary to spinal hyperflexion with exercise. *Spinal Cord*, **44**, 192–195.

Donaldson WF III, Heil BV, Donaldson VP, Silvaggio VJ. (1997). The effect of airway maneuvers on the unstable C1-C2 segment: A cadaver study. *Spine*, **22**, 1215–1218.

Duma A, Novak K, Schramm W. (2009). Tube-in-tube emergency airway management after a bitten endotracheal tube caused by repetitive transcranial electrical stimulation during spinal cord surgery. *Anesthesiology*, **111**, 1155–1157.

Hauswald M, Braude D. (2002). Spinal immobilization in trauma patients: Is it really necessary? *Current Opinion in Critical Care*, **8**, 566–570.

Hauswald M, Sklar DP, Tandberg D, Garcia JF. (1991). Cervical spine movement during airway management: Cinefluoroscopic appraisal in human cadavers. *American Journal of Emergency Medicine*, **9**, 535–538.

Kelleher MO, Tan G, Sarjeant R, Fehlings MG. (2008). Predictive value of intraoperative neurophysiological monitoring during cervical spine surgery: A prospective analysis of 1055 consecutive cases. *Journal of Neurosurgery. Spine*, **8**, 215–221.

Lee YH, Hsieh PF, Huang HH, Chan KC. (2008). Upper airway obstruction after cervical spinal fusion surgery: Role of cervical fixation angle. *Acta Anesthesiologica Taiwan*, **46**, 134–137.

Lennarson PJ, Smith D, Todd MM, et al. (2000). Segmental cervical spine motion during orotracheal intubation of the intact and injured spine with and without external stabilization. *Journal of Neurosurgery*, **92**, 201–206.

Lewandrowski KU, McClain RF, Lieberman I, Orr D. (2006). Cord and cauda equina injury complicating elective orthopaedic surgery. *Spine*, **31**, 1056–1059.

Manoach S, Paladino L. (2009). Laryngoscopy force, visualization and intubation failure in acute trauma: Should we modify the practice of manual in-line stabilization? *Anesthesiology*, **110**, 6–7.

Mason RA, Fielden CP. (1999). The obstructed airway in head and neck surgery. *Anaesthesia*, **54**, 625–628.

McCleod AD, Calder I. (2000). Direct laryngoscopy and cervical cord damage – the legend lives on. *British Journal of Anaesthesia*, **84**, 705–709.

McGuire G, el-Beheiry H. (1999). Complete upper airway obstruction during awake fibreoptic intubation in patients with unstable cervical spine fractures. *Canadian Journal of Anaesthesia*, **46**, 176–178.

Mercieri M, Paolini S, Mercieri A, et al. (2009). Tetraplegia following parathyroidectomy in two long-term haemodialysis patients. *Anaesthesia*, **64**, 1010–1013.

Miller SM. (2008). Methylprednisolone in acute spinal cord injury: A tarnished standard. *Journal of Neurosurgical Anesthesiology*, **20**, 140–142.

Miller RA, Crosby G, Sundaram P. (1987). Exacerbated spinal neurological deficit during sedation of a patient with cervical spondylosis. *Anesthesiology*, **67**, 844–846.

Morris CG, McCoy W, Lavery GG. (2004). Spinal immobilization for unconscious patients with multiple injuries. *British Medical Journal*, **329**, 495–499.

Nolan JP, Wilson ME. (1993). Orotracheal intubation in patients with potential cervical spine injuries. An indication for the gum elastic bougie. *Anaesthesia*, **48**, 630–633.

Robitaille A, Williams SR, Tremblay MH, et al. (2008). Cervical spine motion during tracheal intubation with manual in-line stabilization: Direct laryngoscopy versus GlideScope videolaryngoscopy. *Anesthesia and Analgesia*, **106**, 935–941.

Sagi HC, Beutler W, Carroll E, Connolly PJ. (2002). Airway complications associated with surgery on the anterior cervical spine. *Spine*, **27**, 949–953.

Segebarth PB, Limbird TJ. (2007). Perioperative acute upper airway obstruction secondary to severe rheumatoid arthritis. *Journal of Arthroplasty*, **22**, 916–919.

Terao Y, Matsumoto S, Yamashita K, et al. (2004). Increased incidence of emergency airway management after combined anterior-posterior cervical spine surgery. *Journal of Neurosurgical Anesthesiology*, **16**, 282–286.

Tokunaga D, Hase H, Mikami Y, et al. (2006). Atlantoaxial subluxation in different intraoperative head positions in patients with rheumatoid arthritis. *Anesthesiology*, **104**, 675–679.

Urakami Y, Takennaka I, Nakamura M, et al. (2002). The reliability of the Bellhouse test for evaluating extension capacity of the occipitoatlantoaxial complex. *Anesthesia and Analgesia*, **95**, 1437–1441.

Appendix – Terminology, anatomy, spinal cord injury

Terminology

An anaesthetist unaccustomed to cervical spine surgery may find the jargon confusing. Table 26.3 contains common definitions. The term 'instability' is particularly difficult to deal with as it may mean anything from pain on movement, being more at risk in a fall, or developing a deformity in months or years to come, to gross movement or angulation on small provocation. See Table 26.4 for some definitions.

Cervical spine anatomy

The anatomy of the spine will be familiar to most anaesthetists, but the special characteristics of the occipito-atlanto-axial complex deserves study (Figure 26.7).

The head weighs about 6 kg, so the ligaments and joints of the cranio-cervical junction have to be powerful; the transverse portion of the cruciate ligament of the axis is said to be as strong as the cruciate ligament of the knee. Airway management is influenced by cranio-cervical movement, since extension is required for both basic life support and direct laryngoscopy. In addition, mouth opening is limited if cranio-cervical extension is impaired. Persistent airway obstruction has been reported after cranio-cervical fixation when the fixation resulted in excess flexion. The range of motion between complete flexion and extension is about 24 degrees, but in clinical practice it is very difficult to identify reduced cranio-cervical movement because compensatory movement occurs at lower levels. Curiously, a test of mouth opening such as the Mallampati, may be a better indicator of cranio-cervical rigidity than observation of cranio-cervical movement.

The spinal cord: It descends to L1/2 but in 2–3% it descends as far as L2/3. The spinal cord is intolerant of retraction so that the significance of perhaps

Table 26.3. Glossary of spinal terms

Spondyl(o): word element [Gr], vertebra; vertebral column. The term spondylosis is used to describe degenerative changes, commonly osteophytic projections encroaching on spinal or root canals, and spondylolisthesis to describe loss of vertebral alignment.

Myelopathy: any functional disturbance and/or pathological change in the spinal cord, such as transverse myelopathy (extending across the spinal cord), central cord syndrome, anterior cord syndrome, posterior cord syndrome, Brown-Séquard syndrome.

Radiculopathy: any functional disturbance and/or pathological change in a spinal nerve root.

Spinal stenosis: reduction in the calibre of the spinal canal and hence the space available for the cord; due to disc protrusions, osteophytes, tumours and instability.

Instability: instability of the spine is a spectrum of clinical situations, ranging from complete disruption to slowly worsening deformity. It is not easy to define, and the anaesthetic implications range from considerable to slight. A 'two column' concept of spinal integrity is commonly employed. The anterior column comprises the ligaments and bones back to the posterior longitudinal ligament and the posterior column the elements posterior to the PLL (see Table 26.2 and Figure 26.2).

Subluxation: a significant structural displacement, visible on static imaging, such as subluxation of the atlanto-axial joint caused by rheumatoid arthritis, Down's syndrome or infection of the occipito-atlanto-axial complex. Can be anterior, posterior or vertical in direction. Rotatory subluxation of the atlas on the axis can occur in infection – Grisel's disease.

Table 26.4. Some definitions of instability

Symptomatic

'Loss of the ability under normal physiologic loads to maintain relationships between vertebrae in such a way that there is neither initial nor subsequent damage to the spinal cord or nerve roots, and there is neither development of incapacitating deformity or severe pain' White and Panjabi 1990.

However instability can be asymptomatic, as in rheumatoid arthritis, where up to 50% of patients with anterior atlanto-axial subluxation (AAS) may be unaware of the abnormality. Symptoms of AAS include neck, occipital, and facial pain, sometimes lancinating (L'Hermitte's phenomenon). Neurological impairment as a result of AAS is characteristically subtle, although sudden death has been described. The question is often asked as to whether symptomless rheumatoid patients should have flexion/extension radiographs before anaesthesia. Although there is no evidence of benefit in terms of outcome it is sensible to get the radiographs, because of 'outcome bias' and because current opinion recommends early fixation of AAS.

Radiological measurements

a) Translation

  C1–2: Anterior Atlanto Dental Interval > 5 mm, Posterior ADI < 13 mm.

  C2–T1: >3.5 mm between points on adjacent vertebrae

b) Angulation

  >11 degrees between vertebrae

These values have been widely used but there is poor correlation between radiographic abnormality and neurological symptoms and signs.

Integrity of anterior and posterior spinal columns

The spine can be thought of as two columns (anterior and posterior); anterior column disruption tending to make the spine unstable in extension and posterior column damage favouring instability in flexion.

The Cranio-Cervical Junction or
The Occipito - Atlanto - Axial Complex

Figure 26.7. The relevant anatomy of the cranio-cervical junction.

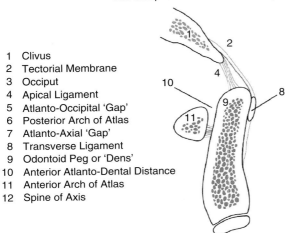
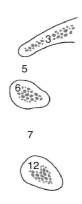

1 Clivus
2 Tectorial Membrane
3 Occiput
4 Apical Ligament
5 Atlanto-Occipital 'Gap'
6 Posterior Arch of Atlas
7 Atlanto-Axial 'Gap'
8 Transverse Ligament
9 Odontoid Peg or 'Dens'
10 Anterior Atlanto-Dental Distance
11 Anterior Arch of Atlas
12 Spine of Axis

the commonest indication for spine surgery, disc protrusion, is considerably different at different spinal levels in terms of the simplicity of surgical approach, because of the anatomical structures that surround the spine. At lumbar levels, disc protrusions can be approached posteriorly because the cauda equina can be retracted to allow extraction of disc fragments. At thoracic levels the approach must be lateral, either through a thoracotomy, or costotransversectomy (removing the head of a rib). At cervical levels the approach can be anterior, but the oesophagus and great vessels are hazarded. Anterior lesions above C2 can require a mandibular or maxillary split.

Blood supply: The cord derives its blood supply from anterior and posterior longitudinal arteries arising from the vertebral arteries, and radicular arteries arising from the aorta. The main vessels form a plexus around the cord, and perforating vessels enter the cord. Spinal cord blood flow is believed to be governed by the same mechanisms that apply to cerebral blood flow. There are characteristic patterns of neurological impairment due to ischaemia; the commonest are the syndromes of central and anterior cord ischaemia (Figure 26.8).

The vertebral arteries are well-protected, but also vulnerable to damage in cervical trauma and surgery, as their course is within the bone. There is often a relatively large radicular vessel, which is known as the artery of Adamkiewicz.

Spinal cord injury

SCI can be complete or incomplete. In complete SCI there is loss of motor, sensory and autonomic function below the lesion. The commonest pattern of incomplete SCI is the central cord syndrome. Anterior and Brown-Séquard syndromes are recognised, as well as the Cauda Equina syndrome due to damage to the neuraxis below the conus of the spinal cord. It is characterised by a lower motor neurone type palsy with loss of bladder and bowel function.

Demographics and associations: Youth, male sex, intoxication with alcohol or drugs are important factors, but there is also an association with falls in the elderly. There is a strong association between severe head or facial injury and SCI, and unsurprisingly, between the finding of a focal neurological deficit and SCI.

Causation: Trauma is the major cause of non-operative SCI. Vertebral fracture or dislocation is frequently present but SCI can occur when there is no radiographic abnormality (Spinal Cord Injury Without Radiographic Abnormality – SCIWORA). Operations on the spine carry a risk of SCI, which increases with the complexity of the surgery and is more likely if a myelopathy is already present. SCI occurs during non-spinal operations, presumably due to a combination of relative malposition and hypotension, and many of these patients are subsequently found to have spinal stenosis. SCI has been described

Central Cord Syndrome

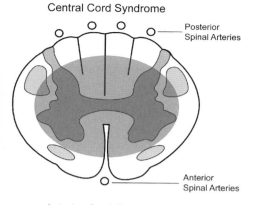

Anterior Cord Syndrome

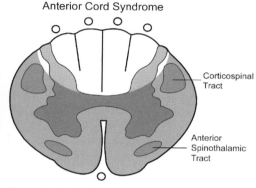

Figure 26.8. The diagram illustrates the areas of cord ischaemia associated with central and anterior cord syndromes. Central cord syndrome is characterised by relative sparing of the lower limb function (the axons supplying the legs descend more peripherally in the cortico-spinal tracts), bladder dysfunction and variable sensory loss. Anterior cord syndrome is characterised by complete motor paralysis below the level of the lesion due to interruption of the corticospinal tract; loss of pain and temperature sensation at and below the level of the lesion due to interruption of the spinothalamic tract; preserved proprioception and vibratory sensation due to intact dorsal columns.

in conscious individuals with normal spines who have adopted, or been forced to adopt, an abnormal posture. It is important to realise that the phenomenon of SCI during anaesthesia is not confined to the cervical region, but also occurs in the thoracic and lumbar (cauda equina) regions. There are many reports of SCI below the cervical level during anaesthesia; the three patients described by Lewandrowski et al are examples. The reports of these cases do not, of course, attempt to ascribe causation to airway management, but when a SCI occurs in the cervical region airway management is nearly always indicted, although the two cases recently described by Mercieri et al (SCI following parathyroidectomy in patients with spinal stenosis) suggest that this may be changing.

Prolonged relative malposition and hypotension seem likely causative factors in at least some cases of SCI during anaesthesia.

Autonomic consequences: Impairment and imbalance between sympathetic and parasympathetic supply (autonomic dysreflexia) can result in cardiovascular instability. Hypotension and bradycardia are common but not invariable in the acute phase, the term 'spinal shock' is often used. Postural hypotension and instability of blood pressure can be a persistent problem. Autonomic dysreflexia can cause dangerous hypertensive crises. Urological manipulation is a common cause and problems are most often seen with lesions above T6. Treatment is postural (sit the patient up), pharmacological with sub-lingual captopril or nifedipine, or anaesthetic with sevoflurane or isoflurane. Neuraxial block is an effective prophylactic measure.

Prevention of secondary cord injury

Hypoxia: This must be prevented; possible aggravations of SCI by airway management manoeuvres are of secondary importance compared with the primacy of maintaining oxygen supply to damaged cord. No method of intubation has been shown to be associated with an improved outcome.

Spinal cord perfusion: Perfusion must be maintained, and a mean blood pressure of 85 mmHg has been recommended for the first week after injury, but hypertension may be inappropriate since in experimental models cord swelling after trauma can be aggravated by severe hypertension. Fluid overload may aggravate cord swelling. Vasoconstrictor drugs are often needed to maintain perfusion pressure. Hyperglycaemia (and hypoglycaemia) should be avoided.

Immobilisation: After suspected spinal injury immobilisation is a standard. Whilst the concept does seem a priori to be a sensible one, it is also certain that there are hazards. Immobilisation methods may force the patient into a position they would not voluntarily adopt, and cause ischaemic pain and tissue damage over pressure points. Collars can increase ICP and contribute to airway obstruction in patients with obtunded consciousness. A Cochrane analysis found no evidence of improved outcome and Hauswald et al reported a worse outcome in patients who were immobilised after blunt cervical injury. Manual In Line Stabilisation (MILS) is recommended during airway management, but there is no evidence of improved outcome, and as with cricoid pressure MILS should be adjusted or released if necessary to achieve ventilation.

Detection of injury: Observational studies have found that there is a higher incidence of later neurological impairment in patients who did not have early diagnosis of spinal injuries. However it is also accepted that a proportion (about 5%) of patients with a spinal injury will suffer a neurological deterioration despite all care. This can occur hours to weeks after the initial injury (subacute post-traumatic ascending myelopathy). The reasons for late deterioration are uncertain but vertebral artery damage is common and it may reflect circulatory instability. This uncomfortable fact should be borne in mind whenever a patient with a history of a spinal injury requires an anaesthetic.

Pharmacological methods: High-dose methylprednisolone after SCI is controversial, and much less used. Many practitioners believe that convincing evidence of benefit that justifies an increased risk of infection, hyperglycaemia, and psychosis is lacking. Magnesium is successful in experimental models, but not at doses that would be tolerable in vivo.

Hypothermia: The debate about the possible benefit of 'moderate' ($33\,^{\circ}$C) hypothermia continues.

The advent of efficient intravascular cooling devices makes hypothermia an achievable goal. However whether any benefit exceeds the disadvantages, the duration necessary, and how slowly hypothermia should be reversed remain uncertain. As with traumatic brain injury hyperthermia should be avoided.

Spinal cord monitoring: Sensory and motor evoked potentials have not been proved to improve outcome. Both false positive and false negative results occur; Kelleher et al found that sensory potentials had poorer sensitivity but higher specificity (52 and 100%) than motor potentials (100 and 96%). Nevertheless, since evoked potentials are sensitive to hypotension, they offer some guide to what level of blood pressure can be allowed. For both sensory and motor potentials the best results can be gained with propofol infusions, though sensory recordings can be elicited in the presence of volatile agents. Motor potentials are abolished by volatile agents, and muscle-relaxant drugs, so that propofol and remifentanil infusions are the most convenient anaesthetic technique. Motor evoked potentials cause muscular contraction and tongues and tracheal tubes have been badly bitten. An effective bite-block must be used.

Airway management: see text.

Chapter 27

Thoracic anaesthesia

Adrian Pearce

Thoracic surgical operations require the anaesthetist to be able to cease ventilation and allow deflation of the operative lung, to protect the lower lung from contamination with blood, tumour or infective material and to continue ventilation of the non-operative, dependent lung. Without the ability to separate and independently ventilate the lungs, thoracic surgery is hazardous. The first planned pulmonary resection by Block on a young female relative in 1883 was a disaster. She died on the operating table and Block committed suicide. A major component of safe thoracic anaesthesia is the appropriate use of endobronchial tubes, double-lumen tubes and bronchial blockers. Indications for their use are not restricted to pulmonary surgery, and there are other clinical indications for lung separation (Table 27.1).

Endobronchial tube

The first attempts at selective lung ventilation were with endobronchial tubes. These long, single-lumen tubes were placed in the bronchus of the dependent, non-operative lung. The classical technique, devised by Magill, was to load the tube onto a rigid intubating bronchoscope and place the tube under direct bronchoscopic view. It was possible to ventilate both lungs at the end of surgery by withdrawing the endobronchial tube into the trachea. The technique of one-lung ventilation by endobronchial placement of a single-lumen tube is still in practice in specialised circumstances, usually with blind or fibreoptic positioning into the appropriate bronchus.

The next development was of a combined tracheal tube and bronchial blocker (Macintosh–Leatherdale). This tube consisted of a standard tracheal tube and a cuffed blocker limb which entered the bronchus of the operative lung. Both lungs could be ventilated when the blocker cuff was deflated, and subsequent

Table 27.1. Indications for lung separation

- Open pulmonary or pleural surgery
- Thoracoscopic procedures
- Unilateral pulmonary haemorrhage
- Unilateral pulmonary infection
- Thoracic vascular or gastrointestinal (GI) surgery
- Thoracic spine surgery (anterior approach)
- Bronchopleural fistula
- Tracheobronchial airway disruption
- Unilateral pulmonary lavage
- Independent lung ventilation in intensive care unit (ICU)

inflation of the cuff would isolate the operative lung. A long narrow channel through the blocker limb allowed egress of air and suctioning of blood or pus from the operative bronchus.

Double-lumen tube (DLT)
Design

The first DLT was designed in 1949 by Carlens (1908–1990) for differential broncho-spirometry, prior to thoracic surgery. Carlens made a tube with two lumens, one longer tube passed into the left main bronchus and the other ended in the lower trachea. A carinal hook engaged the carina to allow and maintain correct placement. In his first study, Carlens inserted the DLT into 60 patients in the awake state under topical anaesthesia. His surgical colleagues at the Sabbatsberg Hospital, Sweden, were so impressed that it was used in thoracic surgery with the first publication of its use in 500 lung resections in 1952.

Core Topics in Airway Management, Second Edition, ed. Ian Calder and Adrian Pearce. Published by Cambridge University Press.
© Cambridge University Press 2011.

Table 27.2. Eponymous equipment for thoracic anaesthesia

Endobronchial blocker

    Magill

    Vernon Thompson

Combined bronchus blocker and tracheal tube

    Macintosh–Leatherdale

Endobronchial tubes

    Magill

    Machray

    Green–Gordon

    Brompton (Pallister)

    Vellacott

DLTs

    Carlens

    Bryce–Smith

    Bryce–Smith–Salt

    White

    Robertshaw

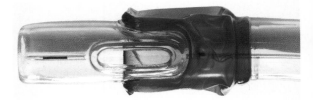

Figure 27.2. Opening in right bronchial limb cuff for upper lobe.

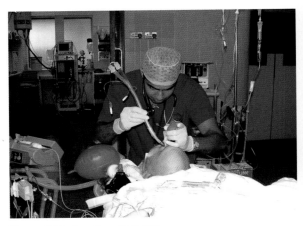

Figure 27.3. Insertion of left DLT.

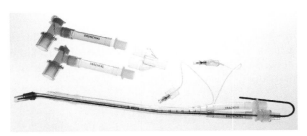

Figure 27.1. Portex right-sided DLT. *Note:* Blue bronchial limb, cuff and pilot balloon.

There have been several designs over the years (Table 27.2) and a number of them (including the original Carlens) are available in single use or disposable, red-rubber or polyvinyl chloride (PVC) material. The Robertshaw design proved particularly popular. Modern DLTs (Figure 27.1) are available as either left- or right-sided (indicating the endobronchial component) in different sizes. Robertshaw ones are available in small, medium and large sizes, and the single use PVC tubes are sized in French gauge (external circumference in mm) with 35 and 37 Fr being suitable for women and 39 and 41 Fr for males. The external diameter of a tube is obtained by dividing its French gauge by π ($\sim$ 3.14).

DLTs are substantially larger than single lumen tubes, and it is not surprising that minor morbidity such as sore throat and temporary hoarseness is more common. There is also the possibility of severe laryngeal trauma such as arytenoid dislocation.

Right-sided tubes have an orifice or slit (Figure 27.2) in the endobronchial portion (often in the cuff) which allows ventilation of the right upper lobe which arises usually 2.5 cm from the carina. No such orifice is needed on the left-sided tubes, as the left upper lobe arises approximately 5 cm from the carina.

Insertion

Pre-insertion checks are to select the appropriate *size* and *side* tube, check inflation/deflation of the bronchial and tracheal cuffs and prepare the special Y-connector that allows connection of a twin-lumen tube to the breathing system. Insertion requires a good technique of direct laryngoscopy (picking up the epiglottis as required) to get the best view of the larynx, with a left-sided tube being introduced with a 90 degrees clockwise orientation to position the angulated tip anteriorly (Figure 27.3).

Table 27.3. Indications for right-sided DLT

- Tumour in the left bronchus
- Left pneumonectomy
- Left lung transplantation
- Left tracheobronchial disruption
- Left bronchial stent in situ
- Distorted left bronchial anatomy

Once the tube is through the larynx, the stylet is removed and the tube advanced such that the lumens are side-by-side in the lower trachea to allow the endobronchial portion to enter the correct bronchus. Insertion depths are 29 cm at the teeth in the average male and 27 cm in the average female.

There is some correlation between depth of insertion and height with one study devising the formula depth of insertion (cm) = $12 + (0.1 \times$ height in cm$)$. Clamping one limb of the connector will stop ventilation of the lung on that side and opening of the cap will allow the lung to deflate when the pleura is open. The open cap allows a route for suctioning and placement of a flexible fibrescope for positioning purposes. It is generally easier to insert a left-sided DLT because of the difficulty presented by the position of the right upper lobe bronchus, but there are specific indications for a right-sided DLT (Table 27.3).

Checking position

Initially it should be confirmed that the DLT is in the respiratory, rather than the gastrointestinal (GI), tract by the methods described in Chapter 16. Then observations of chest movements are made when both lumens are patent and when, in turn, each limb of the Y-connector is clamped. Auscultation of the chest over the lobes should confirm the observation that clamping a limb leads to ipsilateral loss of ventilation with normal ventilation of all lobes of the contralateral lung. A suitable fibrescope should be available for checking or adjusting position of the DLT. Passing the fibrescope first through the tracheal limb allows the anaesthetist to confirm that they have intubated the correct bronchus and that the depth of the tube is correct when a small amount of the blue bronchial cuff can be seen at the carina. With a right-sided DLT, the fibrescope should be placed also through the bronchial limb to make

Table 27.4. Good practice recommendations for DLT placement

- Choose the largest PVC tube that will fit
- Remove the bronchial limb 'stylet' once the tip is past the cords
- Advance the DLT to an appropriate distance (based on height)
- Check position clinically and with fibrescope
- Inflate cuffs slowly and carefully
- Keep intracuff pressures < 30 cm H_2O
- Use a 3-ml syringe for bronchial cuff
- If N_2O used, fill cuffs with saline or N_2O/O_2 mix
- If N_2O used, check cuff pressures intermittently
- Deflate both cuffs before removing or repositioning the tube
- Deflate bronchial cuff when not needed

certain that the right upper lobe is aligned with the appropriate orifice in the tube.

There are a number of published reports of tracheo-bronchial tears due to DLTs, often due to initial overinflation or overdistension of the cuffs with nitrous oxide (N_2O). A review of the world literature published in 1999 identified 33 reports involving 46 patients. The authors made recommendations for safe placement of a DLT (Table 27.4).

Bronchial blocker

A bronchial blocker is effectively a small balloon on a long catheter with a central lumen which, when placed endobronchially, occludes ventilation on that side and allows egress of gas from the isolated lung. It is placed within the bronchus of the operative lung, and early designs were described by Magill in 1936. Fogarty catheters may be used but there are a number of modern blockers. Examples include the Univent tube (tracheal tube with a built-in adjustable blocker, Figure 27.4a and 27.4b; the wire-loop guided Arndt blocker Figure 27.5a and 27.5b) and Coopdech blocker (Figure 27.6). The Univent tube comes in paediatric and adult sizes, and the blocker itself (Uniblocker) is available separately. The Arndt and Coopdech are both inserted through a multiport adapter which has ports for the blocker, flexible fibrescope and breathing system. The Arndt blocker comes

257

(a)

(b)

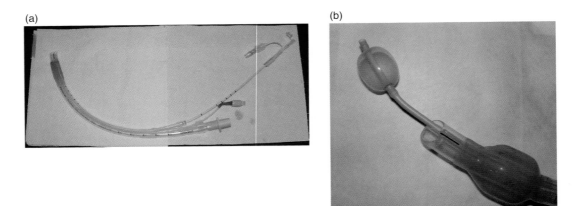

Figure 27.4. (a) Univent tube with torque-control blocker. (b) Tip of Univent tube showing blocker advanced, balloon inflated.

(a)

(b)

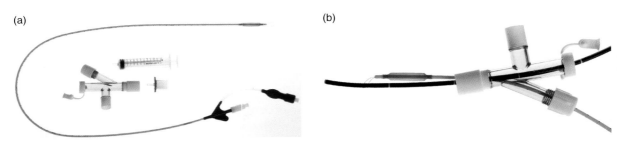

Figure 27.5. (a) Arndt bronchial blocker kit: blocker with wire loop, multiport adapter. (b) The fibrescope passing through the wire-loop of the Arndt blocker.

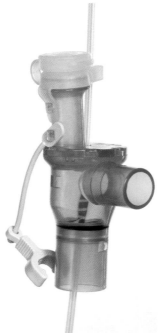

Figure 27.6. Multiport of the Coopdech blocker.

in three sizes for paediatric and adult use, 5 Fr (smallest recommended tracheal tube 4.5 mm), 7 Fr (6.5 mm) and 9 Fr (7.5 mm), each with a low pressure, high volume balloon. The largest adult size comes with either a spherical or elliptical balloon with the spherical being more suited to blockade of the right main bronchus or bronchus intermedius. The steps in placement of an Arndt blocker are given in Table 27.5. User information on the various blockers is invariably available on the Internet.

DLTs are considerably more popular and convenient than bronchial blockers in thoracic anaesthesia, but there are a number of indications (Table 27.6) where a bronchial blocker is preferable and there is a resurgence of interest in them. This is partly due to the design of modern blockers which allows easy placement under vision with a fibrescope but also due to the advantage of continual ventilation through the tracheal tube whilst placement is in progress. It is possible to make a cogent case for the use of a blocker in preference to DLT in non-pulmonary thoracic surgery (e.g., oesophagectomy) where there is no risk

Table 27.5. Steps in placement of Arndt bronchial blocker

- Check which size tracheal tube needed
- Intubate with appropriate single-lumen tube
- Attach multiport connector
- Ventilate patient through breathing port
- Place fibrescope through its port
- Place blocker through its port
- Thread fibrescope through blocker loop (Figure 27.5)
- Pass fibrescope into appropriate bronchus
- Slide blocker off fibrescope into position
- Withdraw fibrescope into trachea and check blocker position
- Inflate cuff to occlude bronchus under fibreoptic vision
- Remove blocker loop only when correctly placed
- Loop may be re-inserted in 9Fr blocker only

Table 27.6. Relative indications for bronchial blocker over DLT

- Abnormal tracheo-bronchial anatomy
- Difficult intubation
- Tracheostomy tube in situ
- Paediatric patients
- When post-operative ventilation planned
- When patient ventilated pre-operatively

Table 27.7. Advantages of DLT over bronchial blocker

Easier and quicker to position

Can often be placed clinically without fibrescope

More rapid lung collapse (DLT has much larger lumen than blocker)

Less likely to be displaced during surgery

Better protection of non-operative lung from gross soiling

Allows suctioning of each lung separately

CPAP easily applied to operative lung

Allows independent lung ventilation

Use of introducer

The introducer is a useful aid to intubation with single lumen tube by direct laryngoscopy but the normal introducer is too short to place a DLT in the same manner. An adaption (Figure 27.7) is to load the introducer through the bronchial limb of the DLT prior to laryngoscopy with 10–15 cm introducer protruding (as in the first recorded use of a gum-elastic bougie in the late 1940s). At direct laryngoscopy the introducer guides the tube through the glottic aperture. Only the larger 39 and 41 Fr DLTs can accommodate a standard introducer in the bronchial limb.

Tube exchange catheter

A single lumen tube can be placed by an alternative to direct laryngoscopy (e.g., flexible or rigid indirect laryngoscopy) and a long narrow tube exchange catheter (100–110 cm) inserted through this. One catheter made specifically by Cook for DLT exchange is 100 cm long, extra firm with a soft-tip. The single lumen tube is removed and the bronchial limb of the DLT advanced over the tube exchange catheter. The catheter should not be inserted beyond the lower trachea (24–25 cm at the teeth) to avoid carinal or bronchial damage, and it is helpful to retract the tongue with a rigid laryngoscope blade during intubation. The tube exchange catheters are supplied with rapi-fit connectors to allow low or high pressure ventilation in case of difficulty or desaturation during the tube exchange. Low-pressure ventilation is much preferred because of the high risk of barotrauma with high pressure ventilation.

of lung soiling, but bronchial blockers do have limitations and Table 27.7 lists some of the advantages of double lumen tubes.

Lung isolation and the difficult airway

Placement of a DLT is more awkward than a single lumen tube and a difficult airway produces additional complexity. Anticipated and unexpected difficult direct laryngoscopy or the presence of a tracheostomy may preclude the normal method of insertion of a DLT. An abnormally narrowed or deviated tracheo-bronchial tree may obviate placement of a DLT. A post-laryngectomy tracheal stoma will readily admit a DLT (short DLTs are produced for this purpose) but only if the stoma is of normal caliber. One of the following options will usually be suitable for a difficult airway.

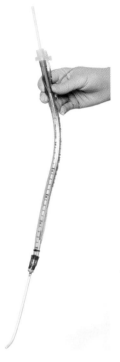

Figure 27.7. Standard introducer placed through endobronchial limb.

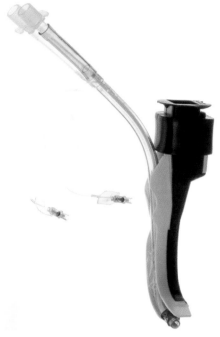

Figure 27.8. Airtraq loaded with DLT.

Flexible or rigid indirect laryngoscopy

Oral flexible fibreoptic intubation with a DLT is a possible solution (in the awake or anaesthetised patient), and the fibrescope can be used to place it in the correct bronchus. It is a more difficult (or at least awkward) technique than with a single lumen tube. A number of the newer rigid indirect laryngoscopes have been used to place a DLT. One model of Airtraq is specifically designed to insert a double lumen tube (Figure 27.8).

Single lumen tube and bronchial blocker

The most versatile solution to the difficult airway is placement of a single lumen tube through the nose or mouth (often by flexible fibreoptic intubation) and subsequent use of a bronchial blocker through this tube. A bronchial blocker can also be used through a tracheostomy.

Supraglottic airway and bronchial blocker

There have been several descriptions, in unusual circumstances such as abnormal tracheobronchial narrowing, where a laryngeal mask has been used to ventilate the patient with the blocker placed through the supraglottic device to achieve lung isolation.

Key points

- Lung isolation is useful in pulmonary and non-pulmonary surgery.
- DLTs are usually simple, quick and effective.
- DLT placement should be confirmed clinically and endoscopically.
- Bronchial blockers (an old technique) are increasingly popular.
- Bronchial blockers have several advantages over DLTs.

Further reading

Arndt blocker on http://www.cookmedical.com/cc/dataSheet.do?id=3988.

Bird GT, Hall M, Nel L, Davies E, Ross O. (2007). Effectiveness of Arndt endobronchial blockers in pediatric scoliosis surgery: A case series. *Paediatric Anaesthesia*, **17**, 289–294.

Brodsky JB. (2009). Lung separation and the difficult airway. *British Journal of Anaesthesia*, **103(Suppl 1)**, i66–i75.

Campos JH. (2010). Lung isolation techniques for patients with difficult airway. *Current Opinion in Anaesthesiology*, **23**, 12–17.

Cohen E. (2008). Pro: The new bronchial blockers are preferable to double-lumen tubes for lung isolation. *Journal of Cardiothoracic and Vascular Anesthesia*, **22**, 920–924.

Ehrenfeld JM, Mulvoy W, Sandberg WS. (2009). Performance comparison of right- and left-sided double-lumen tubes among infrequent users. *Journal of Cardiothoracic and Vascular Anesthesia*, [Epub ahead of print].

Fitzmaurice BG, Brodsky JB. (1999). Airway rupture from double-lumen tubes. *Journal of Cardiothoracic and Vascular Anesthesia*, **13**, 322–329.

Klein U, Karzai W, Bloos F, et al. (1998). Role of fiberoptic bronchoscopy in conjunction with the use of double-lumen tubes for thoracic anaesthesia. *Anesthesiology*, **88**, 346–350.

Narayanaswamy M, McRae K, Slinger P, et al. (2009). Choosing a lung isolation device for thoracic surgery: A randomized trial of three bronchial blockers versus double-lumen tubes. *Anesthesia and Analgesia*, **108**, 1097–1101.

Roscoe A, Kanellakos GW, McCrae K, Slinger P. (2007). Pressures exerted by endobronchial devices. *Anesthesia and Analgesia*, **104**, 655–658.

Russell WJ. (2008). A logical approach to the selection and insertion of double-lumen tubes. *Current Opinion in Anaesthesiology*, **21**, 37–40.

Slinger P. (2008). Con: The new bronchial blockers are not preferable to double-lumen tubes for lung isolation. *Journal of Cardiothoracic and Vascular Anesthesia*, **22**, 925–929.

Slinger P. (2010). The clinical use of right-sided double-lumen tubes. *Canadian Journal of Anaesthesia*, **57**, 293–300.

Vitaid. *Univent Tube.* Available at: www.vitaid.com/usa/univent/index.htm.

Weng H, Xu ZY, Liu J, Ma D, Liu DS. (2010). Placement of the Univent tube without fibreoptic assistance. *Anesthesia and Analgesia*, **110**, 508–514.

Wexler S, Ng JM. (2010). Use of the proseal laryngeal mask airway and Arndt bronchial blocker for lung separation in a patient with a tracheal mass and aspiration risk. *Journal of Cardiothoracic and Vascular Anesthesia*, **24**, 215–216.

Andrew R. Bodenham and Abhiram Mallick

Introduction

Intensive care units (ICUs) were originally developed more than 50 years ago to offer patients short-term respiratory support. Despite advances in other organ support, the fundamental principles of assisted ventilation and airway management have not changed greatly since these beginnings.

Airway care can be very challenging in the critically ill, both to establish the airway and maintain it safely over days, weeks or even longer. With advances in training and equipment, elective airway management in the operating theatre is associated with very low rate of complications. In contrast, in the critically ill patients this is often performed in emergency settings, and complications including a failed airway, hypoxia and cardiovascular collapse are frequent due to the limited physiological reserve of the patient. There may be inadequate time to perform a thorough evaluation of the airway. Skilled airway management with knowledge of airway devices and rescue strategies will avoid or minimise such risks.

Required skills include a) recognising and assessing potentially difficult airways, b) formulating a plan and alternatives for airway management, c) outlining a sequence to maintain ventilation, oxygenation and patient safety according to national guidelines and d) using airway adjuncts, e.g., supraglottic airway devices particularly in unanticipated problem cases.

In this chapter we review tracheal intubation, choice of induction agents and muscle relaxants, safe tracheal extubation, tracheostomy and bronchoscopy in the critically ill patients. The basic patient machine interfaces used in continuous positive airway pressure (CPAP) and non-invasive ventilation (NIV) will also be summarised.

Tracheal (translaryngeal) intubation

Indications

In the ICU, the core indication for tracheal intubation is severe respiratory distress or failure, when CPAP or NIV are considered inappropriate or have failed. Many patients are admitted with a tracheal tube already in situ from the operating theatre, pre-hospital settings, A & E dept, or ward areas.

Indications can be broadly classified into three groups, which may coexist (Table 28.1): a) relieving airway obstruction, b) protection of the airway from aspiration and c) provision of artificial ventilation.

Other indications include control of carbon dioxide in brain-injured patients, investigations (e.g., bronchoscopy, CT or MRI scan) and patient transfers. Most patients with multiple organ failure will require tracheal intubation and assisted ventilation.

Route of intubation

Orotracheal intubation is generally preferred in both elective and emergency settings. Nasal tubes, although considered more comfortable than oral tubes, are associated with a significant risk of nasal bleeding and sinusitis, plus more difficult tracheal suction. They are contraindicated in patients with basal skull fractures, bleeding tendencies and nasal polyps. However they may be useful in patients who are difficult to settle, and are more commonly used in children.

Types of tubes

A full description of tracheal tubes is given in Chapter 10. Particular considerations in critical care are to minimise aspiration past the cuff, and tracheal/ laryngeal damage. There is currently significant

Table 28.1. Indications for tracheal intubation (these may coexist)

Airway obstruction

    Airway oedema

    Tumours

    Head and neck trauma

    Epiglottitis

    Surgery

Risks of aspiration

    Obtunded conscious level

    Brain injury

    Bulbar palsy

    Impaired cough reflexes

Facilitation of IPPV

    Cardiopulmonary resuscitation

    Respiratory failure

    Cardiac failure

    Multiple organ failure

    Major trauma chest injury

Table 28.2. Criteria suggestive of impending need for mechanical ventilation

- Tidal volume < 3 ml/kg
- Respiratory rate > 35 /min
- Vital capacity < 15 ml/kg
- $FEV_1 < 10$ ml/kg
- $P_aO_2 < 8$ kPa
- $P_aCO_2 > 8$ kPa

interest in suctioning systems above the cuff to avoid pooling of secretions and in developing newer cuff designs and the control of cuff pressure.

Decisions to perform tracheal intubation

Patients with respiratory failure, who are not in extremis, may benefit from CPAP or NIV. Decisions to perform tracheal intubation and ventilation should be made primarily on clinical grounds with other objective criteria as a guide (Table 28.2). For example, patients with chronic respiratory or neuromuscular disease may normally have hypercapnia or hypoxaemia, but do not necessarily require assisted ventilation. Consider the underlying diagnosis, possibility of improvement with CPAP or NIV, the clinical trend and serial arterial blood gases. Clinical observations of respiratory rate and depth, conscious level, the ability to cough and talk whole sentences are just as important as arterial blood gases or chest X-rays. If the patient is becoming exhausted then intervention is likely to be required. Tracheal intubation should ideally be performed in a deteriorating patient in a timely fashion during daylight hours, in a safe environment, when skilled assistance is available rather than in a hurry out of hours.

Ethical considerations

In emergency situations tracheal intubation must be performed immediately as part of resuscitation. However in many situations it is possible to delay for a short time, to allow further assessment of the patient and their wishes, and give relatives time to visit. Even a brief opportunity to talk in private can be very important to the families of non-surviving patients.

It may be difficult to withhold tracheal intubation for several reasons: a) there may be little time in which to act; b) by the time the question of intubation arises patients are often not competent to make decisions; c) an order to withhold intubation is likely to result in death, and may be open to later criticism; and d) it is difficult to predict non-survival or futility with absolute certainty.

Some patients will refuse such interventions. However, any decision not to intervene should follow discussion with the patient, family members, intensive care staff and referring teams. It is common for patients and families, who initially insist on such interventions, to change their decision once they understand the burdens of ICU support, and the potentially low probability of survival or good quality of life longer term. There is no requirement for staff to undertake such interventions if they believe it is not in the patient's best interests due to extensive co-morbidities or the fatal nature of underlying disease processes. Nevertheless unless a consensus is reached, any decision to withhold resuscitation is likely to be questioned later. Unless decisions are obvious, the majority of physicians would err on the side of caution, offering the patient the chance of a period of assisted ventilation and revisiting decisions over time.

Any decision to withhold intubation and ventilation should be clearly documented with reasoned arguments in the medical notes. A general DNR and non-escalation order should also be issued to cover other aspects of resuscitation.

Airway assessment

This is described in detail in Chapter 7. Multiple scoring systems have been described to identify the difficult airway, but their value is uncertain in the critically ill. Assessment may be virtually impossible in patients with severe respiratory distress. A focused and brief examination influences the choice of invasive or non-invasive ventilatory support. If a patient needs the former, physical examination of the airway may reveal the risk of difficult mask ventilation and intubation.

The difficult airway

All patients in the ICU should be viewed initially as a potentially difficult airway, when a conventionally trained intensivist would experience difficulty in face-mask ventilation and tracheal intubation. There are numerous conditions associated with difficult airways (Chapter 7), and some will be more common in the ICU patient. These include head and neck trauma and infection, cervical immobility, pharyngeal and laryngeal swelling and morbid obesity. As a result of patient instability there is likely to be far less time for assessment and a much more rapid deterioration in oxygenation.

The difficult airway in this setting includes a) the anticipated difficult airway, b) the unanticipated difficult airway and c) the difficult airway resulting in a 'cannot intubate and cannot ventilate' scenario. Physicians should be able to deal with the latter two rare scenarios. There are issues in relation to initial control of the airway and subsequent management as tubes may get dislodged or blocked on a frequent basis, plus the degree of intubation difficulty may change over time (Figure 28.1).

Preparation for tracheal intubation

Conditions for intubation should be made as safe as possible, within the constraints of the clinical area, and should include an appropriately skilled and experienced person, skilled assistance, optimal patient positioning, lighting, suction, and all other necessary

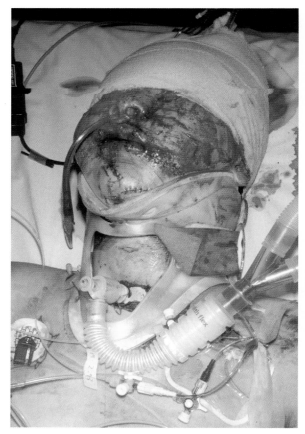

Figure 28.1. This patient has extensive facial and other injuries requiring a few days assisted ventilation. An early open tracheostomy was performed before facial swelling made any requirement for subsequent translaryngeal intubation impossible.

equipment (see Chapter 6). Ideally the same standards should apply as in an elective operating theatre. A supply of 100% oxygen, a well-fitting mask with an attached bag-valve device, suction equipment, Magill forceps, airways (nasal and oral) and bougies should be immediately available. If time allows it may be safer to transfer to the ICU or theatre complex to perform airway interventions. Most ICUs have a mobile pack containing equipments required for tracheal intubation and assisted ventilation, plus portable monitors including capnography. Most ICUs will have a limited range of difficult intubation equipment available with access to more specialised kits from the operating theatres (see Chapters 13, 14, 15). The correct balance of such kits should be determined by the individual unit.

The majority of critically ill patients requiring tracheal intubation should be considered to have a full stomach. Therefore securing the airway with a rapid sequence induction seems logical. In a rapid sequence induction (Chapter 18) the priority is to achieve tracheal intubation and airway protection as rapidly as possible, but with the potential disadvantages of excessive doses of anaesthetic drugs and the routine use of suxamethonium (see below). In contrast a slower controlled sequence induction consisting of titrated doses of induction agents, a non-depolarising muscle relaxant, bag and mask ventilation may offer greater haemodynamic stability, albeit it at a greater risk of pulmonary aspiration. There is no evidence base to support either approach but it is well documented that many emergency intubations in the critically ill are followed by circulatory collapse.

Even with small doses of induction agents critically ill patients can become haemodynamically unstable and vasopressor agents should be readily available. Volume loading the patient, insertion of central venous and arterial cannulae and starting an infusion of vasopressor drugs prior to tracheal intubation may help to control sudden cardiovascular collapse.

Choice of drugs for intubation

Tracheal intubation may be possible without the use of anaesthetic drugs or muscle relaxants in patients following cardiorespiratory arrest or deep coma. In all other situations drugs will be required to anaesthetise the patient, and to obtund airway and cardiovascular reflexes. Patients with an obvious difficult airway, e.g., dental abscess/cervical spine fracture are likely to require an awake fibreoptic intubation or a surgical airway in a theatre environment.

Induction agents including propofol (1–2 mg/kg), etomidate (0.1–0.2 mg/kg), ketamine (0.5–2 mg/kg) and midazolam (2–10 mg) are used to facilitate intubation in critically ill patients. In obtunded patients smaller doses will be sufficient. All agents should be cautiously administered due to inherent risks of cardiovascular collapse.

Muscle relaxants are usually required to facilitate intubation. Suxamethonium, (1 mg/kg) provides excellent intubating conditions in less than a minute and is the traditional drug of choice for rapid sequence induction. However it has a number of side effects very relevant to critical care (Table 28.3):

- Bradycardia, hypotension, and increased salivation/bronchial secretions can be blocked by atropine.

Table 28.3. Contraindications to suxamethonium

Absolute	Relative
Recent significant burns or crush injuries	Severe overwhelming sepsis
Spinal injury (after 24 hours of injury)	Prolonged immobility
Raised K^+, usually renal failure	Neuromyopathies, including critical illness neuropathy
Myasthenia gravis	Cholinesterase deficiency
Dystrophia myotonica and other muscular dystrophies	
History of malignant hyperpyrexia	
History of previous allergy	

- All patients suffer small increases (0.5–1 mmol/L) in serum potassium; avoid suxamethonium in patients with hyperkalaemia.
- Unpredictable rise in serum potassium concentration can occur in patients with major acute burns, prolonged immobility, upper or lower motor neurone lesions, massive crush injuries and various myopathies resulting in ventricular arrhythmias and asystole.
- We believe suxamethonium is probably over-used by trainees and discourage its reflex use in critical care as it is easy to inadvertently use it in unexpectedly susceptible patients. Consider the risk benefits on an individual patient basis.

Non-depolarising agents are the alternatives. Rocuronium has the fastest onset of action, and a dose of 0.8–1.2 mg/kg provides good intubating conditions within 60 seconds. It may be necessary to reverse its action soon after its administration, especially in a 'cannot intubate or ventilate' scenario. Sugammadex, a cyclodextrin compound, rapidly reverses rocuronium (and vecuronium), even after administration in full dosage. It is likely that rocuronium and vecuronium will be increasingly used for tracheal intubation when suxamethonium is contraindicated. Atracurium and cisatracurium offer the most predictable kinetics in patients with renal failure and are the usual maintenance drugs. Atracurium causes histamine release and should be avoided in asthma/COPD.

Intubation sequence

It is important to be prepared for unforeseen complications with or without facemask ventilation dependent on the degree of hypoxaemia and risk of aspiration during tracheal intubation in the critically ill patients. Pre-oxygenation by administration of 100% O_2 via a non-rebreathing mask increases the margin of safety in the event of difficulties. However in such patients there may be loss of lung volumes, diffusion problems, V/Q mismatch, hypercarbia and high metabolic rates, such that pre-oxygenation may not always prevent rapid desaturation.

Following pre-oxygenation, rapid sequence induction is advocated with an assistant applying cricoid pressure. Following tracheal intubation cricoid pressure is maintained until the cuff is inflated and a capnograph trace is confirmed. The cuff pressure should be measured and adjusted frequently thereafter using a standard pressure gauge to less than 25 mmHg, or the lowest pressure compatible with IPPV, to reduce the risks of tracheal mucosal injury from prolonged intubation. A chest x-ray identifies inadvertent endobronchial intubation and lung collapse.

Complications

Complications of tracheal intubation are discussed in Chapter 11. Long-term complications include mucosal oedema and erosion, granuloma formation, cartilage infection/collapse/destruction, in both the trachea and larynx. These may present as voice changes, or airway obstruction and stridor following extubation. Such injuries may be partly responsible for failed trials of extubation. Such complications are minimised by close attention to the choice of tubes and cuff, careful regular adjustment of cuff pressure, timely conversion to tracheostomy and early decannulation of the trachea.

Sedative and analgesic agents to maintain longer term intubation and IPPV

Sedative and analgesic drugs are required for patients to tolerate endotracheal intubation and assisted ventilation, particularly in patients with poor gas exchange. These drugs also reduce awareness of a frightening or noisy environment, provide amnesia for unpleasant procedures including insertion of invasive catheters and analgesia for painful wounds. In addition, sedation may play a therapeutic role by reducing cerebral and systemic oxygen consumption or myocardial work.

Many units use infusions of midazolam or propofol as sedative agents in combination with an opioid including morphine, fentanyl, alfentanil or remifentanil. There is limited evidence base to choose one over another. The choice of agents will depend on local protocols and condition of patients.

The longer term use of muscle relaxants should be restricted. They may be helpful in patients with acute brain injury to prevent surges in intracranial pressure on coughing or those with critical cardiovascular or respiratory insufficiency, where oxygen consumption may be reduced by paralysis. Use of these drugs can be associated with awareness, especially when surgical procedures are carried out (e.g., bedside percutaneous tracheostomy), hypoxia due to accidental unnoticed ventilator disconnection and possibly critical illness neuromyopathies.

Humidification

Adequate humidification is essential to prevent drying and thickening of secretions in the airway and tracheal tube. This is generally provided by a heated water system on the inspiratory limb of the ventilator circuit.

Physiotherapy and tracheal suction

The presence of a tracheal tube and the effects of analgesia and sedation impair the ability to cough and clear secretions. Regular physiotherapy and suction of the airway is essential to prevent accumulation of secretions.

Airway obstruction in the intubated patient

This is common in the ICU and may be due to biting, kinking or dislodgement of the tracheal tube or the effects of thick secretions, blood clot or occasionally a foreign body. Adequate humidification, regular suctioning and careful fixation of tracheal tubes avoids most problems, but these may still arise particularly if the tracheal tube is small in diameter.

It is important to recognise and act on these problems immediately. Typical clues are increased airway pressures, falling tidal volumes, inability to inflate the chest manually, hypoxaemia, raised $PaCO_2/EtCO_2$ ratio or an absent $EtCO_2$ trace. Attempt to ventilate with 100% oxygen with a self-inflating bag. If ventilation is impossible, remove the tracheal tube and manually ventilate the patient with a bag and mask via oral airway or LMA, before re-intubation. If ventilation is possible, pass suction catheters via the tracheal tube. Saline up to 10–20 ml instilled down the tracheal tube helps to loosen thick secretions. In 'ball valve' obstruction the chest can be inflated but exhaled gas is trapped by a plug of mucus or blood impinging on the end of the tracheal tube. If suction catheters or bronchoscopy are unhelpful, apply suction directly to the tracheal tube to aspirate secretions or remove it with suction applied dragging the plug out at the same time. Do not be afraid to replace the tube early; it may be life saving – 'if in doubt take it out'.

Weaning from assisted ventilation

As the patient's condition improves, mechanical ventilation can be gradually reduced until breathing is unassisted. The decision to wean is largely clinical, based on improving respiratory function and resolving underlying pathology. Typical criteria for successful weaning are shown in Table 28.4. A number of studies have shown that weaning is often delayed unnecessarily and the use of sedation holds and weaning protocols may reduce the time to extubation. Some patients, particularly post-operative elective surgical cases, will tolerate weaning well and can be rapidly extubated. Others, particularly those who have been ventilated for some time, or who have significant lung damage, neurological injury or muscle wasting, may take longer and benefit from a tracheostomy.

Some patients tolerate a trial of extubation and a brief period of NIV. However others fail to manage even with CPAP and pressure support before getting tired, as indicated by poor cough, sweating, increasing pulse and respiratory rate (rapid shallow breaths). These patients will need rest periods on the ventilator between periods of CPAP and pressure support and weaning is often protracted.

Tracheal extubation

This is covered in detail in Chapter 17. Particular issues are the potential need to re-intubate following a trial of extubation or accidental extubation. Re-intubation may be unexpectedly difficult as patients may be hypoxic, distressed and uncooperative and have multiple risk factors including airway oedema, which is common after prolonged intubation.

Table 28.4. Typical criteria for successful weaning

Neuromuscular	Awake and cooperative
	Good muscle tone and function
	Intact bulbar function
Haemodynamic	No dysrhythmias
	Hb greater than 8.0gm/litre
	Minimal inotrope requirements
	Optimal fluid balance
Respiratory	FiO_2 <0.4
	PEEP < 10 cmH_2O
	No significant respiratory acidosis (pH< 7.3 or $PaCO_2$ <6.5 kPa)
	Good cough
Metabolic	Normal pH
	Normal electrolyte balance
	Non-distended abdomen
	Adequate nutritional status
	Normal CO_2 production
	Normal oxygen demands

Some patients will extubate without difficulty, others will rapidly deteriorate as a result of inadequate respiratory effort or clearance of secretions. These patients will require re-intubation, ventilation and another period of optimisation and consideration for tracheostomy. Some patients will benefit from weaning straight onto mask CPAP or NIV.

Extubation of a patient with a known difficult airway requires careful planning in anticipation for potential re-intubation. If there are doubts about airway patency prior to extubation then direct laryngoscopy, fibreoptic bronchoscopy, assessment of leak upon cuff deflation are useful checks. Patients who are considered likely to be difficult to re-intubate, can be extubated with an airway exchange catheter in situ, to allow rapid re-intubation. Intravenous dexamethasone, nebulised adrenaline and Heliox have been used with variable success in such circumstances.

Tracheostomy
Indications and timing

Most critically ill patients tolerate short-term translaryngeal tracheal intubation with minimal complications but prolonged use of this route (longer than 1–2 weeks) may be associated with increased risk. Tracheostomy is indicated in patients who require prolonged weaning, have failed extubation, are unable to protect their airway or require prolonged tracheo-bronchial toilet. It limits laryngeal injury secondary to extended translaryngeal intubation and is used for prolonged mechanical ventilation. Emergency tracheostomy/cricothyroidotomy is required for critical upper airway obstruction or the lost airway in the 'can't ventilate, can't intubate' scenario.

Tracheostomy is more comfortable than translaryngeal intubation and this can reduce the undesirable effects of sedation and analgesia to improve cough, respiratory drive, gut function and overall mobility. The timing of tracheostomy remains variable due to a lack of early objective criteria to identify patients most likely to benefit and relies on professional judgement. However the current trend seems to be 'early' tracheostomy, within the first week of tracheal intubation in patients thought likely to be slow to wean.

The recently completed Tracman study which investigated outcomes following early (4 days) versus late (>10 days) tracheostomy in ventilated patients in ICUs, failed to show a benefit from either approach. This study followed smaller underpowered studies with various design weaknesses, which supported 'early' tracheostomy.

Open versus percutaneous tracheostomy

Tracheostomy can be performed by conventional open surgery in the operating theatre or at the bedside. The increased popularity of bedside percutaneous dilational tracheostomy (PDT) has relegated open tracheostomy to a back-up technique in many centres; for patients with a failed or predicted difficult PDT, abnormal anatomy or emergency situations.

Irrespective of technique, tracheostomy carries inherent risks of bleeding, airway obstruction, hypoxia, hypercarbia, pneumothorax and other life-threatening complications. In the critically ill there is little margin for error, and all procedures should be performed or directly supervised by competent operators.

PDT had been found safe in terms of immediate and late complications. The reported complications are summarised in Table 28.5. The advantages of bedside PDT over surgical tracheostomy are mainly

Table 28.5. Complications after tracheostomy

Immediate

- Bleeding
- Puncture of the tracheal tube cuff
- Needle damage to the fibreoptic bronchoscope
- Dislodgement of the tracheal tube
- Anaesthetic awareness
- Hypoxia and hypercapnia
- Increased intracranial pressure
- Damage to the trachea
- Damage to the oesophagus
- False passage of tracheostomy tube
- Pneumothorax/ pneumomediastinum
- Airway obstruction due to blood clot

Early

- Collapsed lung
- Surgical emphysema
- Dislodgement of the tracheostomy tube
- Tension pneumothorax
- Tube blockage from mucus plugs

Late

- Tube blockage from mucus plugs
- Minor bleeding from erosion of small local vessels
- Major bleeding (for example, erosion into the innominate artery/vein)
- Local stomal infection
- Subglottic/tracheal stenosis
- Tracheo-oesophageal fistula or persistent tracheocutaneous fistula
- Permanent voice changes or difficulty in swallowing
- Scarring and tethering of the trachea

of convenience and timing. Nevertheless, the ability to offer most patients a safe, rapid bedside tracheostomy without delay has increased the range of patients to whom it may be offered and has an important advance (Table 28.6).

The number of patients needed for a randomised trial of sufficient power to compare surgical versus

Table 28.6. Indications for tracheostomy

1. Failed trials of extubation and weaning from assisted ventilation

2. Prolonged mechanical ventilation

3. Tracheal access to remove thick pulmonary secretions (easier suction than with trans-laryngeal intubation)

4. Airway protection and prevention of pulmonary aspiration (for example, patients with laryngeal incompetence, bulbar dysfunction such as cerebrovascular accidents, severe brain injury, high spinal cord injury)

5. Bypass of upper airway obstruction (for example, patients with trauma, infection, malignancy, laryngeal or subglottic stenosis, bilateral recurrent laryngeal nerve palsy, severe sleep apnoea)

6. Trauma or surgery in the face/neck region

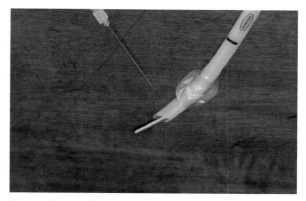

Figure 28.2. Bonfils semi-rigid scope passing through an endotracheal tube. The smooth metal casing protects the scope from the needle damage, and minimises obstruction of airflow and ventilation.

PDT, or indeed the various PDT kits, would be so large and expensive that it is unlikely to be performed. Hence debate over the relative merits of each technique will continue. However a few points can be made with reasonable certainty:

- The skill and experience of the operator and the anaesthetist are paramount irrespective of techniques used. PDT now has established safety data.
- The stomal infection rate from PDT is lower than from open tracheostomy, presumably due to a smaller incision and less devitalised tissues.
- PDT is more difficult if anatomy is unfavourable (i.e., landmarks obscured by adipose tissue or large thyroid, low lying cricoid, large veins overlying puncture site). A small proportion of patients will be anatomically unsuitable for PDT.

Control of the airway during tracheostomy

This is important irrespective of the insertion technique due to the potential for inadvertent extubation and misplacement during the procedure. Separate skilled operators should manage a) the airway and ventilation, anaesthesia and endoscopy and b) the tracheostomy procedure. Airway exchange catheters can be passed via a bronchoscope connector to aid re-intubation if the translaryngeal tube is dislodged. The use of a supraglottic airway device may be helpful if high ventilatory pressures are not required.

Endoscopy is used during PDT in most centres to confirm correct placement of the needle and guidewire and to exclude puncture of the posterior tracheal wall (and oesophageal passage of the guidewire). Endoscopes obstruct the tracheal tube to produce loss of tidal volume, hypoxia and hypercarbia (see bronchoscopy section below), this is reduced with narrow diameter scopes. Expensive needle damage to the flexible scope is avoided by using a semirigid metal scope such as the Bonfils (Figure 28.2.) or using an LMA to keep the flexible scope tip out of the trachea. Capnography connected to the introducer needle can also confirm tracheal placement.

PDT techniques

Various techniques for PDT are described in detail elsewhere. All rely on the placement of an introducer needle and guidewire, ideally between the first/second, and second/third tracheal rings. Higher placement risks damaging the cricoid ring and lower placement risks bleeding from intrathoracic blood vessels and more difficult tube changes. An appreciation of the differences in applied tracheal anatomy between the young and old is important, as in the elderly the trachea may slope backwards at a steeper angle.

High resolution ultrasound scanning of the neck is helpful to identify tracheal rings, the thyroid isthmus and blood vessels (Figure 28.3). Some operators perform an initial blunt dissection of pre-tracheal tissues, and use palpation via the incision to identify pulsatile vessels and the orientation of the anterior tracheal wall before passage of the needle.

269

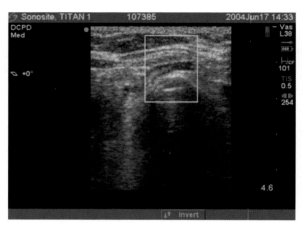

Figure 28.3. Doppler ultrasound scanning of the neck reveals pulsatile vessels in front of the trachea near the potential tracheostomy site.

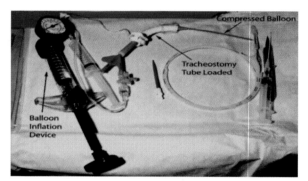

Figure 28.4. Cook Blue Dolphin single step balloon dilation percutaneous tracheostomy kit.

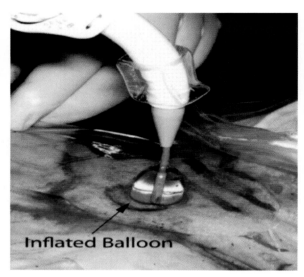

Figure 28.5. Inflated fluid filled balloon dilating stoma during percutaneous tracheostomy, see Figure 28.4 for full kit.

A number of techniques have developed over the last decade using either multiple or single plastic dilators, or forceps, to form a stoma. Most recently balloon dilation has been introduced (Figures 28.4 and 28.5). Following dilation, a tracheostomy tube is inserted with the help of a loading dilator.

Single dilator techniques are the most popular due to the following reasons:

- The single dilator has a hydrophilic coating, which reduces friction to allow smooth rapid dilation of the stoma.
- The faster technique reduces the time during which dilators and bronchoscope obstruct the airway, reducing the risk of hypercarbia and hypoxia.
- The single-step dilator is flexible, tapering to a soft malleable tip, which will bend to the required

angle to follow the direction of the guide wire down the trachea.
- The single dilator reduces aerolisation of blood and secretions compared to a multi-dilator technique.
- The continuous tamponade effect reduces bleeding during the procedure.

Tracheostomy tubes

There are multiple considerations for choice of a tracheostomy tube (Table 28.7). The depth of the stoma should be approximately assessed in each case either by ultrasound, palpation of the stoma, or the lengths of inserted needles or dilators. Endoscopy after insertion, from above via the glottis and through the tracheostomy tube confirms appropriate positioning of the tube and inflated cuff. The stomal section of standard tubes is comparatively short and is only suitable for thin necks (Figure 28.6). A tube which is too short or long will not lie comfortably and will increase the risk of accidental decannulation and damage to the trachea and surrounding structures. Longer adjustable flange tubes should be considered as an option in all cases, particularly where the stoma site is abnormal (Figure 28.7). Such tubes are now available for percutaneous insertion kits and inner cannulae.

Table 28.7. Design considerations for choice of tracheostomy tubes

- Inside and outside diameter
- Stomal and intratracheal component length
- Angle between stomal and intratracheal segments
- Cuff design, Low pressure high volume
- Suction port above the cuff
- Pliability of tube material
- Speaking fenestration
- Inner liners/cannullae
- Tip design for easy passage during PDT
- Soft flange for easy fixation (not causing pressure necrosis on sternal skin)

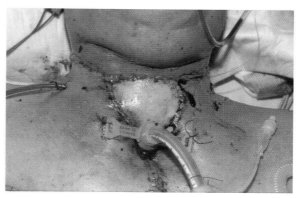

Figure 28.7. An adjustable flange armoured tracheostomy tube passes into a trans-sternal tracheostomy stoma following complex reconstructive surgery for tumour recurrence in the trachea. Innovative solutions to tube placement may be required and there are difficulties in getting cuffs to seal the airway for IPPV.

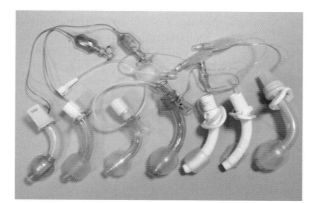

Figure 28.6. Selection of available standard 8 mm internal diameter tracheostomy tubes. Note differences in the lengths of the different sections of the tube.

Changing tracheostomy tubes

Changing a tracheostomy tube in the first 5–7 days before a stable tract has formed can be problematic, particularly after PDT where the tract is tight, and should be avoided if possible. If an early tube change is necessary, it should always be performed by someone who can rescue the airway. The patient should always be pre-oxygenated. A full range of intubating equipments, bougies, tracheal dilators and surgical instruments must also be available at the bedside.

Changing a tracheostomy tube after 1 week is usually straightforward. Nevertheless, care should be taken to suction oropharyngeal secretions pooled above the cuff and to perform thorough tracheal suctioning as the tube is removed. False passage formation can be prevented by railroading a tracheostomy tube over a bougie or suction catheter. A range of smaller tubes should be immediately available.

Removal of tracheostomy tube (decannulation)

Tracheostomy tubes should be removed as soon as possible to regain the normal physiological functions of active coughing, upper airway warming and humidification. There is a tendency to leave tracheostomy tubes in for too long, whilst clinicians await the perfect time to decannulate, and make time consuming referrals to speech therapy. Intensivist-led teams performing a post-ICU tracheostomy review result in timely decannulation, and potentially reduced hospital lengths of stay.

Decannulation should be considered when patients demonstrate a satisfactory respiratory drive, a good cough and the ability to protect their own airway. Patients who show no signs of tiring on CPAP or a T-piece with a low FiO_2 for 12–24 hours are potentially suitable. Coughing secretions up into the tracheostomy tube is a good sign. Generalised weakness, e.g., an inability to hold the head up and an impaired conscious level reduce the chances of success.

Following decannulation, most tracheostomy stomas are allowed to granulate without suturing. They achieve a functional seal within 2–3 days. These partially healed wounds can be quickly re-opened with artery forceps in the first few days after closure, if necessary. Occasional patients will require ENT referral for obstruction, tethered scars or an unhealed

271

sinus. At long-term follow-up, clinicians should be aware of the rare but significant complication of laryngeal or tracheal stenosis giving rise to respiratory symptoms of stridor, persistent cough and voice changes.

Long-term respiratory support

An increasing number of patients are being weaned to nocturnal NIV, where the patient is gradually converted from 24-hour ventilation (often with a deflated cuff) to pressure support ventilation at night with spontaneous breathing during the day. Before removal of the tracheostomy tube nocturnal nasal/facial NIV can be started while tape is placed over the tube and tracheal stoma to prevent gas leakage. Ideally all patients requiring long-term respiratory support would be transferred to a specialist long-term weaning/support unit, with the eventual aim of transfer to home care.

CPAP and NIV

Over the last decade there has been an increased use of CPAP and NIV in acutely ill patients with hypoxemia, COPD, type II respiratory failure secondary to chest wall deformity or neuromuscular disorders, cardiogenic pulmonary oedema, weaning from IPPV, and obstructive sleep apnoea.

Success is dependent on the interface between the patient and circuit. Mask fit is important for comfort and effective support. The correct selection and fitting of the standard facemask, nasal mask, half facemask or a head hood can improve patient compliance and reduce claustrophobia (Figure 28.8). However up to 25% of patients will be unable to tolerate NIV.

Recent improvements in mask design include sophisticated masks which employ cushioned gel and comfort flaps to limit air leakage. Individually moulded masks employing heat sensitive plastic and large masks which enclose the whole face are also now available. Hoods which avoid claustrophobia are increasingly becoming popular for administration of CPAP.

Practical considerations in initiating NIV

Care should be taken to ensure that there are no contraindications. The patient should be able to maintain their airway; there should be minimal oral secretions and no history of recent facial or upper gastrointestinal surgery. In the acute situation a full

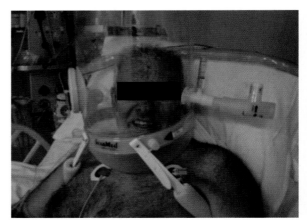

Figure 28.8. CPAP hood (Star Med Spa, Italy, www.starmedspa.com).

facemask of the appropriate size is selected and time should be taken to hold the mask in place to familiarise the patient. Ventilatory support should be increased gradually from an initial setting of 5 cmH$_2$O expiratory peak airway pressure (EPAP) and 12 cmH$_2$O inspiratory peak airway pressure (IPAP) up to 20 cmH$_2$O.

A reduction in respiratory rate and correction of acidosis within a few hours suggests NIV is helpful. As the patient gradually improves, consideration can be given to converting to a nasal mask and gradually reducing the periods and degree of ventilatory support. If the technique fails then the patient should be considered for invasive ventilation or a limitation of care order.

Bronchoscopy

Fibreoptic bronchoscopy is increasingly used for diagnosis and therapy, performed in ventilated patients via a tracheal tube. Common indications include lung collapse, clearance of retained secretions, removal of blot clot, diagnosis of ventilator-associated pneumonia by bronchoalveolar lavage (BAL), detection of airway lesions (e.g., tumour) and visualisation of instruments during PDT. Contraindications are relative and include high airway pressures, critical oxygenation, cardiovascular instability and raised ICP. Careful assessment of risk benefits is required in individual patients.

Management of the airway for bronchoscopy

Separate operators should manage the airway and ventilation, and the bronchoscopy. The bronchoscopist should be prepared to interrupt the procedure immediately if there is destabilisation. Patients are pre-oxygenated, anaesthetised, paralysed and ventilated on 100% O_2. Positive end expiratory pressure (PEEP) should be maintained. Impairment of gas exchange is common due to tube obstruction and when suction is applied through the scope.

Tracheal tubes smaller than 8 mm internal diameter may be significantly occluded by the scope and impair ventilation and oxygenation. A lubricated swivel connector with a fitted rubber cap prevents loss of tidal volume. If pressure controlled ventilation is used, peak pressure setting should be increased to compensate for loss of tidal volume. Suction periods should be limited to 5 seconds or less. Thick secretions often require instillation of saline (10–20 ml) down the injection port to loosen them. During BAL a sputum trap should be used between bronchoscope and wall suction.

Key points

- Full monitoring and the presence of appropriately experienced staff are as important in the ICU as in the operating theatre when managing the airway and performing tracheal intubation.
- Rapid sequence induction is commonly performed in critically ill patients as they are considered to be at risk from aspiration, however suxamethonium should not be used in all patients.
- Slower sequence induction with titrated doses of induction agents and the use of non-depolarising muscle relaxants may be safer in the unstable patient.
- Extubation of a known difficult airway requires careful planning in anticipation of the need for re-intubation.
- Percutaneous tracheostomy is safe provided the operator is trained and patients are selected carefully.
- Tracheostomy tube change in the first 5–7 days should be avoided where possible.
- Tracheostomy tubes are frequently too short for the depth of stoma and should have an internal cannula.

- Bronchoscopy is increasingly performed in ventilated patients both as a diagnostic and therapeutic tool.
- Choice of mask and hood are crucial to the success of CPAP and NIV.

Further reading

Buehner U, Oram J, Elliot S, Mallick A, Bodenham A. (2006). Bonfils semirigid endoscope for guidance during percutaneous tracheostomy. *Anaesthesia*, **61**, 665–670.

Griffiths J, Barber VS, Morgan L, Young JD. (2005). Systematic review and meta-analysis of studies of the timing of tracheostomy in adult patients undergoing artificial ventilation. *British Medical Journal*, **330**, 1243.

Grillo HC. (2004). *Anatomy of the Trachea. Surgery of the Trachea and Bronchi.* Lewiston, NY: BC Decker.

Gromann TW, Birkelbach O, Hetzer R. (2009). Balloon dilatational tracheostomy: Initial experience with the Ciaglia Blue Dolphin method. *Anesthesia and Analgesia*, **108**, 1862–1866.

Intensive Care Society, London. *ICS Guidelines on 'Standards for the Care of Adult Patients with a Temporary Tracheostomy.'* Available at: www.ics.ac.uk.

Kress JP, Pohlman AS, O'Connor MF, Hall JB. (2000). Daily interruption of sedative infusions in critically ill patients undergoing mechanical ventilation. *New England Journal of Medicine*, **342**, 1471–1477.

Lavery GG, McCloskey BV. (2008). The difficult airway in adult critical care. *Critical Care Medicine*, **36**, 2163–2173.

Mallick A, Bodenham A, Elliot S. (2008). An investigation into the length of standard tracheostomy tubes in critical care patients. *Anaesthesia*, **63**, 302–306.

Paw HGW, Bodenham AR. (2004). *Percutaneous Tracheostomy: A Practical Handbook.* Cambridge, UK: Cambridge University Press.

Reynolds SF, Heffner J. (2005). Airway management of the critically ill patient. *Chest*, **127**, 1397–1412.

Schwartz DE, Matthay M, Cohen NH. (1995). Death and other complications of emergency airway management in critically ill adults: A prospective investigation of 297 tracheal intubations. *Anesthesiology*, **82**, 367–376.

Tracman Trial. Available at: www.tracman.org.uk.

Walz JM, Zayaruzny M, Heard SO. (2007). Airway management in critical illness. *Chest*, **131**, 608–620.

Introduction

The anaesthetic literature contains numerous guidelines for airway management, but many of these require the use of expensive equipment which may not be available in a resource constrained environment. Anaesthesia providers in such settings need to rely not only on skill but ingenuity and imagination in the absence of a flexible fibreoptic scope!

The guidelines from organisations such as the Difficult Airway Society and the American Society of Anesthesiologists do contain universal principles which apply as much in resource constrained settings as anywhere else in the world.

- Assess the airway of every patient and formulate a plan of airway management.
- Always have a back-up plan (plan B) in case the first plan fails.
- If confronted with a difficult airway, get help early.
- Maintenance of oxygenation takes priority over other interventions.

Anaesthesia providers in hospitals with limited resources should be familiar with the equipment they have available and be willing to use their ingenuity to improvise alternative airway equipment. All locations where anaesthesia is provided should prepare an emergency airway box and an airway resource cart containing emergency airway equipment. The difficult airway box and/or cart should be checked regularly and users should be familiar with its contents before it is needed in an emergency.

This chapter discusses examples of airway management techniques which do not rely on expensive equipment.

Spontaneous breathing under ketamine anaesthesia

Ketamine is extensively used in the developing world because of its advantages:

- Spontaneous breathing is maintained more reliably than with most other anaesthetic drugs.
- If a patient was able to maintain their own airway awake, they will usually be able to do so under ketamine.
- Airway reflexes are maintained, reducing the risk of aspiration.
- A single drug can produce analgesia and hypnosis.

These advantages of ketamine need to be balanced against the disadvantages including emergence delirium, delayed emergence and copious secretions. Patients anaesthetised with ketamine alone will frequently move and vocalise during surgery. Ketamine anaesthesia can therefore be supplemented with other drugs to reduce these unwanted effects while maintaining the benefits of airway protection. Ketamine alone is not suitable for laryngoscopy. Airway reflexes are maintained and the patient will not tolerate instrumentation of the airway.

Ketamine anaesthesia with spontaneous breathing is a particularly useful anaesthetic for patients with facial burns requiring debridement and skin grafting (Figure 29.1). In such patients intubation and securing the tracheal tube may be difficult but intubation can be entirely avoided with ketamine.

The following is an example of suitable anaesthesia for a burns patient which will maintain spontaneous breathing on room air.

- Ketamine 2 mg/kg IV bolus followed by an infusion of 4 mg/kg/hr

Core Topics in Airway Management, Second Edition, ed. Ian Calder and Adrian Pearce. Published by Cambridge University Press.
© Cambridge University Press 2011.

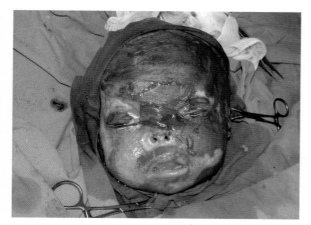

Figure 29.1. Patient with facial burns for split skin graft is anaesthetised with ketamine infusion + midazolam + morphine while breathing room air.

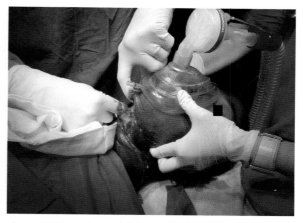

Figure 29.2. Incision and drainage + debridement of neck sepsis. Airway management with a facemask is feasible provided that the surgery is quick and mask ventilation is adequate. A suitable 'plan B' must be considered in advance.

- Diazepam 20 µg/kg or midazolam 50 µg/kg will improve sedation and reduce emergence hallucinations
- Morphine boluses of 50–100 µg/kg titrated to the respiratory rate up to a maximum of about 500 µg/kg
- Propofol boluses of 500 µg/kg if there is still movement or vocalisation despite the ketamine + morphine.

Facemask anaesthesia with spontaneous and assisted ventilation

Laryngoscopy and the muscle relaxation used for laryngoscopy can both be hazardous. The act of unsuccessful laryngoscopy may cause laryngospasm, swelling or bleeding in the airway and may create a 'can't intubate, can't ventilate' situation. In a patient where laryngoscopy has been identified as difficult but no difficulty with a facemask is anticipated, a facemask anaesthetic may be used as the primary plan of airway management. This is particularly useful in short cases which do not require muscle relaxation (Figure 29.2).

Oropharyngeal and nasopharyngeal airways should be immediately available to facilitate mask ventilation. A secondary intervention must be immediately available for airway salvage ('Plan B') in case facemask ventilation becomes impossible. Depending on the clinical situation, appropriate alternate plans may include laryngoscopy, laryngeal mask airway, or a surgical airway.

Features which make mask ventilation difficult or impossible

In the pre-operative airway examination, the patient must be examined for features which may make mask ventilation difficult or impossible (see Chapter 7).

If any of the following features are present, an alternate management plan must be considered.

- Airway obstruction while awake.
- Unable to lie down flat due to airway obstruction.
- Facial hair.
- Other facial abnormality making it difficult to get a good seal with a mask. Edentulous patients with depressed cheeks are difficult to mask ventilate, as are neonates and infants, and patients with trauma or sepsis on the face (including the eyes).
- Unable to protrude the mandible forwards (upper lip bite test).
- Swelling in the neck obscuring the angle of the mandible. The jaw thrust manoeuvre relies on being able to palpate the angle of the mandible and push it forwards.

Limited mouth opening is not necessarily a contraindication to using a facemask. It is possible to maintain a good airway with a facemask using a nasopharyngeal airway. One is more concerned if the mandible cannot move forwards and if the angle of the mandible is not palpable.

Awake laryngoscopy or awake insertion of LMA

If the airway anatomy is abnormal and a difficult laryngoscopy under anaesthesia is anticipated, it is important to maintain spontaneous breathing until the airway is secure. In such cases one may consider laryngoscopy or insertion of an LMA in the awake or lightly sedated patient.

Topical anaesthesia for awake laryngoscopy

The mouth and pharynx is topically anaesthetised with 10% lidocaine spray as far as possible. After 1–2 minutes, the laryngoscope can be introduced to the extent of the topical anaesthesia. Further lidocaine spray can now be applied more distally. The laryngoscope is removed and re-introduced a little further after 1–2 minutes. In this manner it is possible to spray as you go deeper until the glottis is visible. The glottis should be anaesthetised with 2–4% IV formulated lidocaine to avoid laryngospasm that may result from application of the 10% oral spray.

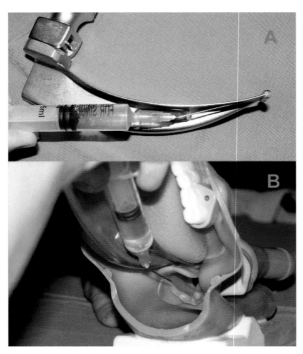

Figure 29.3. A method of applying local anaesthetic spray to the larynx. (A) The needle is bent slightly and will be guided into the mouth along the metal of the laryngoscope blade to avoid accidental trauma to the patient's mouth. (B) The needle is carefully moved away from the metal to spray the larynx under direct vision.

After a further 1–2 minutes, it is possible to intubate the patient. If a syringe and needle is used to apply the local anaesthetic, care must be taken to avoid accidentally pricking the patient's mouth which will bleed profusely. Figure 29.3 illustrates a method of applying local anaesthetic solution to the larynx.

Alternative methods of providing topical anaesthesia include:

- Gargling: a cooperative patient may be asked to gargle with 4% lidocaine. The ability to gargle should be assessed with water first. As the patient gargles, the pharynx will be progressively anaesthetised until local anaesthetic solution is aspirated, resulting in a cough. After the cough, gargling should be maintained for a further 90 seconds to ensure adequate anaesthesia of the larynx.
- Glossopharyngeal nerve blocks: the main factor limiting the success of awake laryngoscopy is the gag reflex, that can be completely abolished by performing bilateral glossopharyngeal nerve blocks.

Laryngoscopy under anaesthesia while maintaining spontaneous breathing

If an endotracheal tube is needed and the patient has features suggesting a difficult laryngoscopy but not difficult mask ventilation, it may be safer to confirm that it is possible to visualise the vocal cords before giving muscle relaxants (see Chapter 6). In such cases anaesthesia can be induced while maintaining spontaneous breathing. Once the patient is deeply enough anaesthetized to tolerate laryngoscopy, the anaesthetist can perform a 'quick look'. It is dangerous to touch the vocal cords with a laryngoscope or tracheal tube at this stage as the stimulus is likely to cause laryngospasm. If the glottis is visible, there are two options:

- The cords can be sprayed with 2–4% IV lidocaine and the tube passed during the same laryngoscopy within 20 seconds (see Figure 29.3).

TAKE NOTE: The 10% spray used for pharyngeal anaesthesia *SHOULD NOT* be used on the cords as it may cause laryngospasm.

- The laryngoscope may be removed. Muscle relaxants and short-acting opiates may then be administered safely while mask ventilation is maintained. Laryngoscopy can then be repeated in a fully anaesthetised and paralysed patient and the patient intubated.

An inhalational induction may be preferable to using intravenous agents which are more likely to cause apnoea. If the inhalational induction is combined with intravenous agents such as midazolam, ketamine, propofol or fentanyl, these must be given cautiously in small doses to avoid apnoea.

Halothane is preferable to sevoflurane for inhalational induction due to favourable onset and offset characteristics:

- Sevoflurane induction is frequently associated with breath-holding.
- The rapid onset and offset of action of sevoflurane means that patients may wake up during the laryngoscopy.
- Conversely, should anaesthesia be deepened to the point of apnoea, recovery from halothane anaesthesia may still occur as the drug is metabolised, while sevoflurane will remain active as the drug can only be excreted by breathing.

The authors do not have personal experience with ether, but inhalational induction with ether may also be quite suitable for laryngoscopy.

If it is not possible to visualise the glottis, spontaneous breathing is maintained and 'plan B' is used. Depending on the clinical situation, plan B may involve any of the following: waking the patient up, continuing with a facemask or LMA, alternate methods of intubation such as blind, light wand, retrograde intubation or a surgical airway.

Lighted stylet intubation

A lighted stylet consists of a malleable stylet with a bright light at the tip which is adjusted to illuminate at the distal end of the tracheal tube. It is placed blindly via the mouth or nose and transillumination is visible in the neck to show the position of the tube. This relatively inexpensive reusable device is a valuable item to keep in the difficult airway cart. See Chapter 14.

Reverse transillumination

In a non-emergency situation, where mask ventilation remains possible, the location of the larynx can be improved by transillumination through the cricothyroid membrane. The brightest possible light source should be used, preferably the output from a cold light source for a bronchoscope. The theatre should be darkened as far as possible. The light is placed over the cricothyroid membrane and laryngoscopy performed. The location of the larynx will be revealed by the glow of transmitted light from the light through the cricothyroid membrane, allowing intubation to be performed.

Blind nasal intubation (awake or under anaesthesia)

Blind nasal intubation was previously popular, but is unfortunately becoming a lost art. Blind nasal intubation remains a valuable technique especially in resource constrained environments without access to a fibreoptic scope. Blind nasal intubation can be performed awake or under anaesthesia. Usually spontaneous breathing is maintained as the air movement though the tube helps to identify the correct position.

The procedure is explained in detail to the patient to encourage good cooperation. Fentanyl 1–2 µg/kg and/or midazolam is given intravenously titrated with care to avoid apnoea. The nostril via which the greatest flow is felt while occluding the contralateral nostril is selected.

Topical anaesthesia for blind nasal intubation

1. Vasoconstrictor drops are inserted into the nostril to reduce bleeding and shrink the nasal mucosa.
2. Transtracheal injection of local anaesthetic. The cricothyroid membrane is identified and punctured with a small IV cannula on a syringe containing 4 ml of 2% lidocaine solution. Air is aspirated to confirm the position of the needle tip in the airway. The needle is removed, leaving the plastic cannula tip in the larynx. Air is again aspirated and the lidocaine is injected through the flexible cannula into the airway. The patient coughs the local anaesthetic up onto the vocal cords and down the trachea.
3. Local anaesthetic gel in the nose. Lidocaine 2% sterile urethral gel is inserted into the chosen nostril. This is a simple effective method of anaesthetising and lubricating the nostril and pharynx. The local anaesthetic gel is inserted into the nostril with the patient lying supine. As the gel warms, it runs backwards and more is inserted to fill the nostril again. In this way

(a)

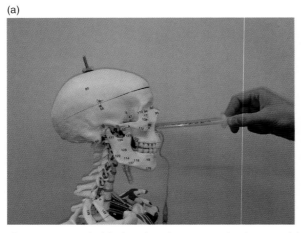

(b)

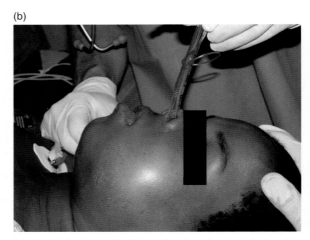

Figure 29.4. Awake blind nasal intubation. Note the direction of the tube is at 90 degrees to the face so that the tube passes below the inferior turbinate and along the top of the hard palate.

10–20 ml of gel is inserted and allowed to run back all the way to the pharynx.

4. Wait at least 3 minutes for the topical anaesthesia to work.

Guiding the tube into the nasopharynx

1. A tube size 0.5–1 mm smaller than for oral intubation is selected. Size 6.5 or 7 is usually suitable for adults. The tube may be softened slightly in warm water according to individual preference. Softening the tube helps insertion into the nose but can make manipulation into the larynx more difficult. The tube should not be softened excessively in hot water.

2. The tube is inserted gently but firmly into the chosen nostril. The direction is at 90 degrees to the face so the tube passes along the top of the hard palate and down behind the soft palate. The tube must not be pushed up into the brain! (Figure 29.4).

3. If the tube does not curve down into the oropharynx easily, the following manoeuvres can help guide the tube downwards:

   - Cephalad distraction of the tube while advancing it firmly but gently
   - Rotation of the tube through 180 degrees and back or through 360 degrees
   - Malleable introducer shaped to a curve
   - Suction catheter passed through the tube and brought out of the mouth to railroad the tube over.

Care must be taken to ensure that the tube has not dissected submucosally behind the oropharynx.

Guiding the tube into the larynx

Position the patient with a small pillow under the occiput to flex the neck but extend the head. Watch for misting in the tube as the air moves through it with spontaneous breathing. The presence of a capnograph tracing is also useful. If air stops moving through the tube, it has most likely gone into the oesophagus and must be withdrawn slightly and repositioned. Advance the tube during inspiration only, as the vocal cords open maximally during inspiration. Watch or palpate the larynx, and observe the movement of the skin caused by the tip of the tube. In patients with significant respiratory pathology and desaturation, oxygen may be insufflated through the tube.

If the tube gets stuck ('hangs up') at any point, make minor adjustments to the head position and/or try rotating the tube. Jaw lift by an assistant or slight flexion of the head helps to get the tube past the epiglottis. Gentle traction on the tongue using fingers or a gentle tissue holding forceps (Allis forceps) is also useful to lift the epiglottis.

If the tube tip is in the piriform recess, a bulge will be visible in the neck on one side of the larynx. Withdraw the tube slightly and rotate it towards the other side, then advance again during the next inspiration. External manipulation of the thyroid cartilage to align the glottis with the tube may be attempted.

If the tube passes into the oesophagus it will lift the larynx and the tube will advance easily to its full length. Withdraw the tube until air movement in the tube is detected. Apply external laryngeal pressure with your other hand and, while feeling for the movement caused by the tube, advance the tube again with the next inspiration.

If the tube does not pass easily into the trachea, the following manoeuvres may be helpful:

- Inflation of the cuff in the pharynx to lift the tip of the tube forwards into the larynx.
- A suction catheter, gum elastic bougie or airway exchange catheter can be inserted through the tube into the larynx and trachea to help direct the tube into the trachea.
- If the tube keeps going into the oesophagus leave it there and put another tube in the other nostril (see section on 'Double tube' below).
- Repositioning of the head: either flexion of the neck if the tube snags on the epiglottis or anterior aspect of the thyroid cartilage, or extension of the head if the tube enters the oesophagus.
- Palpate the larynx yourself – do not allow an assistant to manipulate the larynx. It is possible to feel the position of the tube tip as it displaces the larynx. External laryngeal manipulation can be coordinated with your other hand advancing the tube.

Blind nasal intubation should be accomplished without excessive force.

Good topical anaesthesia is vital for awake intubation. The patient must breathe comfortably without crying, grunting or speaking. Any form of vocalisation involves closing the vocal cords and prevents the tube from entering the larynx. Vocalisation also confirms that the tube has *not yet* entered the larynx. If the patient is uncomfortable and vocalising, efforts to intubate him will be futile. Topical anaesthesia should be reapplied to cover the point of discomfort before further attempts are made. Take note of the maximum safe dose of local anaesthetic (8 mg/kg).

Once the tube enters the trachea, coughing through the tube without any vocalisation confirms correct placement. A capnograph trace will also be present. If the tube goes beyond the extent of the topical anaesthetic and touches the carina, this is a very potent stimulus to the awake patient. Have an assistant ready to inject propofol or other intravenous induction agent immediately before the patient's hand

comes up to pull the tube out! Confirm the correct tube position clinically and with capnography before securing it.

Submental intubation

Patients who require facial reconstruction may have severe maxillary damage, precluding nasal intubation. However oral intubation may not be suitable due to surgical access requirements. Procedural airway management may be achieved by means of tracheostomy, which may be an appropriate technique if multiple operations over an extended period of time will be required. Safe, short-term airway management may be achieved by submental intubation. This carries fewer potential complications than tracheostomy. In addition it provides a better cosmetic scar than a tracheostomy scar.

After routine oral intubation with a reinforced tube, a 1.5-cm skin incision is made medial to and parallel to the inferior border of the mandible in the submental area. A passage for the endotracheal tube is then created through the mylohyoid muscle to the floor of the mouth by blunt dissection with a curved haemostat. The pilot balloon is first grabbed with the haemostat and pulled through the passage. Next, the tracheal tube is briefly disconnected from the breathing circuit and the tube connector is separated from the tracheal tube. While being secured in the mouth the reinforced tube is pulled extraorally with the haemostat. The tracheal tube is reconnected to the tube connector and to the anaesthesia breathing circuit, and the position confirmed clinically and with capnography. The tube comes to lie on the floor of the mouth in the sulcus between the tongue and the mandible. The tube is secured to the skin with silk sutures.

Blind oral (digital) intubation

Blind oral intubation can be performed in awake or anaesthetised patients. However it is less well tolerated by awake patients than nasal intubation and may be impossible if the patient refuses to open their mouth or bites down unexpectedly. Many of the principles, such as adequate topical anaesthesia and the methods of guiding the tip of the tube into the larynx, are similar to blind nasal intubation. A malleable introducer is inserted into the tube and bent to a 90 degree angle ('hockey stick') to guide the tip of the tube around the curve of the tongue and forward into the larynx. Jaw lift and tongue retraction are used to lift the epiglottis and get the tube behind the epiglottis and into the laryngeal aditus. Observation and palpation of the larynx are vital to ascertain the position of the tip of the tube and make minor adjustments to guide the tube into the larynx.

Digital intubation is possible in anaesthetised patients. With the anaesthetist facing the patient's head and standing at the level of the shoulders, two fingers are inserted into the patient's mouth and directed backwards over and behind the tongue. The epiglottis is usually easily palpated and trapped by the fingers against the base of the tongue. The tube is then guided into the larynx between the two palpating fingers for a digitally guided blind intubation. Insertion of the anaesthetist's fingers into the patient's mouth carries a significant personal danger and should thus be reserved for anaesthetised patients who will not bite.

Double tube

The natural alternative path for a tube that fails to enter the larynx during an intubation attempt is into the oesophagus. Recognition of an oesophageal intubation most commonly leads to removal of the oesophageal tube. However the oesophageal tube may be left in place as it provides two valuable functions:

- Inflation of the cuff of the oesophageal tube will occlude the oesophagus and allow safe regurgitation of gastric contents outside the airway.
- The position of the oesophageal tube provides a guide to the position of the larynx – anterior to the oesophageal tube.

A second laryngoscopy is performed with the oesophageal tube in place. A tracheal tube with an introducer, a bougie or an airway exchange catheter can be passed gently anteriorly to the oesophageally placed tube. In the event of resistance being encountered, force should not be applied but withdrawal and gentle redirection and/or rotation of the tube attempted. If the tube is not accurately placed within 90 seconds or the patient shows any signs of desaturation, the attempt should be abandoned and oxygenation maintained with a facemask. Repeated attempts to pass the tube blindly should be avoided as bleeding, swelling or creation of a false passage may occur.

Intubation through Laryngeal Mask Airway (LMA)

The LMA Classic™ or other supraglottic airway devices (SGAs) are available in reusable and disposable forms and have become ubiquitous, even in resource constrained environments. The LMA™ is recommended by the ASA and DAS as the initial rescue device for management of both emergency and non-emergency failed intubations. Other SGAs have also been used successfully as rescue devices.

After successful placement of an SGA, a tracheal tube, bougie or airway exchange catheter may be passed into the trachea if required. An LMA Classic™ tends to direct any flexible device passed through it posteriorly but successful passage of an ETT via the LMA has been well described.

The intubating LMA (iLMA™) is now available in a disposable form that may be affordable in resource constrained environments. The design of this device results in a much improved success rate for tracheal tube placement compared with the Classic LMA™ See Chapter 9.

Rigid bronchoscopy and intubation with bougie/airway exchange catheter

When the mouth is too small to allow conventional laryngoscopy, the glottis may be visualised with a rigid bronchoscope. Care must be taken to avoid damage to the teeth. A retromolar approach with the rigid bronchoscope angled from the angle of the mouth and passing behind the right molar teeth may provide a superior view to a midline approach. A gum elastic bougie or airway exchange catheter is inserted through the rigid bronchoscope and into the glottis. The bronchoscope is carefully removed, keeping the bougie in place. A lubricated tracheal tube is passed over the bougie and into the trachea. A smaller size cuffed tracheal tube (size 6) will pass more easily than a larger size.

Retrograde intubation using guide wire through cricothyroid membrane

Retrograde intubation is useful in three scenarios:

- Elective awake intubation in patients that would be candidates for awake fibreoptic intubation where scopes are available. Topical anaesthesia as for awake blind nasal/oral intubation will be required.

- Intubation in the non-emergency failed intubation pathway (Can't intubate; Can ventilate).
- Intubation after airway rescue in the emergency failed intubation pathway (Can't intubate, Can't ventilate).

Retrograde intubation is preferred to tracheostomy if the cause of airway obstruction is likely to resolve in 72 hours and/or there is a fresh surgical incision in the neck or upper chest (sternotomy).

Retrograde intubation is possible with commercially available kits and is described in the relevant chapter in this book (see Chapter 14).

In the absence of the relevant kit, an alternative is to use a single lumen central venous line kit. The trachea is punctured at the level of the cricothyroid membrane, or lower if the trachea is easily palpable. The bevel of the needle should be directed upwards to allow the guide wire to exit superiorly, via the mouth or nose. Attempting to pass an endotracheal tube over the wire is more likely to be effective if the wire is first covered with the central venous catheter fed over the tip of the wire which has emerged from the mouth or nose, to stiffen it and increase its diameter. The catheter should have all protrusions, such as fixation hubs, removed or cut off (without reducing the length) before use.

The smallest tube of adequate length should be used for initial access as the discrepancy in tube lumen and catheter diameter is minimised. The most appropriate tube is an intubating LMA (iLMA™) tube or a Flex-Tip™ (Parker Medical) tube. If these are not available, a silicone reinforced tube is preferred to a PVC tube, which will have to be used if this is the only tube available.

The chosen tube should be advanced over the guide wire and catheter until the bevel is palpable at the puncture site in the neck. The wire *and catheter* are then withdrawn through the mouth or nose with gentle forward pressure on the tube until the wire is retracted into the tube and the tube advanced into the trachea. Care must be taken to avoid leaving the catheter inside the tube as it would be aspirated. The position of the tube should be confirmed by capnography and clinical signs. If a larger tube is required, tube exchange may be performed over a bougie or airway exchange catheter once the patient is adequately anaesthetised.

Cricothyroidotomy using scalpel

For emergency surgical airway access, cricothyroidotomy is preferable to tracheostomy for the following reasons:

- It is quicker and easier to identify the cricothyroid membrane.
- The airway is more superficial at this point. It is therefore easier to get into the airway instead of the pre-tracheal space.
- It avoids dissection through and thus bleeding from the strap muscles, isthmus of the thyroid gland and the blood vessels surrounding the thyroid gland.

Many suitable kits are available for cricothyroidotomy. However in hospitals with limited resources, these may not be available and if they are, the staff may not be familiar with their use. It is therefore preferable to use simple equipment which is readily available. The following items are needed:

- Scalpel blade and handle. A short rounded blade, e.g., size 20, should be used.
- Size 5 or 6 cuffed endotracheal tube or tracheostomy tube.
- Malleable introducer.
- Tracheal hook (if rapidly available).
- Local anaesthetic with adrenaline.

The cricothyroid membrane is identified, and the skin is infiltrated with local anaesthetic and adrenaline solution (Figure 29.5). The local anaesthetic is omitted to save time if the patient is unconscious in an emergency (Can't intubate, Can't ventilate) scenario.

The scalpel is held vertically with the blade on the skin over the cricothyroid membrane. The scalpel is pushed down so that a small transverse stab incision is made through the skin and cricothyroid membrane into the airway. The blade should be inserted about 1 cm and not more to avoid damage to the back of the larynx.

The scalpel is removed and turned around. The scalpel handle is then inserted into the stab incision and rotated to dilate the stab incision slightly.

The cuffed tracheal tube is inserted next to the scalpel handle into the airway. A malleable introducer bent close to the tip of the tube helps direct the tube down the trachea. A tracheal hook may be used to apply caudal traction on the cricoid cartilage. As soon as the cuff is completely below the skin, do not advance the tube any further. Air entry and capnography are checked and the tube is secured.

281

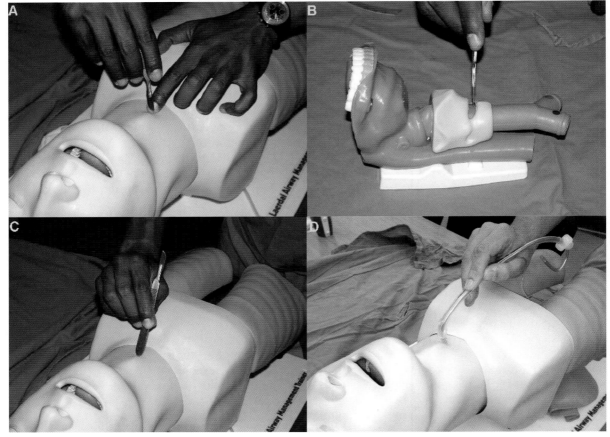

Figure 29.5. Cricothyroidotomy. (A and B) The cricothyroid membrane is identified and a transverse stab incision is made. (C) The stab incision is dilated with the scalpel handle which is rotated. (D) The tracheal tube is inserted with the aid of a malleable introducer.

Tracheostomy

Open tracheostomy is a surgical technique that should be performed in an operating theatre by a surgeon experienced in the technique. A surgeon, scrub nurse and instruments should be available if a patient with a difficult airway unsuitable for an awake technique is to be anaesthetised. The anaesthetist may assist the surgeon with local anaesthesia, particularly skin infiltration incorporating a vasoconstrictor and transtracheal local anaesthetic injection.

Tracheostomy may be required for:

- Elective awake airway control in patients that would otherwise be candidates for awake fibreoptic intubation where scopes are available. Tracheostomy is preferred to retrograde intubation where the cause of airway obstruction is unlikely to resolve in 72 hours.

- Airway control in the non-emergency failed intubation pathway (Can't intubate, Can ventilate).
- Airway control after airway rescue in the emergency failed intubation pathway (Can't intubate, Can't ventilate), particularly after cricothyroidotomy.

Tracheostomy may be performed percutaneously using a variety of commercial kits and has increasingly become a bedside procedure in the ward and ICU. Percutaneous tracheostomy may be performed by intensivists and/or anaesthetists familiar with the technique, as well as surgeons. Fibreoptic visualisation of needle puncture, wire insertion and dilation of the tracheo-cutaneous tract has been recommended. Where a fibreoptic scope is not available percutaneous tracheostomy remains feasible using one of the following techniques to maintain ventilation during the procedure:

- The existing tracheal tube may be pulled back under direct vision with a laryngoscope. The cuff is inflated above the vocal cords but with the tip of the tube still through the glottis. The tube is held in position, the inflated cuff being pushed down onto the larynx to create a seal and allow ventilation during cannulation of the trachea below the level of the cuff. In this way cuff puncture is avoided. However reliable ventilation cannot be ensured by this means and the patient must be carefully monitored for adequacy of ventilation during the procedure.

- Exchange of the existing tracheal tube for an LMA™ or supraglottic airway device (SGA). This is only possible if inflation pressure required for oxygenation is <25 cmH$_2$O. The devices allowing the highest inflation pressure are the LMA Proseal™ or Supreme™.

- A technique that does not require fibreoptic control has been described where the tracheal tube already in place is exchanged for a size 5 microlaryngeal tube. The cuff of this tube is placed as close to the carina as possible, while maintaining bilateral ventilation. The patient is ventilated using volume control, accepting the higher airway pressures for the same tidal volumes achieved with the previous tube as a result of increased resistance of the smaller tube. This allows tracheal puncture, wire passage, dilation and tube placement with the airway maintained by the size 5 tracheal tube. Once the tracheostomy tube is placed, tracheal placement is confirmed by inflating the tracheostomy tube cuff and deflating the tracheal tube cuff. Ventilation will follow the path of least resistance and 'blow' out of the tracheostomy tube. Further confirmation is achieved by attaching the breathing system to the tracheostomy tube. Ventilation will 'blow' from the tracheal tube lumen. This technique has the advantage of maintaining ventilation throughout the procedure and partial posterior tracheal wall protection by the size 5 tracheal tube.

- The existing tracheal tube may be advanced by 4–6 cm. After skin incision and prior to tracheal puncture the tracheal tube cuff is deflated. The cuff is re-inflated for guidewire advancement and initial dilatation. After insertion of the main dilator the tube is partially withdrawn, dilatation completed and the tracheostomy tube inserted. The posterior tracheal wall is protected throughout, and the tracheal tube is only withdrawn completely after clinical and capnographic confirmation of tracheal placement of the tracheostomy tube.

Surgical and percutaneous (if kits are available) tracheostomy are thus feasible options for patients in resource constrained settings where fibreoptic intubation scopes are not available.

Suggested items for difficult airway cart

Comprehensive guidelines for equipment that should be considered in operating theatres have recently been published in South Africa. These guidelines suggest that health facilities should provide:

- An emergency airway box with a limited amount of essential equipment for emergency management of failed intubation. This must include supraglottic airway devices and cricothyroidotomy equipment.

- An airway resource cart with equipment for elective management of an identified difficult airway. This will include a greater variety of airway equipment and alternate devices. A comprehensive list is beyond the scope of this chapter, but is available in the quoted reference (Hodgson RE).

Key points

- Certain principles of airway management apply equally in well resourced and resource constrained environments. These include the need to evaluate the airway of every patient, to plan airway management including alternate plans (plan B) and to ensure oxygenation of the lungs at all times.

- In the absence of expensive airway equipment, anaesthesia providers must be willing to use their skill and imagination to manage a difficult airway. This may at times include the use of unconventional techniques.

- All anaesthesia providers should have quick and easy access to emergency airway equipment and should be familiar with the airway management equipment available in their setting.

Further reading

American Society of Anesthesiologists Task Force on Management of the Difficult Airway. (2003). Practice guidelines for management of the difficult airway. *Anesthesiology*, **98**, 1269–1277.

Amin M, Dill-Russell P, Manisali M, Lee R, Sinton I. (2002). Facial fractures and submental tracheal intubation. *Anaesthesia*, **57**, 1195–1212.

Arora MK, Karamchandani K, Trikha A. (2006). Use of a gum elastic bougie to facilitate blind nasotracheal intubation in children: A series of three cases. *Anaesthesia*, **61**, 291–294.

Batra YK, Mathew P. (2005). Airway management with endotracheal intubation (including awake intubation and blind intubation). *Indian Journal of Anaesthesia*, **49**, 263–268.

Bein B, Scholz J. (2005). Supraglottic airway devices. *Best Practice & Research. Clinical Anaesthesiology*, **19**, 581–593.

Cattano D, Abramson S, Buzzigoli S, et al. (2006). The use of the laryngeal mask airway during guidewire dilating forceps tracheostomy. *Anesthesia and Analgesia*, **103**, 453–457.

Chung DC, Mainland PA, Kong AS. (1999). Anesthesia of the airway by aspiration of lidocaine. *Canadian Journal of Anaesthesia*, **46**, 215–219.

Collins PD, Godkin RA. (1992). Awake blind nasal intubation – a dying art. *Anaesthesia and Intensive Care*, **20**, 225–227.

Craven R. (2007). Ketamine. *Anaesthesia*, **62**(Suppl 1), 48–53.

Davis L, Cook-Sather SD, Schreiner MS. (2000). Lighted stylet tracheal intubation: A review. *Anesthesia and Analgesia*, **90**, 745–756.

Dimitriadis JC, Paoloni R. (2008). Emergency cricothyroidotomy: A randomised crossover study of four methods. *Anaesthesia*, **63**, 1204–1208.

Doerges V. (2005). Airway management in emergency situations. *Best Practice & Research. Clinical Anaesthesiology* **19**, 699–715.

Fisher L, Duane D, Lafreniere L, Read D. (2002). Percutaneous dilational tracheostomy: A safer technique of airway management using a microlaryngeal tube. *Anaesthesia*, **57**, 253–255.

Gold MI, Buechel DR. (1960). A method of blind nasal intubation for the conscious patient. *Anesthesia and Analgesia*, **39**, 257–263.

Helm M, Gries A, Mutzbauer T. (2005). Surgical approach in difficult airway management. *Clinical Anaesthesiology*, **19**, 623–640.

Henderson JJ, Popat MT, Latto IP, Pearce AC. (2004). Difficult Airway Society guidelines for management of the unanticipated difficult intubation. *Anaesthesia*, **59**, 675–694.

Hodgson RE, Milner A, Alberts A, Barrett D, Joubert I, Hold A. (2007). Airway management resources in operating theatres. Provisional recommendations for South African hospitals and clinics. *South African Journal of Anesthesiology and Analgesia*, **13**, 17–23.

Kheterpal S, Han R, Tremper KK, et al. (2006). Incidence and predictors of difficult and impossible mask ventilation. *Anesthesiology*, **105**, 885–891.

Latorre F, Otter W, Kleemann PP, Dick W, Jage J. (1996). Cocaine or phenylephrine /lidocaine for nasal fibreoptic intubation? *European Journal of Anaesthesiology*, **13**, 577–581.

Lenfant F, Benkhadra M, Trouilloud P, Freysz M. (2006). Comparison of two techniques for retrograde tracheal intubation in human fresh cadavers. *Anesthesiology*, **104**, 48–51.

Lim SL, Tay DH, Thomas E. (1994). A comparison of three types of tracheal tube for use in laryngeal mask assisted blind orotracheal intubation. *Anaesthesia*, **49**, 255–257.

Meyer RM. (1989). Suction catheter to facilitate blind nasal intubation. *Anesthesia and Analgesia*, **68**, 701.

Morgan JP III, Haug RH, Holmgreen WC. (1994). Awake blind nasoendotracheal intubation: A comprehensive review. *Journal of Oral and Maxillofacial Surgery*, **52**, 1303–1311.

Nekhendzy V, Simmonds PK. (2004). Rigid bronchoscope-assisted endotracheal intubation: Yet another use of the gum elastic bougie. *Anesthesia and Analgesia*, **98**, 545–547.

Nafiu OO, Coker N. (2007). A rather unconventional use of the laryngeal mask airway. *Pediatric Anesthesia*, **17**, 998–1000.

Owens VF, Palmieri TL, Comroe CM, et al. (2006). Ketamine: A safe and effective agent for painful procedures in the pediatric burn patient. *Journal of Burn Care & Research*, **27**, 211–217.

Raath R. (2004). *Innovative Techniques for Airway Management*. (Abstract). Proceedings of the 2nd South African Airway Management Congress, Durban.

Regan K, Hunt H. (2008). Tracheostomy management. *Continuing Education in Anaesthesia Critical Care & Pain*, **8**, 31–35.

Sarner JB, Levine M, Davis PJ, Lerman J, Cook DR, Motoyama E. (1995). Clinical characteristics of sevoflurane in children: A comparison with halothane. *Anesthesiology*, **82**, 38–46.

Schwartz DE, Wiener-Kronish JP. (1991). Management of the difficult airway. *Clinics in Chest Medicine*, **12**, 483–495.

Sharma B, Sood J, Kumra VP. (2007). Uses of LMA in present day anaesthesia. *Journal of Anesthesia in Clinical Pharmacology*, **23**, 5–15.

Simmons ST, Schleich AR. (2002). Airway regional anesthesia for awake fiberoptic intubation. *Regional Anesthesia and Pain Medicine*, **27**, 180–192.

Stemp LI. (2004). 'Quick Look' direct laryngoscopy to avoid cannot intubate/cannot ventilate inductions. *Anesthesia and Analgesia*, **98**, 1815.

Szmuk P, Ezri T, Evron S, Roth Y, Katz J. (2008). A brief history of tracheostomy and tracheal intubation, from the Bronze Age to the Space Age. *Intensive Care Medicine*, **34**, 222–228.

Timmerman A, Russo SG. (2007). Which airway should I use? *Current Opinions in Anaesthesiology*, **20**, 595–599.

Weksler N, Klein M, Weksler D, et al. (2004). Retrograde tracheal intubation: Beyond fibreoptic endotracheal intubation. *Acta Anaesthesiologica Scandinavica*, **48**, 412–416.

Wilson WC, Minokadeh A, Benumof JL, Frass M, Barbieri P. (2007). Definitive airway management. In: Wilson WC, Grande CM, Hoyt DB (Eds.), *Trauma: Emergency Resuscitation, Perioperative Anesthesia, Surgical Management.* Vol. I. Boca Raton, FL: CRC Press. pp. 155–196.

Section 4
Chapter

Ethics and the law

30

Ethical issues arising in
airway management

Andrew D.M. McLeod and Steven M. Yentis

In this chapter we discuss some aspects of airway management that may present ethical dilemmas. Medical ethics and law are distinct fields, yet their extensive overlay leads to frequent confusion between them. Some situations that might appear clear cut from a legal perspective may actually have more complex ethical issues attached to them. Chapter 31 will discuss the medicolegal aspects of similar airway management issues.

Consent and refusal relating to specialist airway techniques

Seeking a patient's informed consent is grounded in the ethical principle of respect for autonomy, and supported in Western societies by the value placed on an individual's right to liberty and self-determination. Ideally, consent for medical treatment should be a 'substantially autonomous authorisation', and as such requires the three elements of competence, information and voluntariness to be fully realised. The concept of valid consent has been extensively explored, as have the challenges of achieving it in practice. Recent guidance by the General Medical Council (GMC) represents an official ethical standard for the practice of consent within the UK, and this is supplemented by specific guidance from professional bodies such as The Association of Anaesthetists of Great Britain and Ireland (AAGBI).

Being ill or undergoing treatment is a stressful and confusing time, and exercising full autonomy in these circumstances can be difficult. Patients may also have misconceptions about the role of consent, and the rights they have to make decisions. Consent for anaesthesia remains particularly problematic. The time allocated for anaesthetists to talk to their patients pre-operatively is frequently brief, and usually occurs only *after* patients have decided to proceed with surgery. Information given during the pre-operative period can easily be disregarded or forgotten, as much of it may be technically unfamiliar and hard to understand. Many patients find mathematical expressions of risk difficult to comprehend, and their perceptions can be affected by a number of well known biases. Although the expression of risk can be made more intelligible for patients, actual complications can be hard to predict for individuals, making it difficult to convey risks and benefits with great certainty.

A second fundamental difficulty is that consent for anaesthesia is usually subsumed within a patient's overall consent for surgery, which is normally viewed as a composite 'procedure'. The required level of detail about anaesthesia can be hard to judge, as is the issue of whether patients must give consent to each individual aspect of the anaesthetic. The so-called sectionalisation of consent (where every last component of a procedure must be described) is not advocated. However where a specific sub-procedure might involve material risk or a 'different invasion of bodily integrity', patients might feel entitled to be consulted. Thus most anaesthetists would now routinely include consent for epidural catheter insertion, or analgesic suppositories. It has been argued that the use of techniques such as fibreoptic intubation or use of the intubating laryngeal mask airway during general anaesthesia would not require individual discussion and agreement if these were a routine part of the anaesthetist's practice, although there may be a divergence between the airway techniques that anaesthetists consider 'routine', and those which the public would expect to be consulted about.

Core Topics in Airway Management, Second Edition, ed. Ian Calder and Adrian Pearce. Published by Cambridge University Press.
© Cambridge University Press 2011.

The role of consent for 'awake' airway techniques

As a basic principle, patients must be given all the information that might be significant to their choice. Providing this information can also give patients an enhanced sense of control, reassure them that they are being kept informed and help in the preparation for anaesthesia. Furthermore, information can help clarify more basic issues such as the role of anaesthetist and foster a relationship of trust. Thus, explaining the conduct of fibreoptic intubation would be good practice both ethically and also clinically by helping to reduce patients' anxiety and uncertainty.

Consent for awake fibreoptic intubation should include a summary of its benefits and risks, a description of the procedure, and the reassurance that it is a safe and routinely performed one, which can be made comfortable with local anaesthesia and possibly some sedation. Supplementary information such as leaflets or even video presentations may be helpful too, and the patient should ideally be counselled before their admission for treatment.

Refusal of a specific airway technique

If patients have been asked for their consent to a specialised airway technique, the corollary is that they have the right to refuse. Although the rights of the competent patient to refuse medical treatment are well established, an ethical dilemma can arise when a specific refusal changes the risks of anaesthesia dramatically. If a patient with a very difficult airway should decline awake tracheostomy or fibreoptic intubation, our ethical duty to respect his/her autonomy comes into direct tension with a second duty to prevent harm.

> Clinical example: A patient who is morbidly obese and has severe rheumatoid arthritis affecting her cervical spine, is scheduled for shoulder replacement. Due to her past experience she adamantly refuses to undergo awake fibreoptic intubation or regional anaesthesia. What is the right thing to do?

One would hope that sympathetic counselling and a reassuring description of fibreoptic intubation can avoid a stalemate. Some degree of persuasion could also be acceptable providing it does not become coercion. At the very least we should feel able to recommend a plan and say why we are doing so. A record of all these conversations is important and may also be useful to the patient if they wish to reflect on their decision.

Where a patient remains steadfast that they will refuse any awake procedure, an ethical dilemma remains. Similar decisions have led to harm or even death after induction of anaesthesia. We might have legitimate fears that this could be a choice that the patient (or her family) bitterly regrets afterwards. For the anaesthetist too there can be difficulty in proceeding with a course of action which feels acutely uncomfortable. As Webster and McKnight have argued, performing such actions can lead to a 'moral residue' which is detrimental to anaesthetists (and their profession). Practically speaking a number of options should be explored:

- Referral to a trusted senior colleague for a second opinion would always be good practice. That colleague might even feel they have the skills and confidence to deal with this challenge.
- Some institutions provide a clinical ethics team who at the very least can help to clarify the arguements and considerations, and may shed light on new options for resolution.
- In the elective situation, it could be argued that the patient has committed herself to a course where the risks now greatly outweigh the benefits, and thus is not entitled to demand care.

In an emergency, where a difficult airway is deteriorating there is little time for deliberation. All anaesthetists will be faced with situations in their career where they simply have to try to do their best.

Patients may also make advance refusals of treatment. The legal aspects of these decisions will be covered in the next chapter, but there are also ethical dimensions to consider. The problem of precedent autonomy questions the extent to which a person can make decisions on behalf of their *future* self. More practically, it can be difficult for a patient to envisage reliably what their future condition might be like, and which specific treatments would be unacceptable in very different circumstances.

> Example. A patient with terminal lung cancer expects 6–9 months of reasonable quality life. He has refused intubation in the event of cardio-respiratory arrest, but has just suffered an anaphylactic reaction to antibiotics given during placement of a pleural drain. (Casarett D, Ross LF. *N Engl J Med*, 1997;**336**:1908–1910)

In this scenario the patient has made a reasonably well thought-out refusal of intubation, but now is in circumstances that he had probably not foreseen. It might feel very hard to honour his request, particularly if this reaction is the result of a medication error. The key question may be whether honouring the patient's refusal in this eventuality is truly in accordance with his deeper intentions. If a brief period of resuscitation could restore the patient back to being able to enjoy some months of quality life, then intubation for a short period could be ethically justified. This decision will need to be made quickly however, and possibly with incomplete information, and as such might be vulnerable to reassessment in hindsight.

Patients with 'do not attempt resuscitation' (DNAR) decisions may also present for anaesthesia to allow palliative procedures to be performed, or feeding tubes to be placed. This can present a dilemma to anaesthetists regarding the extent to which the normal requirements of safe anaesthesia and airway management might contravene specific details of the DNAR decision. Although these might be circumstances that the patient would not have originally considered, it would also be unethical to suspend their decision unilaterally. Any DNAR or advance decision should therefore be reviewed individually before anaesthesia, and be redrafted if necessary. In a procedure orientated approach, it would be appropriate to explore whether tracheal intubation is indicated, and if so whether the patient would accept it in order for their treatment to proceed. In a goal orientated approach, limits to airway management would be considered more in the light of a patient's longer term goals, e.g., avoiding long-term ventilation. Either of these frameworks can help formulate an airway management plan where resuscitation has previously been refused, or deemed inappropriate. The AAGBI has issued specific guidance to assist in the peri-operative management of patients with DNAR decisions in place.

Making decisions on behalf of incompetent adults

Anaesthetists and critical care clinicians may have to perform airway procedures such as percutaneous tracheostomy on incapacitated patients. Although the legal requirements for making this decision are reasonably clear, some ethical dilemmas are more complex.

> Clinical example – a young woman is unconscious after a road traffic accident, and has sustained thoracic injuries. Her lungs remain ventilated via an endotracheal tube, but she requires a tracheostomy to help her wean from ventilation. Her family and boyfriend are adamant that she 'would not want one'.

Substituted decision making involves judging whose opinion most validly represents the patient's overall best interests, and whether the patient's own views of their best interests can be reliably ascertained and practically incorporated into a decision. In this example, the patient's family may be correctly expressing the patient's view that she would rather have more prolonged ventilation than a scar at the front of her throat, even if she is actually finding the oral tracheal tube distressing to tolerate. Conversely a prolonged period of oral intubation may cause physical damage to her larynx and subglottis as well as the possible psychological consequences of long-term sedation.

Teaching, training and research

Doctors have a firm ethical duty to develop and maintain their skills, participate in the training of colleagues and students, and contribute to safer healthcare. Although this is required by the GMC, doctors are also obliged to make the individual patient's care their first concern. When involving patients directly in training, an obvious tension can exist, but it is not always clear how to resolve this. Our impression is that this issue is frequently fudged or concealed in practice.

> Clinical example: A patient with rheumatoid arthritis and extensively crowned teeth has previously had difficult intubations and dental injury. The patient is happy for awake fibreoptic intubation, but does not wish to be 'trained on'.

Current guidance from the GMC states that you *must* [our italics] give patients information about 'the people who will be mainly responsible for and involved in their care, what their roles are and to what extent students will be involved'. Patients should also be aware of 'their right to refuse to take part in teaching or research'. This does not however resolve the issue of how doctors should acquire and maintain skills such as airway management techniques.

Trainee doctors should initially develop skills as far as is reasonably possible on part task trainers, manikins, or simulator systems. The use of recently deceased human cadavers has a very limited role, and the ethical acceptability of this has decreased steadily. Use of the deceased person is now specifically covered by the Human Tissue Act 2004, which expressly requires consent for (amongst other purposes) 'education or training relating to human health'. Further training must therefore be acquired through supervised practice on living human subjects. Clinical staff and course delegates have been proposed as appropriate subjects for training in techniques such as fibreoptic bronchoscopy. Although medically qualified participants might be able to give more informed consent than most patients, the potential for subtle forms of coercion still exist, which indicates that local ethical approval of such training courses is advisable.

Most practical training however will require the participation of patients. It can be argued that because most patients benefit from the altruism of previous patients who have participated in teaching and training, from a principle of justice they should be equally willing to take part themselves. Patients' consent is still required however, and one approach suggests that consent for training should be obtained as if for research. However unlike a research protocol, airway procedures performed during training are done for that patient's expected benefit, and would also be the same as indicated in routine practice. The following checklist can be followed when considering employing a particular procedure on a patient for teaching or training purposes.

- Recognise the patient's rights to autonomy
- Assess the magnitude of benefits and harms to the patient from performing this particular procedure (including whether the technique can be considered 'routine')
- Consider how the benefits could be maximised, and the potential harms minimised
- Actively consider the alternatives
- Follow existing professional guidance or other relevant standards as far as possible
- Consider the need for specific consent – this will depend on the circumstances as outlined above
- Educate other staff to be aware of these issues, and base training within efficient and structured programmes.

Research

Like any other type of medical research, investigations into airway management must be conducted to rigorous ethical standards. Beauchamp and Childress have summarised the ethical conditions required to justify research involving human subjects as follows:

- The knowledge gained should be of value
- There is a reasonable prospect that the research will generate this knowledge
- The use of human subjects is necessary for this research
- The balance of benefit over risk is acceptable
- The privacy and confidentiality of subjects is protected
- The selection of subjects is fair and does not involve exploitation
- Autonomous subjects must give fully valid consent.

The declaration of Helsinki states more specifically how these conditions should be met, and although we cannot provide a fuller discussion in this chapter, ethical aspects of conducting and publishing research in anaesthesia have been covered by a number of writers.

The duty to contribute to safety and good standards

The GMC's Good Practice guide states that 'If you have good reason to think that patient safety is or may be seriously compromised by inadequate premises, equipment, or other resources, policies or systems, you should put the matter right if that is possible'. The Tavistock working group also identified the duty to contribute to safety as a shared ethical obligation for all healthcare staff. Although this could be covered by the ethical duty to avoid harm, it may be overlooked when our focus is usually on the individual patient. The broader duty to be safe would obligate doctors to take part in risk management programmes, and actively identify unsafe factors, or inadequate resources (Table 30.1).

Wise use of resources can also be considered as an ethical duty when viewed from a principle of justice. In a publicly funded healthcare system, many decisions to purchase a particular item of equipment could deny another patient somewhere else a different aspect of care. Thus enthusiasm to purchase a new

Table 30.1. Examples of activities to improve patient safety relating to airway management

- Anticipating where airway emergencies might occur and providing appropriate training and equipment, e.g., a difficult airway trolley, CO_2 monitoring etc

- Organising teaching in airway management for trainees and other colleagues

- Following up of patients whose airways proved difficult, such as letters, entries in notes, medic-alert bracelets, and anaesthetic databases

- Devising local protocols and guidelines for the management of airway emergencies, such as paediatric epiglottitis, or failed obstetric intubation

- Identifying latent system errors and taking active measures to limit their potential for harm, e.g., blocked tubes, oxygen disconnection points etc

- Instituting effective critical incident recording – and responding to critical incidents and near misses, with effective learning programmes

- Assisting or even reporting colleagues whose clinical skills could pose a significant risk to patients.

item of airway equipment should be balanced against its clinical value, and its cost implications, although these calculations can admittedly be hard to make.

Key points

- Seeking consent for anaesthesia should include a discussion of any specialist or non-routine airway techniques. Providing good information about procedures such as awake fibreoptic intubation and its intended benefits shows respect for patients' autonomy, and can help allay their anxiety.

- A patient's refusal of awake tracheostomy or fibreoptic intubation may occasionally present an ethical dilemma. While the competent patient's rights must be respected, there are occasionally situations where a clinician cannot be compelled to provide care when the risks would greatly outweigh the benefits.

- Do Not Attempt Resuscitation (DNAR) decisions may place difficult constraints on safe airway management for some patients. They should be individually reviewed before proceeding with anaesthesia.

- Exposing patients to extra procedures purely for airway management training or research

must be done with their informed consent, and anaesthetists must weigh up the possible benefits, harms and alternative methods available.

- Anaesthetists have a duty to maintain their skills and contribute to patient safety and risk management programmes, for example developing failed intubation procedures and setting up difficult airway management resources.

Further reading

Adams AM, Smith AF. (2001). Risk perception and communication: Recent developments and implications for anaesthesia. *Anaesthesia*, **56**, 745–755.

Beauchamp T L, Childress J F. (2009). *Principles of Biomedical Ethics.* 6th ed. Oxford: Oxford University Press.

Bray J K, Yentis S M. (2002). Attitudes of patients and anaesthetists to informed consent for specialist airway techniques. *Anaesthesia*, **57**, 1012–1015.

Buchanan A E, Brock D W. (1990). *Deciding for Others: The Ethics of Surrogate Decision Making.* Cambridge: Cambridge University Press.

Casarett D, Ross L F. (1997). Overriding a patient's refusal of treatment after an iatrogenic complication. *New England Journal of Medicine*, **336**, 1908–1910.

Davis J K. (2002). The concept of precedent autonomy. *Bioethics*, **16**, 114–133.

Frerk C. (2003). Training course in local anaesthesia of the airway and fibreoptic intubation using course delegates as subjects. *British Journal of Anaesthesia*, **90**, 258.

General Medical Council. (2006). *Good Medical Practice.* London. Available at: http://www.gmc-uk.org/guidance/ good_medical_practice/GMC_GMP.pdf.

General Medical Council. (2008). *Consent: Patients and Doctors Making Decisions Together.* London. Available at: http://www.gmc-uk.org/guidance/ethical_guidance/ consent_guidance/Consent_guidance.pdf.

Harmer M. (2003). Clinical research. In: Draper H, Scott W E (Eds.), *Ethics in Anaesthesia and Intensive Care.* London: Butterworth Heinemann.

Hunter J M. (2000). Ethics in publishing; are we practising to the highest possible standards? *British Journal of Anaesthesia*, **85**, 341–343.

Maclean A R. (2002). Consent, sectionalisation and the concept of a medical procedure. *Journal of Medical Ethics*, **28**, 249–254.

McKnight D J, Webster G C. (1997). Refusal of treatment and moral compromise. *Canadian Journal of Anesthesia*, **44**, 239–242.

Office of Public Sector Information. (2004). *Human Tissue Act.* Available at: http://www.opsi.gov.uk/ACTS/ acts2004/ukpga_20040030_en_1.

Patil V, Barker G L, Harwood R J, Woodall N M. (2002). Training course in local anaesthesia of the airway and fibreoptic intubation using course delegates as subjects. *British Journal of Anaesthesia*, **89**, 586–593.

Smith R, Hiatt H, Berwick D. (1999). Shared ethical principles for everybody in healthcare: A working draft from the Tavistock Group. *British Medical Journal*, **318**, 248–251.

The Association of Anaesthetists of Great Britain and Ireland. (2006). *Consent for Anaesthesia*. London: Association of Anaesthetists of Great Britain and Ireland.

The Association of Anaesthetists of Great Britain and Ireland. (2009). *Do Not Attempt Resuscitation (DNAR) Decisions in the Perioperative Period*. London:

Association of Anaesthetists of Great Britain and Ireland.

Waisel DB, Burns JP, Johnson JA, Hardart GE, Truog RD. (2002). Guidelines for perioperative do-not-resuscitate policies. *Journal of Clinical Anesthesia*, **14**, 467–473.

White SM. (2004). Consent for anaesthesia. *Journal of Medical Ethics*, **30**, 286–290.

World Medical Association Declaration of Helsinki. (2008). *Ethical Principles for Medical Research Involving Human Subjects*. Available at: http://www.wma.net/en/30publications/10policies/l3/17c.net.

Yentis SM. (2005). The use of patients for learning and maintaining practical skills. *Journal of the Royal Society of Medicine*, **98**, 299–302.

Chapter 31

Legal and regulatory aspects of airway management

Andrew D.M. McLeod and Steven M. Yentis

In this chapter we discuss some aspects of airway management where medicolegal considerations may apply. Most examples have been drawn from English law but these rulings have 'persuasive authority' in Scotland and Northern Ireland and are generally followed there. No laws apply solely to airway management, but areas of common law (e.g., assault and negligence) and statutory law (e.g., The Mental Capacity Act 2005) may both be relevant. In addition, bodies such as the General Medical Council (GMC) are legally empowered to regulate medical practice, and as such their requirements carry greater force than other professional guidelines.

Consent and refusal for airway management techniques

In English law (and most jurisdictions) touching a person without their consent represents a battery, *even* if no harm arises. To avoid this charge a clinician must first seek a patient's consent by explaining 'in broad terms' the nature and purpose of an investigation or procedure. They should also ensure that the patient has capacity to give valid consent, and is doing so voluntarily. For children under 16 years, a parent (or person with parental responsibility) must give consent on their behalf, unless the child is specifically deemed Gillick competent. Most disputes about consent concern the quality of information provided, and whether certain risks should have been disclosed. Such claims will normally be dealt with as negligence (see below) rather than battery. The following issues will be critical.

What *should* patients be warned of?

Law requires that patients must be provided with any significant facts that may influence their decisions about healthcare. However it offers little prospective guidance as to the specific information and risks that should be disclosed. Instead, responsibility is placed on the clinician to judge what an individual patient would wish to know. The Association of Anaesthetists of Great Britain and Ireland (AAGBI) has issued guidance on the risks that should be disclosed before anaesthesia, including 'specific risks or complications that may be significant to the patient's decision, for example the risk of vocal cord damage if the patient is a professional singer'. Rare risks such as death and serious disability 'should be provided in written information' although it is not customary to discuss them with every patient unless they ask. However it would be important to warn patients when there is an increased likelihood of airway management problems, particularly if they have alternative options such as awake intubation or regional anaesthesia.

The GMC's more stringent 2008 guidance requires that doctors *must* (author's italics) give patients the information they want or need about their treatment options, including 'the potential benefits, risks and burdens, and the likelihood of success for each option'. This is echoed by the recent judgement in *Birch,* where a patient had not been informed about the comparative risks of other available procedures. In relation to risk, doctors must include failures of technique as well as side effects and complications, and patients *must* be told about the possibility of serious adverse outcomes, even if the likelihood is 'very small'.

Applying these requirements to consent for airway management remains problematic. Reciting a full litany of hazards is not warranted for every patient, nor would it be good practice ethically. Rather, specific warnings should be appropriate to the intended

Core Topics in Airway Management, Second Edition, ed. Ian Calder and Adrian Pearce. Published by Cambridge University Press.
© Cambridge University Press 2011.

Table 31.1. Specific risks from airway management techniques that might warrant discussion pre-operatively

Dental injury, particularly to capped and crowned teeth

Sore throat, oral and vocal cord or laryngeal injury

Nasal injury, epistaxis and sinusitis

Injuries to the jaw or temporomandibular joint pain

Aspiration of gastric contents

Pulmonary or tracheo-oesophageal injury

Hypoxia

Emergency procedures, e.g., cricothyrotomy

Abandonment of technique

Prolonged intubation and ventilation

technique, the likelihood of complications, and the significance of certain risks to an individual patient (Table 31.1).

Was the patient adequately warned?

To defend a claim of negligent consent, a doctor must be able to demonstrate that a patient was warned of a particular risk or outcome. Although written consent is not obligatory in law for most procedures, good documentation remains paramount as patients' memories can be unreliable for warnings given before treatment. Current guidance from the AAGBI is that a separate consent form is not usually required for anaesthesia, but all conversations and disclosures of risk should be documented in the notes or anaesthetic record. However even if a specific risk was recorded, a patient could legitimately claim that a complication was not explained fully. Patients who are asked to consent on the day of surgery may also feel that they had inadequate time to reflect or were under some pressure to proceed. Patients with particular challenges like a difficult airway should ideally be seen in anaesthetic clinics, and given information well before their admission for treatment.

Would the patient have proceeded had they been warned?

A successful negligence claim must also satisfy the legal test of causation, i.e., the patient would not have gone ahead had they been warned. Now that the patient has actually experienced the complication, this claim may appear to be blessed by hindsight, although it has traditionally been distrusted for this same reason. However in *Chester v Afshar*, the Courts have shown that the principle of causation may not be so rigorously applied, and that the patient's right to have adequate information is paramount.

Refusal of a proposed airway technique by a competent patient

In Israel, a competent patient's refusal of life-saving treatment can be overridden, providing a physician is confident that they will give consent *retrospectively*. No such legal avenue exists in the UK or other Western jurisdictions, where the competent patient's rights to refuse treatment are firmly established. Providing they are not acting under duress and have been informed of the risks and benefits of all available options, their refusal must be respected 'notwithstanding that the reasons for making the choice are rational, irrational, unknown or even non-existent'. Patients who refuse specific airway techniques present a dilemma to the anaesthetist. Refusal of awake intubation may lead to harm or even death. Could a doctor be criticised for acceding to a patient's refusal?

In such a situation, it would be important initially to establish that the patient has sufficient capacity to make this decision and clearly understands its possible consequences. Although an 'unwise' choice does not alone imply lack of capacity, it might indicate some disorder of thinking or temporary impairment. Capacity to make medical decisions is now defined by the Mental Capacity Act 2005 (or the Adults with Incapacity Act 2000 in Scotland), and its requirements must be followed. All conversations should be documented clearly, and second opinions from senior colleagues are advisable. If a satisfactory resolution cannot be found, a clinician may have a final right not to offer treatment, provided he or she believes that the risks now overwhelmingly outweigh the benefits to the patient. This step however may require legal advice. All trusts should have access to emergency legal support and medical defence organisations normally provide 24-hour access.

Advance refusals and end of life care

Competent patients may refuse certain treatments in anticipation of losing capacity. These directives are now referred to as advance decisions under the

Mental Capacity Act. For potentially life-saving treatments such as intubation, the decision must be signed, witnessed and include words to the effect that *the decision applies even if life is at risk*. These decisions are sometimes difficult to implement, but an advance decision that is valid and applicable to the present circumstances must be followed. Conversely patients cannot legally demand particular treatments that a medical team believes would be futile or against their overall interests. As we have discussed in Chapter 30, all advance decisions and 'do not attempt resuscitation' orders should be carefully reviewed before anaesthesia.

The incapacitated adult

Traditionally no one could give consent on behalf of another adult. The Mental Capacity Act now allows persons endowed with Lasting Power of Attorney (LPA) *for welfare* to make medical decisions on behalf of incompetent patients. LPA holders cannot refuse life-saving treatment however, unless clearly authorised by a previous advance decision. The Act and its code of practice requires that all decisions made on behalf of incompetent adults should be in the fullest sense of their best interests, taking into account any previously expressed wishes as well as the contributions of family and other interested parties. If relatives should refuse treatment such as tracheostomy adamantly, or conversely insist on intubation that would not benefit the patient, legal advice should be sought and potentially a court order could be needed.

Regulation of airway products and practice

Competence to practice

The GMC requires doctors to be competent and up to date, although the precise competencies required of specialists are not yet defined. Airway management standards are currently published by the Royal College of Anaesthetists as competency requirements for training, but have also been proposed for professional development, and may play a role in future specialist recertification. GMC guidance requires doctors to participate in the maintenance of safety and good standards and this is also an ethical duty (see Chapter 30).

Product regulation

A medical device can be any product related to healthcare except a medicine, and thus would include airway management devices. The Medicines and Healthcare Products Regulatory Agency (MHRA) regulates the manufacture, licensing and use of all medical devices in the UK. The Consumer Protection Act 1987 also imposes 'strict' liability (i.e., fault does not have to be proven) on a manufacturer if a patient is injured by a defective product. This area of law is extensive and complex, but three aspects related to airway products can be highlighted:

Developing new products

New products can be developed and used within a hospital trust, but if they are placed (or even advertised) within the wider market, the full force of law and regulations applies. Any anaesthetist hoping to develop an airway device should be fully aware of the legislation. Under the Medical Devices Directive new devices must carry the CE mark which represents the manufacturer's statement that the device complies with all relevant requirements, although this does not necessarily include clinical efficacy. There is current concern regarding the many new airway products introduced on to the market without the rigorous evaluation to which drugs are subjected.

Non-standard use of medical devices

The rules for developing new medical devices also apply to non-standard use of existing ones, such as employing a breathing system filter for oxygen administration. This would be considered a modification under the Consumer Protection Act 1987. If this modification is advertised (or publicly described) outside an individual organisation, liability for harm will pass to the 'designing' anaesthetist, or manufacturing body.

Reusing 'single use' devices

A manufacturer will not be held liable if a patient is harmed through the reuse of a device labelled 'single use', liability instead passing to the user or their employer. Manufacturers are not obliged to prove why a device *must* be 'single use', which has led to allegations of profit motive being a consideration. This issue has been controversial during the evaluation of single use laryngoscope blades, which many anaesthetists felt potentially posed more risk than the theoretical possibility of prion disease transmission.

Standards of care, complications, and forms of legal action

In addition to the natural progress of their illness, patients may suffer harm through accident, negligence or a combination of these factors. For a claim of negligence to succeed, claimants must show that:

- The defendant owed them a duty of care.
- The defendant breached that duty of care.
- Damage occurred as a result.

Standards of care

The *Bolam* principle states that a practice is acceptable if it is supported by a 'responsible body' of medical opinion. Although this has been increasingly under pressure in the Courts (e.g., that opinion must be 'reasonable' and 'withstand logical analysis'), the basic concept still applies in English law.

Role of guidelines

Guidelines may be used by experts to support their opinion in court, and have been employed both as a 'sword' (for the claimant) or as a 'shield' (for the defendant). The Difficult Airway Society and the American Society of Anesthesiologists' (ASA) guidelines could both be seen as authoritative for airway management, while locally produced guidelines may also be relevant. In *Early v Newham* it was argued that the claimant had suffered distress after being woken from an unsuccessful intubation attempt. However the anaesthetic department successfully demonstrated that the anaesthetist had adhered to previously agreed guidelines, and the claim was dismissed. A recent ASA closed claim analysis found that guidelines had played a role in only 18% of airway claims. In future however, it may be required to show that a reasonable body of medical opinion would have departed from recognised guidelines in a specific situation in order to defend a claim of negligence.

Breaches of duty

The standard of care will ultimately be judged on the specific facts of a case. The following are suggested as generic examples of potential breaches of duty in regard to airway management:

- Failure to take an adequate history or consult previous records.
- Failure to make an adequate airway examination.
- Incorrect use of properly working equipment or failure to check.
- Failure to follow accepted practice or guidelines.
- Failure to recognise and/or treat a complication.
- Failing to record airway difficulties adequately.

Damages and settlements

The most common complaints of harm arising from airway management are dental trauma, injury to the airway and hypoxic injury. The ASA closed claim database study found that (excepting dental injuries), damage to the larynx (33%), pharynx (19%), oesophagus (18%), trachea (15%), temporomandibular joint (10%) and nose (5%) were the commonest causes of claims relating to airway injury. However death or hypoxic brain injury accounted for more than half of all claims arising from airway management problems in a parallel analysis.

Most claims are settled outside the courts, and often without an admission of fault. In England, the National Health Service Litigation Authority (NHSLA) handles clinical negligence claims arising in NHS practice. Summary data obtained* reveal that from its inception in 1995, more than 90 claims (excluding dental injuries) arising from complications of airway management are recorded, and specific difficulties with intubation are noted in 33% of claims.* In 63% of these cases, death or hypoxic brain injury had resulted, and where associated damages were paid, these have been as much as £650 000.

Other consequences of a catastrophic outcome

After a death or serious incident there may be an internal hospital inquiry and possibly a coroner's inquest. Measures could be imposed upon a health professional, such as suspension, disciplinary sanctions by the GMC, or even criminal charges (below). After such incidents, families of the patient deserve compassionate counselling and honest explanations

---

* The authors are grateful to the NHSLA for providing these data.

of what happened. The personal stress for a doctor can also be immense. Support from colleagues and good medicolegal representation is essential, and helpful guidance has been issued by the AAGBI.

Gross negligence and manslaughter

Understandably it has been argued that criminal prosecution of doctors who simply make mistakes would not normally be in the public interest. Also, errors in airway management can produce injuries far out of proportion to the initial act or omission. However doctors may be found guilty of criminal negligence where they displayed 'gross negligence', defined as 'recklessness or wilful knowledge of risk which might bring about serious injury or death, but nevertheless a conscious intention to take that risk'.

When death results from gross negligence, a charge of manslaughter could be made. *R v Adomako* remains one of the key cases for defining criminal negligence in English law. In this case, a patient died due to the anaesthetist's failure to notice and make good a tubing disconnection. Prosecutions have been successfully brought against other anaesthetists for causing deaths, but as these are criminal cases, the standard of proof must be 'beyond reasonable doubt' rather than 'on balance of probabilities'. Overall, convictions of doctors for manslaughter are uncommon, but have become more frequent in recent decades.

Corporate manslaughter

The Corporate Manslaughter and Corporate Homicide Act 2007 now allows criminal charges to be brought against an organisation if it has grossly breached its duty of care (for example in attending to safety), and this has caused a death. As yet no medicolegal case law has been generated to indicate how it will be applied.

The consent of competent patients must be gained before performing airway management techniques that depart from routine practice or have risks that may influence the patient's decision.

Key points

- The competent patient's legal right to refuse medical treatment extends to airway management techniques. Procedures such as intubation may also be refused as part of a formal Advance Decision.

- Anaesthetists and intensivists should be familiar with the Mental Capacity Act 2005 (or the Adults with Incapacity Act 2000 in Scotland) when making decisions on behalf of incapacitated patients.
- Anaesthetists intending to develop a new airway device, or publish a modification of an existing device, should be thoroughly familiar with product regulation and consumer protection law.
- Claims of negligence continue to rely on the presence of a responsible body of medical opinion as the test for an acceptable standard of care. However such an opinion must be both logical and reasonable.
- Extreme cases of negligence may be dealt with under criminal law, and where death results could possibly lead to charges of manslaughter.

Further reading

American Society of Anesthesiologists Task Force on Management of the Difficult Airway. (2003). Practice guidelines for management of the difficult airway: An updated report by the American Society of Anesthesiologists Task Force on Management of the Difficult Airway. *Anesthesiology*, **98**, 1269–1277.

Birch v University College London Hospital NHS Foundation Trust [2008] EWHC 2237 (QB).

Bolam v Friern Hospital Management Committee [1957] 2 All ER 118.

Chester v Afshar [2004] 4 All E.R. 587 and [2004] UKHL 41.

Consumer Protection Act 1987. Available at: http://www. opsi.gov.uk/si/si1987/Uksi_19871680_en_1.htm.

Corporate Manslaughter and Corporate Homicide Act 2007. Available at: http://www.opsi.gov.uk/acts/ acts2007/pdf/ukpga_20070019_en.pdf.

Domino KB, Posner KL, Caplan RA, Cheney FW. (1999). Airway injury during anesthesia. *Anesthesiology*, **91**, 1703–1711.

Early v Newham Health Authority [1994] 5 Med LR 214.

Ferner RE, McDowell SE. (2006). Doctors charged with manslaughter in the course of medical practice, 1795–2005: A literature review. *Journal of the Royal Society of Medicine*, **99**, 309–314.

General Medical Council. (2008). *Consent: Patients and Doctors Making Decisions Together*. London. Available at: http://www.gmc-uk.org/guidance/ethical_guidance/ consent_guidance/Consent_guidance.pdf.

General Medical Council. (2006). *Good Medical Practice*. London. Available at: http://www.gmc-uk.org/guidance/ good_medical_practice/GMC_GMP.pdf.

Grant LJ. (1998). Regulations and safety in medical equipment design. *Anaesthesia*, **53**, 1–3.

Gross ML. (2005). Treating competent patients by force: The limits and lessons of Israel's Patient's Rights Act. *Journal of Medical Ethics*, **31**, 29–34.

Henderson JJ, Popat MT, Latto IP, Pearce AC; Difficult Airway Society. (2004). Difficult Airway Society guidelines for management of the unanticipated difficult intubation. *Anaesthesia*, **59**, 675–694.

Hodges C. (2000). The reuse of medical devices. *Medical Law Review*, **8**, 157–181.

McCall-Smith A. (1995). Criminal or merely human?: The prosecution of negligent doctors. *The Journal of Contemporary Health Law and Policy*, **12**, 131–146.

Mental Capacity Act 2005. Available at: http://www.opsi.gov.uk/acts/acts2005/20050009.htm.

Peterson GN, Domino KB, Caplan RA, Posner KL, Lee LA, Cheney FW. (2005). Management of the difficult airway. A closed claims analysis. *Anesthesiology*, **103**, 33–39.

R v Adomako [1995] 1 AC 171, (1994) 19 BMLR 56.

Re T (Adult: Refusal of Treatment) [1993] Fam 95, [1992] 4All ER 649.

Rowley E, Dingwall R. (2007). The use of single-use devices in anaesthesia: Balancing the risks to patient safety. *Anaesthesia*, **62**, 569–574.

Royal College of Anaesthetists. (2005). *Continuing Professional Development*. London. Available at: http://www.rcoa.ac.uk/docs/CPD_guidelines.pdf.

Samanta A, Mello MM, Foster C, Tingle J, Samanta J. (2006). The role of guidelines in medical negligence litigation: A shift from the *Bolam* standard? *Medical Law Review*, **14**, 321–366.

The Association of Anaesthetists of Great Britain and Ireland. 2005. *Catastrophes in Anaesthetic Practice – Dealing With the Aftermath*. London: Association of Anaesthetists of Great Britain and Ireland.

The Association of Anaesthetists of Great Britain and Ireland. (2006). *Consent for Anaesthesia*. London: Association of Anaesthetists of Great Britain and Ireland.

Wheat K. (2005). Progress of the prudent patient: Consent after *Chester v Afshar*. *Anaesthesia*, **60**, 217–219.

White SM, Baldwin TJ. (2004). *Legal and Ethical Aspects of Anaesthesia, Critical Care and Perioperative Medicine*. Cambridge: Cambridge University Press.

Wilkes AR, Hodzovic I, Latto IP. (2008). Introducing new anaesthetic equipment into clinical practice. *Anaesthesia*, **63**, 571–575.

32

Sample structured oral examination questions

During the Structured Oral Examination of the FRCA examination, the examiners are given an answer sheet, which contains the information around which the discussion of the question should proceed. The material here is not taken from the question bank of the FRCA (although some of the authors are past and present examiners). Nevertheless, the detail given is fairly typical of the SOE sheets, and might also be the basis of a written question.

1. An anaesthetised patient has a SpO_2 of 90%. Outline possible causation and management.
2. Three hours after an operation, which was performed through an incision on the anterior aspect of the neck, a patient complains of difficulty in breathing. What are the possible causes?
3. What is Ludwig's angina, how does it present, how does it affect the airway, how is it treated? What is the anaesthetic technique of choice in a patient with this condition?
4. What is epiglottitis and how is it managed?
5. How might a child with an inhaled foreign body present? Describe your anaesthetic management for removal of the inhaled object.
6. Discuss the management of a patient who is bleeding following tonsillectomy.
7. Summarise the peri-operative anaesthetic management of a young man who is going to undergo an ORIF of facial fractures.
8. A 15-year-old male autistic child requires an EUA and probable dental restoration treatment. A previous attempt to anaesthetise him failed due to non-cooperation. How would you proceed?
9. A patient requires surgical fixation of an unstable cervical spine. What might be meant by 'unstable' and what are the implications for airway management?
10. A patient with long-standing rheumatoid arthritis requires a total hip arthroplasty operation. How may rheumatoid arthritis affect the airway and how would you manage the anaesthesia?
11. Describe management of anaesthesia for repair of broncho-pleural fistula.
12. An ethical dilemma.

Core Topics in Airway Management, Second Edition, ed. Ian Calder and Adrian Pearce. Published by Cambridge University Press.
© Cambridge University Press 2011.

Q1 An anaesthetised patient has a SpO_2 of 90%. Outline possible causation and management. (Andrew Farmery and Ian Calder)

Q1 Discussion

Note: the question does not say at what point in the anaesthetic procedure this value of SpO_2 has been recorded, or whether it is changing rapidly.

Possible causes

- False positive reading? Check oximeter position and observe the patient.
- Gas supply problem? Is the F_IO_2 of the fresh gas flow adequate? Are there any disconnects?
- Hypoventilation? Is this an equipment problem (occluded circuit, malfunctioning ventilator) or a patient problem (not breathing, obstructed upper airway, laryngospasm, bronchospasm)
- Is there a ventilation/perfusion mismatch? Possible causes: effect of anaesthesia (diminished hypoxic pulmonary vasoconstriction?), positive pressure ventilation, diminished cardiac output, oesophageal or endobronchial intubation, aspiration, embolus (fat, air, clot), pneumothorax, other lung disease. This could be an iatrogenic causation if one-lung anaesthesia has been initiated.

Management

- Definitive management will depend on the cause (e.g., laryngospasm and bronchospasm will require appropriate treatment), but the initial response will be to check that all equipment is connected, patent, and that the patient's lungs are being ventilated with a suitable concentration of oxygen. Switch to ventilation by hand, observe and feel the bag movement, observe the capnography.
- Increase the inspired fraction of oxygen (F_IO_2). Provided there is a patent airway an increased F_IO_2 should improve the saturation unless there is a large degree (>30%) of ventilation/perfusion mismatch. This should be true even if hypoventilation is still occurring, due to passive absorption of oxygen (Alveolar gas equation for oxygen and carbon dioxide: $P_AO_2 = P_B. F_IO_2 - P_ACO_2/R$).
- If the saturation does not improve despite there being a patent airway, a high F_IO_2 and adequate ventilation, it suggests that a significant degree of ventilation/perfusion mismatch or fixed shunt exists. Remediable causes such as tube malposition or foreign body in the airway, aspiration or pneumothorax must be excluded. A minor degree of mismatch is often encountered after the induction of anaesthesia or initiation of positive pressure ventilation.
- Improving the cardiac output should lessen the impact of ventilation/perfusion mismatch by increasing the mixed venous oxygen saturation. Inotropes and fluid infusions may be required.

Q2 Three hours after an operation, which was performed through an incision on the anterior aspect of the neck, a patient complains of difficulty in breathing. What are the possible causes? (Ian Calder)

Q2 Discussion

What are the possible causes?

- Airway obstruction: haematoma or swelling due to tissue oedema. The airway obstruction is not caused by compression of the trachea – it is caused by swelling of the peri- and supraglottic pharyngeal tissue, presumably due to venous and lymphatic obstruction. Bilateral recurrent laryngeal nerve palsy would be a possibility after a total thyroidectomy. Laryngeal trauma is a possible cause, particularly if there was pre-operative laryngeal pathology (e.g., rheumatoid arthritis or acromegaly).
- Cardiopulmonary pathology.
- Neurological pathology: was the surgery directed towards the spinal canal? Persistence or recrudescence of neuro-muscular block (unlikely at 3 hours).
- Foreign body in the airway (dentures?).
- Anxiety state.

What would be your management if the patient has a haematoma?

- Much will depend on the clinical picture – whether the patient is *in extremis,* or still able to talk and swallow. Management will also be influenced by the grade of laryngoscopy at the preceding operation and whether something has been done that is likely to degrade that appearance apart from the haematoma (e.g., a cranio-cervical fusion).
- If the patient is approaching complete obstruction with loss of consciousness and desaturation the management is to apply oxygen with CPAP via a facemask, whilst the wound is opened to reduce tissue pressure. If those measures reverse the obstruction it may be possible to take the patient to theatre, assemble a team of experienced anaesthetists and surgeons and prepare for a surgical tracheotomy if attempts to intubate fail.
- If the obstruction is still complete, despite opening the wound, an attempt at direct or video-laryngoscopy must be made. The glottis may be obscured by curtains of swollen pharyngeal mucosa. A gum-elastic bougie is often the instrument of choice. If intubation is not achieved a supraglottic airway device (SAD) should be inserted, and if ventilation is not satisfactory a surgical airway must be established.

- If the obstruction is incomplete (the characteristics include: insisting on sitting up, difficulty in speaking, tracheal tug, stridor [not always present]), senior help should be enlisted and the patient moved to theatre. NB SpO_2 is not a good guide to the patency of the airway. It is nearly always advisable to decompress the tissues by opening the wound before moving.
- Temporising measures such as nebulised epinephrine (1 ml 1:1000 in 5 ml of saline) and helium/oxygen may be worthwhile whilst preparations are made in theatre (the staff and equipment for emergency tracheostomy must be assembled).
- Establishing a per-glottic airway may be impossible, so surgeons should be ready to perform a tracheostomy.
- A flexible fibreoptic intubation is often possible, but considerable expertise is required. It is usually impossible to see anything during inspiration and the 'scope must be advanced during expiration. If the 'scope can be placed in the trachea one can give a sleep dose of propofol and railroad a tube. Flexometallic tubes (6 or 6.5 mm) are best and the tube should be constantly rotated (like a drill) during insertion.
- Inhalational induction with sevoflurane in oxygen has the advantage of preserving spontaneous breathing, but depends upon the airway remaining at least partially patent (N_2O must be avoided – effect of density and turbulent flow).
- Intravenous induction and neuro-muscular paralysis may be required to permit ventilation through a SAD or the introduction of a tracheal tube over a gum-elastic bougie. Tracheal intubation can be achieved through a SAD. If per-glottic intubation cannot be achieved a tracheostomy must be performed.
- The wound must be explored, decompressed and closed. The patient should be ventilated in head-up tilt until the swelling has receded (24–48 hours).

Q3 What is Ludwig's angina, how does it present, how does it affect the airway, how is it treated? (Viki Mitchell)

Q3 Discussion

What is the anaesthetic technique of choice in a patient with this condition?

- Ludwig's angina (LA): a bilateral, rapidly spreading sub-mandibular cellulitis, originating from a dental infection (usually the second or third lower molar), which is due to streptococci or mixed oral flora.

Presentation, effect on airway

- LA presents with pain, fever, trismus and dysphagia. Elevation and displacement of the tongue occurs with firm induration of the floor of the mouth and peri-oral oedema.
- The infection may spread posteriorly and cause trismus, occasionally involving the deep cervical spaces and eventually the mediastinum. The patient may have difficulty swallowing or maintaining an airway.
- This is a life-threatening condition with serious anaesthetic implications. The face and neck are swollen and indurated making identification of the bony landmarks (the crico-thyroid ring) difficult or impossible and a tracheostomy under local anaesthesia carries the risk of mediastinitis.
- Bag mask ventilation, direct laryngoscopy and tracheostomy may be difficult.

Treatment

- Antibiotics (metronidazole and amoxicillin) and steroids (dexamethasone) to reduce swelling are first line treatment.

- Surgery to decompress the fascial spaces is indicated if antibiotics fail, usually bilateral incisions parallel and inferior to the mandible with deep dissection into the sub-mandibular triangle through the mylohyoid muscle into sublingual region. Any infected teeth are also removed. Even if no pus is seen, cellulitis resolves faster after decompression. 35% need intervention for airway control. In the pre-antibiotic era death occurred in 40–60% of cases, it still occurs but is now less than 5%.

Anaesthetic technique

- Detailed assessment of the airway is essential.
- Awake fibreoptic intubation is the technique of choice and the patient should give informed consent for this procedure. An antisialogue should be administered beforehand. Sedation is contraindicated if the airway is compromised. Administration of local anaesthesia to the airway via cricothyroid puncture is inadvisable because of the risk of infection; a spray as you go technique is preferable. A nasal tube is not mandatory but provides the best surgical field. A throat pack should be inserted after intubation.
- Patients should remain intubated and ventilated until airway oedema resolves, ITU care should be arranged in advance.

Q4 What is epiglottitis and how is it managed?
(Anil Patel)

Q4 Discussion

Acute and Chronic Epiglottitis

- Acute epiglottitis is an acute inflammatory disease of the epiglottis, arytenoids and aryepiglottic folds which become grossly swollen and obstruct the laryngeal inlet. It is a medical emergency and the onset and progression of symptoms can be rapid and lead to complete upper airway occlusion, hypoxemia and death.
- Chronic swelling of the epiglottis can also occur secondary to infiltrates and tumour extension around the valleculae and tongue base. Chronic swelling of the epiglottis allows the patient to adapt and the typical features of acute presentation are not seen until near total obstruction or an acute or chronic presentation occurs.

Causative organisms

- Acute epiglottitis is usually caused by infectious agents including *Haemophilus influenzae* type b (HiB), group A *Streptococcus pneumoniae*, *Haemophilus parainfluenzae*, *Streptococcus aureus* and β-hemolytic streptococci.
- The introduction of the HiB vaccine in 1992 has dramatically reduced the incidence of acute epiglottitis and it is now rare in children in the UK. Streptococcal epiglottitis can occur in vaccinated children.

Clinical Presentation

- Adults and children present with a sore throat, abrupt onset of fever, dysphagia, drooling, open mouth, muffled voice, stridor and respiratory distress. Patients often assume the tripod position, sitting up with their hands outstretched.
- In children acute epiglottitis typically occurs aged 2–5 years old and the main differential diagnosis is laryngotracheobronchitis (croup). Croup typically occurs in younger children, is associated with a barking cough, has a more gradual onset over 2–3 days and rarely appears toxic.

Management

- The diagnosis is made on the history and examination and an experienced anaesthetist and ENT surgeon should be available. For adults and children preparation for a difficult intubation and emergency tracheostomy should be made.
- **Children:** keep the child and parents calm. Indirect laryngoscopy, placement of intravenous lines, oropharyngeal examination, intramuscular injections and lateral neck radiographs should not be undertaken because further distress may precipitate complete airway obstruction.
- Following urgent transfer to theatre an inhalational induction with sevoflurane or halothane in oxygen is commenced with the child usually sitting or in the preferred position. An experienced surgeon able to perform a tracheostomy should be ready. Nitrous oxide is not used (effect of density in turbulent flow). Further monitoring and intravenous access are established as anaesthesia deepens. Intravenous fluids and atropine may be administered to reduce the likelihood of bradycardia associated with intubation.
- On laryngoscopy, the epiglottis and aryepiglottic folds are swollen and the classic 'cherry-red' epiglottis may be seen. Often, the glottic opening is not seen and the only clue may be a small mucous bubble during spontaneous ventilation or by gentle pressure on the child's chest. An uncuffed tracheal tube usually 1–3 mm smaller than normal is placed. Initially this is an oral tube and once the child is stable this is replaced by a nasal tube which is less likely to become dislodged during the subsequent ventilation on a paediatric intensive care unit.
- Throat and blood cultures are taken, antibiotic therapy commenced and the child transferred to a paediatric intensive care unit. Extubation is normally possible within 48 hours.
- **Adults:** for cooperative adults very careful flexible fibreoptic laryngoscopy, intravenous lines and careful oropharyngeal examination by experienced personnel can be performed.
- Inhalational induction in an adult with a compromised airway is often unfamiliar, difficult, slow, and the depth of anesthesia can be hard to assess. The patient will become more hypoxic and hypercarbic with long periods of instability, arrhythmias and apnoea. The traditional view is that the technique is safe because if the patient obstructs, the volatile agent will no longer be taken up, the patient will lighten and wake up. This frequently does not happen and the technique is often not reliable. Some centres therefore use an intravenous induction technique in adults with epiglottitis. The use of muscle relaxants remains controversial.
- Extubation should be delayed until the condition is clearly settling, and there is a leak around the tube on cuff deflation.

Q5 How might a child with an inhaled foreign body present? Describe your anaesthetic management for removal of the inhaled object. (Anil Patel)

Q5 Discussion

Presentation

- Foreign body aspiration is the commonest indication for bronchoscopy in children aged 1–4 years old.
- Inhaled foreign bodies can lodge in the larynx, trachea, main bronchi or smaller airways and their effects will depend on the duration, degree and site.
- Nuts are common inhaled foreign bodies and as they absorb water they swell, become friable, cause a chemical irritation of the airway and require urgent removal.
- Foreign bodies within the larynx and trachea present with acute dyspnoea, stridor, coughing and cyanosis. This may necessitate the Heimlich manoeuvre to dislodge the obstruction. If the obstruction is in the bronchus, the child is more likely to be wheezy, coughing and dyspnoeic with evidence of decreased air entry on the side of the obstruction.
- The child may present much later if the obstruction does not pose a functional problem with mucosal irritation, oedema and pneumonitis distal to the obstruction.

Investigation

- Chest radiographs may not reveal the lesion as most foreign bodies are radiolucent so a positive history and clinical symptoms of aspiration may be the only guide to the diagnosis.

Management

- Dislodging an inhaled foreign body can convert a partial obstruction to a more severe or even complete obstruction. The general principle of removal of inhaled foreign bodies during laryngoscopy and tracheobronchoscopy is to maintain spontaneous ventilation in the hope of reducing the chances of the foreign body being pushed distally into the airway.

- However in practice maintenance of spontaneous ventilation in a critically obstructed airway can be extremely difficult to sustain and intermittent positive pressure ventilation may be needed with some centres routinely using controlled ventilation and muscle paralysis.

Induction

- Sedative premedication should be avoided because it may precipitate total airway occlusion.
- Induction is usually by an inhalational technique with sevoflurane or halothane in oxygen. At a deep plane of anaesthesia laryngoscopy is performed and topical local anaesthetic (lignocaine) administered. Intravenous anticholinergic agents (atropine 20 µg per kg or glycopyrrolate 10 µg per kg) help reduce secretions and reflex bradycardia associated with airway instrumentation.
- Close observation and monitoring throughout the procedure is required to ensure a correct depth of anaesthesia to prevent movement, coughing and laryngospasm. Because of its shorter duration of effect sevoflurane is often changed to isoflurane once a deep plane of anaesthesia is achieved. Maintenance may be in the form of a propofol infusion.
- Some bronchoscopes allow the attachment of a T-piece to a side arm on the bronchoscope through which oxygen and volatile agent can pass directly into the distal trachea acting in a similar manner to an uncuffed tracheal tube. However some bronchoscopes do not allow T-piece attachment and insufflation or intravenous anaesthesia technique are required.

Post-operative care

- Post-operative care involves a high dependency environment, humidified oxygen and observation for airway oedema. Intravenous steroids are often continued to limit the oedema caused by the trauma of tracheobronchial instrumentation and foreign body removal. If infection is suspected antibiotics are continued until any airway swelling and oedema has resolved.

Q6 Discuss the management of a patient who is bleeding following tonsillectomy. (Anil Patel)

Q6 Discussion

Incidence

- Over 50 000 tonsillectomies are carried out in England every year and it is one of the commonest paediatric ENT surgical procedures.
- The National Prospective Tonsillectomy Audit (over 33 000 tonsillectomies) showed haemorrhage rates were 1.9% in the under 5 age group, 3.0% in the 5 to 15 age group, and 4.9% in the over 16 year olds. The return to theatre rate was 0.8% in the under 5 group, 0.8% in the 5 to 15 age group and 1.2% in the over 16 age group. Haemorrhage rates were higher in males, patients with quinsy and adults.

Clinical presentation

- Primary bleeds usually occur within 6 hours of surgery and may not be obvious in the immediate recovery period as blood is swallowed. The bleeding is usually a venous or capillary bleed rather than arterial and problems arise because of hypovolaemia, aspiration risk and difficult laryngoscopy.
- Signs suggesting haemorrhage are an unexplained tachycardia, excessive swallowing, increased capillary refill time, pallor, restlessness, sweating, and airway obstruction.
- Hypotension is a late feature.

Management

- Anaesthesia for these patients can be challenging (it is still a cause of mortality) and senior help should be sought.
- Patients should be given oxygen, adequately resuscitated, haemoglobin, haematocrit, and coagulation checked, blood typed and cross-matched. Large bore reliable intravenous access should be established (this may be a counsel of perfection in children).
- After resuscitation, options for anaesthesia include a rapid sequence induction which is usually the preferred technique, or an inhalational induction.

- Laryngoscopy can be difficult because of the presence of blood clots, continuous oozing of blood, and reduced venous and lymphatic drainage causing intra-oral swelling and oedema. A patient with an uneventful initial laryngoscopy and tracheal intubation can become difficult very quickly.

Intravenous induction

- For a rapid sequence induction patients should be in a slight head down position, protecting the airway from aspiration of blood. Some patients may not tolerate lying supine and pre-oxygenation, induction and cricoid pressure may have to be applied with patient semi-upright. The advantage of a rapid sequence induction is the rapid induction and control of the airway with less chance of regurgitation during induction. The disadvantages are the potential to inhale blood and cardiovascular depression from induction.
- A difficult laryngoscopy should be anticipated, prepared for and a selection of smaller tracheal tubes may be needed if airway and tracheal oedema is significant. Following tracheal intubation a large bore gastric tube should be placed to decompress the stomach and evacuate swallowed blood at the beginning and at the end of the procedure.

Inhalational induction

- An inhalational induction may be an option for those experienced with the technique but can be challenging in the lateral or head down position. This technique can be slow and blood can be inhaled and precipitate laryngospasm. For the inexperienced tracheal intubation in a lateral position is more difficult.
- Recovery
- At the end of the procedure extubation should be with the patient fully awake. Careful post-operative monitoring with close observations and high quality recovery should be available and haemoglobin levels rechecked.

Q7 Summarise the peri-operative anaesthetic management of a young man who is going to undergo an ORIF of facial fractures. (James Nicholson)

Q7 Discussion

Pre-operative assessment – general

- Definitive surgical management of these fractures is rarely an emergency, and can be planned as a semi-elective procedure in the first 48–72 hours post injury.
- History: usual anaesthetic history with particular reference to the following-
- Timing of injury with reference to last meal – delayed gastric emptying after injury.
- Mechanism of injury. ? Alcohol involved – delayed gastric emptying. ? Drugs involved.
- Associated injuries: head injury – was there loss of consciousness? C-spine injury? Is a CT head/neck indicated pre GA? Chest injuries or evidence of aspiration? CXR may be indicated.
- Circulatory stability: FBC, XM if signs of significant bleeding, or complicated fracture.
- Analgesia (may be poorly controlled if only written up for oral meds, which patients often cannot swallow). Use of NSAIDs pre-op? – For discussion, because of possible inhibition of platelets and fracture healing.
- Start IV maintenance fluids if not drinking well.

Pre-operative airway assessment

- Mouth opening – limited by pain, or physical cause? Mandibular nerve block to differentiate?
- Loose teeth, intra-oral trauma, nasal patency, bleeding?
- Swelling in soft tissues, possible bleeding into tissues – worrying if tongue or floor of mouth.

Discussion with surgeons

- Likelihood of physical obstruction to mouth opening?
- Complexity of fracture with estimate of operating time.
- What access are they going to require – what approach will they use
- Airway choice: nasal/oral/sub-mental tube or tracheostomy?

Anaesthetic

The main issue is what form of airway to use, and which technique for induction, this will depend on the findings from the above assessment. The options include:

- Airway assessed as NOT being problematic: standard IV induction and paralysis followed by nasal intubation.
- Potentially difficult intubation, but not judged to have difficult airway: IV induction, followed by intubation with fibreoptic or video scope.
- Airway potentially difficult ventilation, OR difficult intubation, and risk of reflux: awake fibreoptic intubation. Tracheostomy or TTJV if bleeding prevents view with fibreoptics.
- Suspected midline fracture in body of sphenoid, or nasal trauma that precludes nasal intubation: oral intubation followed by surgical tracheostomy in theatre or conversion to sub-mental intubation.

Other intra- and post-operative care.

- Anti-emetics, IV fluids (likely to have poor intake of oral fluids pre- and post-op)
- Hypotension and hypocapnia should be avoided if any head injury
- Catheter and warming devices (forced air mattress) if complex fracture
- Balanced analgesic regimen – paracetamol, NSAID, opiates
- IV antibiotics and steroids to decrease swelling
- HDU environment if any airway concerns. If swelling is sufficient to endanger airway, consider overnight intubation and ventilation on ICU

*ORIF = open reduction and internal fixation

Q8 A 15-year-old male autistic child requires an EUA and probable dental restoration treatment. A previous attempt to anaesthetise him failed due to non-cooperation. How would you proceed? (Eric Hodgson and Jane Stanford)

Q8 Discussion

Preliminary discussion with parents/carers/dentists/nurses

- Examining the views, and enlisting the support of all concerned is likely to be crucial.
- Do the parents have suggestions and can they say why it went wrong last time? Is there any alteration to the approach that could help? It is best to make the parents feel that they are setting the boundaries.
- This child is likely to be very strong, so the extent of restraint, and who will do it, must be clearly established.
- **Pre-medication**: again this needs to be discussed with his parents or carers. Some children are disinhibited by pre-medicant drugs and behave better without. Intra-nasal midazolam can be very effective.
- If the parents think that no or light pre-medication will be likely to fail, discuss using a mixture of oral ketamine (5 mg/kg) and midazolam (0.2 mg/kg) in 50 ml of juice. This mixture usually produces a well-sedated child. Ketamine is a drug of abuse in the UK, so the discussion may be difficult.
- A written record of the discussion should be made.

Anaesthesia

- Place EMLA or similar over veins.
- When possible administer a sevoflurane mask induction and place an IV cannula.
- Place an appropriate airway; an LMA will often be suitable but a nasal TT may be required.
- If a throat pack is required, safeguards to prevent accidental retention must be instituted.
- Consider paracetomol IV up to 40 mg/kg and dexamethasone 8 mg.
- Leave the patient in the lateral position, observed but if possible undisturbed, whilst awakening.
- Dexmedetomidine: where this available (not in the UK) a sublingual dose of 1 mg/kg added to the above pre-medication will apparently often allow an EUA and possibly the treatment to proceed without the addition of further anaesthesia.

Q9 A patient requires surgical fixation of an unstable cervical spine. What might be meant by 'unstable' and what are the implications for airway management? (Ian Calder)

Q9 Discussion

Cervical instability

- This term encompasses a wide spectrum of abnormalities, which range from complete disruption of all bony, joint and ligamentous structures to asymptomatic radiological abnormalities, which may result in deformity over time, or render the patient at increased risk in an accident.
- There are many causes, some congenital such as trisomy 21 or Morquio's syndrome, and trauma, infection, tumours, and arthritides such as rheumatoid or ankylosing spondylitis.
- There are quoted radiographic limits of angulation (in degrees) and translation (in mm), but correlation with neurological findings is not good.
- A two 'column' (anterior and posterior) concept is often employed to assess stability. A patient with disruption of the anterior column will tend to be unstable in extension.

Implications for airway management

- A major implication is sometimes that the patient is fixed in a device such as a halo-body frame, which renders the spine completely immobile and makes direct laryngoscopy difficult.
- There is always concern that airway management might cause a neurological injury. There is not satisfactory evidence that airway management has ever caused an injury, but there is not clear evidence that it has not. No technique has been shown to be associated with a better outcome.
- It is prudent to employ techniques that are least likely to result in movement at unstable sites. Many practitioners feel that flexible fibreoptic intubation under sedation and topical anaesthesia is suitable. However others point to episodes of serious coughing and bucking, or even airway obstruction, during attempts at fibreoptic intubation, and suggest that this technique should not be regarded as a panacea.
- If direct laryngoscopy is employed it is reasonable to use a gum-elastic bougie, as suggested by Nolan and Wilson, so that minimal exposure of the larynx is required.
- Manual In Line Stabilisation of the head and neck (MILS) is often employed, but there is no evidence of better outcome and, as with cricoid pressure, it should not be the reason for failure to establish an airway.
- It may be felt that positioning the patient for surgery is best done whilst the patient is awake, particularly if the patient is to be prone. This requires awake intubation and careful sedation, so that the patient remains cooperative.

Q10 A patient with long-standing rheumatoid arthritis requires a total hip arthroplasty operation. How may rheumatoid arthritis affect the airway and how would you manage the anaesthesia? (Ian Calder)

Q10 Discussion

- **Airway:** Rheumatoid arthritis is one of the classic causes of difficult intubation because the disease can involve the temporo-mandibular joints (TMJ), the cervical spine and in particular the cranio-cervical junction (CCJ), and the laryngeal joints and tissues, leading to glottic stenosis. Some patients will admit to intermittent stridor. Cervical spine disease can lead to myelopathy with poor respiratory function. Venous and arterial access can be difficult due to tissue abnormality and deformity.

- Better medical management means that the classic cervical spine complications of subluxation are becoming rare. The most frequent subluxation was anterior atlanto-axial (AAS), due to destruction of the transverse ligament of the atlas. Vertical subluxation (where the odontoid peg enters the foramen magnum) could occur due to erosion of the lateral masses of the axis, and rarely posterior AAS followed erosion of the odontoid peg. Anterior AAS can be symptomless although the patient usually complains of pain in the back of the head (C2 root distribution), sometimes lancinating on flexion (L'Hermitte's phenomenon); occasionally patients have fifth nerve symptoms. Flexion/extension lateral radiographs or scans should be obtained if they have not been performed recently (there is no agreed definition of recently).

- **Anaesthesia:** airway assessment should look for CCJ, TMJ and laryngeal involvement (inter-dental distance, jaw protrusion, Mallampati and voice changes or stridor). Spinal or CSE anaesthesia is an attractive approach, but may be technically difficult.

- If laryngoscopy might be difficult, flexible fibreoptic laryngoscopy under topical anaesthesia and sedation would be a sensible option. A small diameter tracheal tube should be used (6.0 mm).

- If AAS is present a regional technique is more attractive. If general anaesthesia has to be induced attention must be paid to positioning during anaesthesia. The position that causes least AAS is with the upper cervical spine (C2 and below) supported and the head and C1 allowed to displace backwards. This is best achieved with a large headring.

- If glottic stenosis is present it may be best to use a SAD and avoid intubation if general anaesthesia cannot be avoided. If intubation is performed, a small tube must be used and all care taken to minimise trauma. Dexamethasone should be given and extubation over an exchange catheter considered.

Q11 Describe management of anaesthesia for repair of broncho-pleural fistula. Describe the clinical features associated with the development of a broncho-pleural fistula 3 days after a right sided pneumonectomy. (Adrian Pearce)

Q11 Discussion

- A bronchopleural fistula (BPF) is a direct communication between the tracheobronchial tree and pleural space.
- Early BPF following pneumonectomy indicates mechanical failure of stump repair.
- Onset of dyspnoea, raised respiratory rate, and hypoxaemia.
- Productive cough, salty fluid (fluid in pneumonectomy space entering trachea).
- Decrease in fluid level in pneumonectomy space on chest radiograph.
- Deterioration due to contralateral lung soiling and infection.
- Possible shift of mediastinum to left.

What is the immediate management on the ward?
- Oxygen by facemask and resuscitation as needed.
- Patient sitting up, leaning to the right (to try to reduce space fluid entering trachea).
- Insertion of chest drain under local anaesthesia.
- Preparation for the patient to return to theatre and ICU post-op.
- Surgery will be thoracotomy and bronchial stump repair +/− initial rigid bronchoscopy.

What are the options for airway management with a large right-sided BPF?
The aim is to protect the lung from aspiration and control the air-leak through the fistula that might follow positive pressure ventilation.

Awake intubation with double-lumen tube (DLT): with the endobronchial limb placed in the left bronchus. Right limb clamped. A text-book answer which maintains spontaneous ventilation (avoiding problems of air-leak with positive pressure ventilation) during placement of a double-lumen tube (which provides isolation of the good lung). Not easy to do and sedation in ASA IV/V patient has its own problems.

Intubation with left DLT under deep inhalational anaesthesia: maintaining spontaneous ventilation. Intubation can be accomplished with direct laryngoscopy but it is helpful then to place the fibrescope through the bronchial limb to guide it into the appropriate bronchus rather than just blindly advancing the DLT. Right limb clamped. Anaesthesia deep enough to allow intubation with DLT and maintain spontaneous respiration is difficult in ASA IV/V patient and this approach may be hazardous.

Standard or rapid sequence IV induction, paralysis and intubation with DLT: is the common practical approach. It is possible to avoid facemask ventilation or, if facemask ventilation is needed, (i) cope with the bronchopleural leak (ii) temporarily clamp the intercostal drain or (iii) place the intercostal drain under 15–20 cm water. Direct laryngoscopy is used to intubate the trachea and a fibrescope is used to advance the DLT or endobronchial tube into position. Right limb clamped.

Place a single lumen tube into the trachea followed by bronchial blocker: this is not the preferred option because the blocker cuff sits in the disrupted bronchus and may neither control the leak nor prevent soiling. In addition it may be impossible to re-suture the bronchus with blocker in place. May be useful for BPF post-lobectomy.

Q12 A 60-year-old man with lymphoma presents with increasing difficulty breathing. On examination he has bulky cervical lymph nodes, and reduced mouth opening. He has some stridor and is anxious, but he is not obviously cyanosed. You are concerned that his airway may deteriorate further. You explain that he could soon need a procedure to help his breathing, but he refuses, saying he has made it plain that he 'does not want to end up in ICU'. His family insists that you 'do something'. What should you do? (Andrew McLeod and Steven M. Yentis)

Q12 Discussion

Quickly try to establish the relevant clinical facts.

- How rapidly is his airway deteriorating?
- What procedures or therapies could improve his breathing?
- To what extent would you need his cooperation?
- What is his overall prognosis and what treatments could change the course of his disease?
- Have any limits been placed on his treatment such as a DNAR order?

Assess whether he currently has capacity to make decisions about intubation, tracheostomy, or end of life treatment.

The Mental Capacity Act (2005) states that an adult's capacity should be presumed, unless they are suffering from some impairment or disturbance of mind or brain. Here this could include hypoxia, hypercapnia, and other disease or drug effects.

Try to correct any reversible disturbance (e.g., hypoxia), and then establish whether he has lost the ability to:

- Understand information
- Retain it for long enough to make a decision
- Weigh it up and arrive at a choice
- Communicate this choice.

If you doubt that he has sufficient capacity, try to establish his prior wishes.

- Has he made any formal advance decision refusing particular treatments 'even if life is at risk'? His wish to avoid ICU is probably too vague alone to countermand tracheostomy, but valid advance decisions must be respected.
- Has he specifically authorised a Lasting Power of Attorney (LPA) holder to decide such matters on his behalf?

- His family can help establish what his wishes might be, but they cannot demand particular treatments.
- Act in what you judge to be his best interests. The Mental Capacity Act gives guidance as to the criteria to use, but this case will remain challenging to resolve.

If he does have capacity, he has the legal right (in most western jurisdictions) to refuse any treatment, even if you believe he is irrational or wrong.

- Treating him against his will would be an assault, and performing any awake airway procedure would also be hard without his cooperation.
- Establish that his refusal is fully voluntary.
- Ensure that he is fully aware of the possible outcome of his decision (i.e. death through airway obstruction) and explain what other options he has.
- Documenting all of the above carefully.

Fear may be contributing significantly to this man's decision. It would be important to address his concerns and correct any erroneous beliefs as far as you can. Explain what options might be possible, and reassure him that:

- Procedures under local anaesthesia should not be particularly distressing.
- He may not need ICU care, but if he did it might only be for a short time.
- Tracheostomy may be temporary, allowing time for medical treatment to help.

If he still adamantly refuses any airway intervention, even to save his life, you must respect his wishes. This will be a difficult and distressing situation to handle.

- Seek advice from colleagues (e.g., an ENT surgeon, and a palliative care specialist) and discuss this case with a medicolegal advisor.
- If this patient's stipulations conflict with your personal values, you can ask another colleague (time permitting) to provide care.
- You must still continue to help him by suggesting other measures that might be acceptable (e.g., Heliox) and being open to continued discussions.
- Given his firmly stated wishes, it would be wrong to wait until he loses capacity and then attempt airway rescue, unless he clearly indicates that he now wants this.

311

Index